EXPLORING ETHICAL DILEMMAS IN ART THERAPY

Exploring Ethical Dilemmas in Art Therapy: 50 Clinicians From 20 Countries Share Their Stories presents a global collection of first-person accounts detailing the ethical issues that arise during art therapists' work. Grouped according to themes such as discrimination and inclusion, confidentiality, and scope of practice, chapters by experienced art therapists from 20 different countries explore difficult situations across a variety of practitioner roles, client diagnoses, and cultural contexts. In reflecting upon their own courses of action when faced with these issues, the authors acknowledge missteps as well as successes, allowing readers to learn from their mistakes. Offering a unique presentation centered on diverse vignettes with important lessons and ethical takeaways highlighted throughout, this exciting new volume will be an invaluable resource to all future and current art therapists, as well as to other mental health professionals.

Audrey Di Maria, MA, LCPAT, ATR–BC is an Adjunct Associate Professor in the Graduate Art Therapy Program in Art Therapy at the George Washington University in Washington, DC, where she has taught since 1978. She has chaired the Education and Publications Committees of the American Art Therapy Association, is a recipient of AATA's Clinician Award, and was secretary of the Art Therapy Credentials Board during the development of the initial version of its code of ethics.

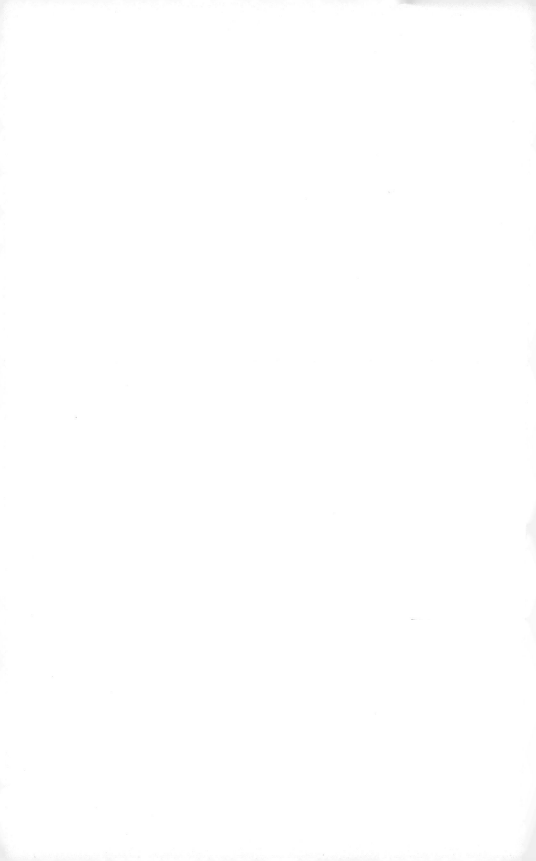

EXPLORING ETHICAL DILEMMAS IN ART THERAPY

50 Clinicians From 20 Countries Share Their Stories

Edited by Audrey Di Maria

COUNTRIES REPRESENTED:
ARGENTINA, AUSTRALIA, CANADA, CHILE, FRANCE, GHANA, HONG KONG, ICELAND, INDIA, JAPAN, JORDAN, LEBANON, THE PHILIPPINES, SOUTH AFRICA, SOUTH KOREA, SWEDEN, UKRAINE, THE UNITED KINGDOM, THE UNITED STATES OF AMERICA, AND THE WEST INDIES

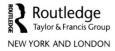
Routledge
Taylor & Francis Group

NEW YORK AND LONDON

First published 2019
by Routledge
52 Vanderbilt Avenue, New York 10017

and by Routledge
2 Park Square, Milton Park, Abingdon, Oxon, OX14 4RN

Routledge is an imprint of the Taylor & Francis Group, an informa business

Library of Congress Cataloging-in-Publication Data
A catalog record for this title has been requested

ISBN: 978-1-138-68189-7 (hbk)
ISBN: 978-1-138-68190-3 (pbk)
ISBN: 978-1-315-54549-3 (ebk)

Typeset in Bembo
by Newgen Publishing UK

This book is lovingly dedicated to
Kenneth James Nankervis,
my husband,

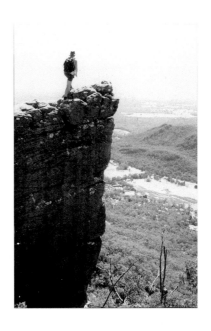

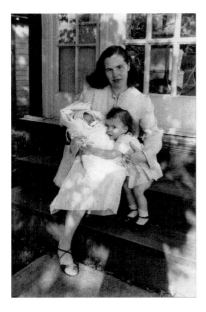

and to the memory of
H. Jane Evans Whitney, my mother,
and Gail Alice Evans, my sister.

There are no ordinary days.

CONTENTS

Contributors   *xiii*
Foreword by Judith A. Rubin   *xxii*
Preface   *xxx*
Acknowledgements   *xxxi*

PART I
Looking Beneath the Surface   **1**

1   Factors That Can Influence the Ethical Decision-Making Process   3
    Audrey Di Maria

2   Informed Consent and More: Positioning the Private Practice
    Contract at the Crossroads of the Art Therapist's Ethical, Clinical,
    Financial, and Legal Responsibilities   12
    Anne Mills

PART II
The Ethical Dilemmas   **23**

Assumptions, Discrimination, Exclusion   **25**

3   After the Typhoon: We Brought Art Materials, They Wanted Coffee   27
    Maria Regina A. Alfonso

 4 Art Therapist? Yes. Minister? That, Too! Ethical Issues That May
   Arise When One Has Dual Roles   36
   Martina E. Martin

 5 Can Biases Ever Be Right? The Ethics of Working Internationally
   as an Art Therapist, a Trainer, and a Professor   43
   Heidi Bardot

 6 Culturally Adaptive Art Therapy Practice: Is It Ethical?   50
   Mercedes Ballbé ter Maat

 7 Do No More Harm: The Ethical Practice of Art Therapy with
   Hospitalized Adults Who Have Severe and Persistent Mental Illness   55
   Deirdre M. Cogan

 8 Not Just Another Old Person: Art Therapy with Those Who Strive
   for Autonomy and Respect within a Culture of Invisibility   62
   Emery Hurst Mikel

 9 Redressing Social Injustice: Transcending and Transforming the
   Borders of Art Therapy Training in South Africa   68
   Hayley Berman

10 Translation of the Therapeutic Language: Can One Teach or
   Practice Art Therapy Ethically Without Considering Culture?   76
   Sojung Park

11 Walking a New Path: Ethical Considerations in Indigenizing Art
   Therapy in Canada   83
   Jennifer Vivian

Confidentiality   **89**

12 A Part of, Yet Separate: Ethical Issues Arising in Art Therapy with
   Combat Service Members and Their Families   91
   Paula Howie

13 'But I Am Understanding That You Mean To Say . . .': The Use of
   Language Interpreters in Art Therapy   97
   Elaine S. Goldberg

14 Ethics and Morality on the Stand: Art Therapist as Expert Witness   104
    David E. Gussak

15 No Man, or Woman, Is an Island—Especially on an Island:
    Practicing Art Therapy in the West Indies   111
    Karina Donald

16 When "Client" Is Plural: Confidentiality in Art Therapy with
    Groups, Families, and Couples   118
    Mary Ellen Ruff

17 Youth Behind Bars: Ethical Issues That Confront Art Therapists
    Who Work in Juvenile Detention Centers   124
    Jane Scott

Conflicting Interests   **131**

18 An American Art Therapist in France: 30 Years of Teaching and
    Supervising European Art Therapists and Practicing Art Therapy   133
    Elizabeth Stone

19 Art for Sale? Using Client Art for Promotional Purposes   140
    Lisa Raye Garlock

20 Art Therapy in Chile: The Ethical Challenges and Dilemmas
    of an Emerging Professional Practice   147
    Pamela Reyes H.

21 'I Am Not Disordered, I Am Special': Ethical Issues Faced by Art
    Therapists in the Evolving World of Children with Special Needs   154
    Laurie Mowry-Hesler

22 If Not for the Grace of God, There Go I: The Ethical Challenges
    of Providing Art Therapy and Other Services to Those
    Who Are Homeless   161
    Gwendolyn M. Short

23 'It's Not Even My Fault': Ethical Issues Encountered in Providing
    Art Therapy for Those Who Have Been Injured on the Job   167
    Donald J. Cutcher

24 My Top Ten Ethical Pet Peeves: An Art Therapist Reflects Upon
A Career Working in Psychiatric Settings 173
Charlotte G. Boston

25 Separation of Church and State: Parochial Politics, Third-Party
Payers, and Art Therapy for an Individual with Complex Trauma,
Eating Disorder, and Dissociative Identity Disorder 181
Michelle L. Dean

Multiple Roles **189**

26 Actually, Hong Kong *Is* a Small Town: Art Therapy and Multiple
Relationships within a Community 191
Jordan S. Potash

27 Avenues and Barriers of Dual Roles: Ethics and the ART Therapist
as Researcher 198
Richard Carolan

28 Hovering Between Art Education and "Art Therapy": The
Ethical Perspective of a Ghanaian Art Educator 204
Mavis Osei

29 It's Not All Academic: Addressing Non-academic Ethical Issues
That Arise in Art Therapy Education 210
Mary Roberts

30 Testifying on the Termination of Parental Rights: Art Therapy
and Case Management in an Early Intervention Program 219
Cheryl Doby-Copeland

31 The Art Therapist/Art Teacher: Practicing Ethically in
Treatment Settings and School Settings 225
Barbara Mandel

Scope of Practice **233**

32 Adapting the Instinctual Trauma Response Model to Meet
the Needs of Clients in Ukraine: Ethical Considerations 235
Iryna Natalushko

33 Apps, Telehealth, and Art Therapy: Online Treatment and Ethical
    Issues for the Digital Age   242
    Ellen G. Horovitz

34 A Safe Space, Standards, and "Gut Feelings": Ethics and Cultural
    Diversity in Art Therapy Training Groups   253
    Diane Waller

35 But Who Really *Is* On First? Art Therapy as Collaborative
    Treatment for Trauma Disorders   259
    Tally Tripp

36 Ethical Concerns When Applying Drawing to Promote Memory:
    Research Conducted in Iceland   266
    Unnur Ottarsdottir

37 My First Year as an Art Therapist in India: Ethical, Cultural,
    Logistical, and Supervisory Issues   273
    Sangeeta Prasad

38 The Mini Art Therapeutic Session Program in a School Setting
    in Japan   279
    Yuriko Ichiki and Mercedes Ballbé ter Maat

39 Traveling without My GPS: Creating the First 100% Online Art
    Therapy Master's Degree Program   285
    Penelope Orr

40 Widening the Lens of Ethical Practice in Art Therapy: Visual Free
    Speech and the Inclusive Studio Environment   292
    Michael A. Franklin

Transference and Counter-transference   **299**

41 An Open Book: How Does a Bereaved Art Therapist Maintain
    Boundaries with Bereaved Clients?   301
    Sharon Strouse

42 Boys Will Be Boys: Men, Ethics, and Art Therapy   308
    Michael Pretzer

43 Coloring Inside the Rooms: Art Therapy in Residential Substance
    and Gambling Addiction Treatment   316
    Todd C. Stonnell

44 Gaza Was Different: Ethical Issues That Arose on an Art Therapy
    Journey in the Middle East   322
    Shirin Yaish

45 Is All Art Making Ethical? Dilemmas Posed in the Making of
    Response Art by Australian Art Therapy Trainees   332
    Patricia Fenner and Libby Byrne

46 Multiple Roles in Art Therapy Supervision: Using *El Duende*
    One-Canvas Process Painting   339
    Abbe Miller

47 Trauma and Displaced Aggression: An Art Therapist Works with
    Refugees in Sweden   352
    Catherine Rogers Jonsson

The Abuse of Power   **359**

48 If You Don't Stand for Something, You'll Fall for Anything:
    Finding Courage When Asked to Do Wrong   361
    Leslie Milofsky

**PART III
Drawing to a Close**   **371**

49 Finishing Art Therapy without the Work Unraveling: Ethical Issues
    in Terminating Long-term Therapy with Children   373
    P. Gussie Klorer

50 When the Art Therapist Is Ready to Leave Before the Client Is:
    The Ethical Challenges of Closing a Clinical Practice   379
    Deborah A. Good

Appendix A: The Private Practice Contract by Anne Mills   *389*
Appendix B: Chapter Writers' Resolutions to Their Ethical Dilemmas *396*
Index   *442*

CONTRIBUTORS

Editor

Audrey Di Maria, MA, LCPAT (MD), ATR-BC, Editor, is an Adjunct Associate Professor in the Graduate Art Therapy Program at the George Washington University in Washington, DC, where she has taught since 1978. She has chaired the Education and Publications Committees of the American Art Therapy Association and received AATA's Clinician Award for her work with children. She was Secretary of the Art Therapy Credentials Board during the development of the initial version of its code of ethics.

Foreword author

Judith A. Rubin PhD, ATR-BC, HLM, author of the Foreword, is a psychologist, psychoanalyst, and board-certified art therapist. A past President and Honorary Life Member of the American Art Therapy Association, she has written six books and created thirteen films. Faculty in Psychiatry, University of Pittsburgh and the Pittsburgh Psychoanalytic Center, she has presented widely in the US and abroad. President of Expressive Media, she is currently working on the creation and dissemination of a Streaming Training Film Library.

The 50 Clinicians

Maria Regina A. Alfonso, MS Ed., MA (Art Therapy), LCPAT, ATR-BC, is a consultant/technical advisor with Save the Children's HEART program, a global psychosocial support program designed for post-conflict/post-disaster contexts. Gina founded Cartwheel Foundation, which provides access to culturally relevant education and health services for the hardest to reach indigenous people in her native Philippines. Advisor to MAGIS Creative Spaces for Therapy and Education and The Learning Child School in the Philippines, Gina is a doctoral candidate at the European Graduate School in Leuk-Stadt, Switzerland.

Mercedes Ballbé ter Maat, PhD, LPC, ATR-BC, is a Professor in the College of Psychology at Nova Southeastern University in Fort Lauderdale, FL, past President of the American Art Therapy Association, and President of the European Branch of the American Counseling Association. She has over 30 years of combined experience as an art therapist, mental health counselor, school counselor, and professor. Humanitarian work has recently taken Mercedes to her native Argentina, Lebanon, and Swaziland.

Heidi Bardot, MA, LCPAT, ATR-BC, is Director of the Art Therapy Graduate Program at the George Washington University in Washington, DC. She is a licensed, board-certified art therapist who has created service-learning programs in India, Croatia, South Africa, and the United Arab Emirates. She trains relief workers in art and trauma in Lebanon. She has published and presented nationally and internationally on war relief, trauma, resiliency, grief, and international education.

Hayley Berman, PhD, is an art psychotherapist registered with the HCPC and the HPCSA, an artist, and a social entrepreneur. Founder of Lefika La Phodiso in Johannesburg, Africa's first psychoanalytically informed Community Art Counselling and Training Institute, Hayley earned her doctorate in psychosocial studies at the University of West of England and is currently Director of the MA in Art Therapy Program at the University of Hertfordshire. Her long-standing research interest lies in developing methodologies that assist in creating long-term psychosocial change.

Charlotte G. Boston, MA, LCPAT, ATR-BC, is an experienced clinician, educator, administrator, and consultant, who has worked with clients aged 5–75. Most of her work has been with psychiatric inpatients, including older adults and members of the military. Charlotte has served on the American Art Therapy Association's Board of Directors, as well as on various AATA committees, and is President-elect of the Art Therapy Credentials Board. She has presented and published locally and nationally.

Libby Byrne, PhD, AThR, teaches and does research in the Master of Art Therapy Program at La Trobe University in Melbourne, Australia. She is an art therapist who has worked with trauma, grief, and loss in public health and ministry settings and has been a practicing and exhibiting artist for the past 20 years. She continues to develop and extend her engagement with art as practice-led theological inquiry with the University of Divinity.

Richard Carolan, EdD, ATR-BC, is a licensed psychologist and board-certified art therapist who designed, developed, and directs the doctoral program in Art Therapy at Notre Dame de Namur University in Belmont, CA, where he has taught for more than 20 years. He served as President of the Art Therapy Credentials Board and received AATA's Distinguished Educator Award. He and Amy Backos edited *Emerging Perspectives in Art Therapy: Trends, Movements, and Developments* (Routledge, 2017). A father of three, he is an active artist and maintains a private practice.

Deirdre M. Cogan, MA, LPC, ATR-BC, ATCS, CCTP, has 30 years of clinical experience in both public and private sectors. She is currently Director of Creative Arts Training at a large public psychiatric facility and a staff member at the Center for Post Traumatic Disorders, both in Washington, DC. Deirdre's research interests lie in designing programs that address the recovery challenges of mentally ill women who face barriers due to poverty, gender inequality, and cultural stigma. Deirdre received AATA's 2015 Distinguished Clinician Award.

Donald J. Cutcher, MA, LCAT, ATR-BC, is a founder and Honorary Life Member of the Buckeye Art Therapy Association (OH), one of the oldest state art therapy associations in the US, and an AATA member since 1973. He has presented on ethics for BATA, AATA, and other professional organizations, providing information on documents and the interface between the codes of various professions. Don is retired from private practice, providing services to clients experiencing physical and/or psychological trauma from workplace injuries.

Michelle L. Dean, MA, ATR-BC, LPC (PA), CGP, is co-founder of The Center for Psyche & the Arts, LLC near Philadelphia, PA. She is Director of the Art Therapy program at The University of the Arts, and Adjunct Professor at Arcadia University, Cedar Crest College, and Drexel University. She is an artist, supervisor, nationally recognized speaker, and author with several publications her credit, including *Using Art Media in Psychotherapy: Bringing the Power of Creativity to Practice* (Routledge, 2016).

Cheryl Doby-Copeland, PhD, LPC, LMFT, ATR-BC, HLM, has over 40 years of art therapy experience and received the AATA Clinician Award in 2003. Dr. Copeland served on the Board of Directors of AATA from 1999–2001 and 2013–2017. She has taught graduate courses in multicultural diversity and family/marital art therapy. Since 1978, Dr. Copeland has actively promoted multicultural competence in the profession of art therapy. In 2018, she was named an Honorary Life Member of AATA.

Karina Donald, MA, ATR-BC, completed her Master's degree in Art Therapy at George Washington University in 2011 and is currently a doctoral candidate in Family Therapy. Most of her clinical work and research on mental illness and trauma has taken place in the Caribbean. Karina is an adjunct faculty member at the University of the West Indies Open Campus and a research consultant at Texas Woman's University in Houston, TX.

Patricia Fenner, Dip. Vis. Arts, Dip. Education, MA (Hochschule Der Kunste, Berlin), MA and PhD (La Trobe University), AThR, is Course Coordinator of the Master of Art Therapy program at La Trobe University, Melbourne, Australia. Besides focusing upon issues relevant to the training of art therapists, her research interests include the role of the material in the therapeutic encounter and art therapy in cancer care and in mental health recovery, both locally and in the Asia Pacific region.

Michael A. Franklin, PhD, ATR-BC, Chair of the Art Therapy Program at Naropa University, Boulder, CO, has practiced and taught in various clinical and academic settings since 1981. Founder of the Naropa Community Art Studio, a research project training socially engaged art therapists, Michael received AATA's Distinguished Educator Award in 2016. An international lecturer, his book, *Art as Contemplative Practice* (SUNY Press, 2017), focuses upon integrating relationships among art, social engagement, yoga philosophy, and meditation.

Lisa Raye Garlock, MS, LCPAT, ATR-BC, ATCS, is Assistant Professor and Clinical Placement Coordinator of the George Washington University Art Therapy Program. She also serves on the Art Therapy Credentials Board. Lisa works with Common Threads Project, an international non-profit that trains therapists in trauma work that includes art therapy and story cloths. She is interested in women's and human rights issues and, in her own artwork, uses a variety of media, including textiles and glass.

Elaine S. Goldberg, PhD, ATR-BC, is an art therapist and clinical psychologist who works with medically ill patients at a children's hospital. She is a Clinical Assistant Professor of Psychiatry, Behavioral Sciences, and Pediatrics, George Washington University School of Medicine and Health Sciences. Elaine began her career working at a public psychiatric hospital where she developed an interest in studying the therapeutic effects of medication as reflected in changes in the artwork of patients participating in schizophrenia research.

Deborah A. Good, PhD, LPAT, LPCC, ATR-BC, ATCS, is a board-certified art therapist and New Mexico Licensed Professional Art Therapist and Clinical Counselor. She has worked in the mental health field for 45 years in outpatient and hospital settings. Deborah is a past President of both the American Art Therapy Association and the Art Therapy Credentials Board. She has authored several book chapters, Forewords, and articles on art therapy and speaks nationally and internationally on various art therapy and counseling topics.

David E. Gussak, PhD, ATR-BC, is Professor of Art Therapy and Chairperson of the Department of Art Education at Florida State University, Tallahassee, FL. He has published numerous articles and book chapters and lectures nationally and internationally on art therapy in correctional settings, working with aggressive and violent clients, and forensic art therapy. He authored *Art on Trial: Art Therapy in Capital Murder Cases* (Columbia University Press, 2013) and, with Marcia Rosal, co-edited the *Wiley Handbook of Art Therapy* (John Wiley & Sons, 2016).

Ellen G. Horovitz, PhD, LCAT, ATR-BC, E-RYT, LFYP, C-IAYT, is Professor Emerita, founder, and former director of the Graduate Art Therapy Program at Nazareth College, Rochester, NY. She has 35 years' experience with myriad patient populations (aged 3–96) as a licensed art therapist, psychotherapist, registered yoga teacher, and certified yoga therapist. She has authored nine books, most recently, *A Guide to Art Therapy Materials, Methods, and Applications: A Practical Step-by-Step Approach* (Routledge, 2017).

Paula Howie, MA, LPC, LCPAT, ATR-BC, HLM, worked in the Art Therapy Service at an Army Medical Center for 25 years and currently lectures at the School of Visual Art and Florida State University. She is a past President of the American Art Therapy Association. Paula is author of *Art Therapy with Military and Veteran Populations: History, Innovations, and Applications* (Routledge, 2017) and co-editor of *Art Therapy with Diverse Populations: Crossing Cultures and Abilities* (Jessica Kingsley Publishers, 2013). She is an avid watercolor painter.

Yuriko Ichiki, PhD, is a certified clinical psychologist who completed her MA in Art Therapy at the George Washington University in 1990. She is Professor of the Teacher Education Center for the Future Generation at Nara University of Education in Japan. She provides training, consultation, and workshops for public school teachers in Japan, using art therapy.

Catherine Rogers Jonsson, MFA, MA, ATR-BC, is an Authorized Art Therapist in Sweden who received her MFA from Columbia University and her MA in Art Therapy from the University of Wisconsin-Superior. Catherine has 25 years of clinical art therapy experience and lectures at Portland State University. A professional artist based in Sweden, she has numerous solo and group exhibitions in the US and Europe to her credit. Her work concerns contemporary issues in spirituality and philosophy.

P. Gussie Klorer, PhD, LCSW, LCPC, ATR-BC, HLM, is author of *Expressive Therapy with Traumatized Children* (Rowman and Littlefield Publishers, 2017), as well as numerous articles and book chapters focused on clinical work. She has served on the Editorial Boards of the *Trauma and Loss Journal, American Journal of Art Therapy,* and *Art Therapy: Journal of the American Art Therapy Association.* She is the 2001 recipient of the AATA Clinician Award and an Honorary Lifetime Member of AATA.

Barbara Mandel, MA, received a BA in Painting/Studio Arts from the University of Rochester and an MA in Art Therapy from George Washington University. She has helped children and adolescents express themselves through art in a wide variety of settings, including hospitals, day treatment centers, community centers, public and private schools, and museums. Barbara is also a painter and volunteers as a School Docent at the National Gallery of Art in Washington, DC.

Martina E. Martin, M. Div., MA, LPC, ATR-BC, is a board-certified art therapist and Licensed Professional Counselor in Washington, DC. She earned a BA in Political Science and a M.Div. from Howard University in 2002 and 2007, respectively, then an MA in Art Therapy from George Washington University in 2011. As a Provisional Deacon in the United Methodist Church, she serves in an appointment beyond the local church as a full-time psychotherapist with a community-based health organization.

Emery Hurst Mikel, MA, LCAT, LCPAT, ATR-BC, is founder and director of Water & Stone, a Creative Arts Therapy PLLC in Brooklyn, NY. Her therapeutic work supports adults dealing with anxiety, grief, loss, dementia, and related issues. She also mentors other therapists, supervises interns, and offers community workshops focused upon creativity, empowerment, mindfulness, and personal or business development. She received her MA in Transpersonal Counseling Psychology–Art Therapy from Naropa University in Boulder, CO.

Abbe Miller, MS, LPC, ATR-BC, has practiced and taught the processes of transformational art and art therapy for more than 35 years, with over 70 workshops and paper presentations. Abbe is an Associate Professor in the Graduate Art Therapy and Counseling Program at Albertus Magnus College in New Haven, CT and a doctoral student in Expressive Therapies at Lesley

University in Cambridge, MA. She maintains a private practice, supervises, and offers weekend intensives on the *el duende* painting process (EDPP).

Anne Mills, MA, LPC, ATR-BC, is in private practice with Art Therapy Services of Washington, DC and is Director of the Diagnostic Drawing Series Archive. Her areas of specialization include supervision/consultation, hypnotherapy, and the treatment of survivors of severe early trauma, particularly those who are highly dissociative. Anne provides resiliency-focused treatment for adolescents and adults who have experienced difficult transitions such as illness, bereavement, and loss of culture (refugees, expatriates, international students, trans-national workers).

Leslie Milofsky, MA, LCPAT (MD), ATR-BC, is an art therapist with the District of Columbia Public School System and an adjunct professor at George Washington University's Art Therapy Program. Leslie believes that organic and found materials are a compelling addition to any art therapist's tool kit and that exposure to children and animals is a humbling and healing blessing in anyone's life.

Laurie Mowry-Hesler, MA, LMFT, ATR-BC, ATCS, is a board-certified Art Therapist, Certified Art Therapy Supervisor, and Licensed Marriage and Family Therapist. Since her career began in 1984, she has worked in therapeutic treatment centers, schools, at-risk community programs, and private practice. She is an adjunct professor in the Graduate Art Therapy Program at George Washington University in Washington, DC. Laurie and her husband have four children.

Iryna Natalushko, MA, CTT, is a teaching art therapist based in Ukraine. Iryna uses the Instinctual Trauma Response model and its adaptations to help adults and families with a history of traumatic experiences that have not been fully integrated and continue to influence their lives. During the 2017–2018 academic year, Iryna was a visiting Fulbright Scholar with the George Washington University Art Therapy Program and the ITR Training Institute, working to support the ITR method training and research.

Penelope Orr, PhD, ATR-BC, ATCS, is program head and developer of the Edinboro University Master's in Art Therapy Program, the first 100% online Art Therapy Master's Degree Program. Her research focus has been on the use of digital media in art therapy over the past 20 years. She has written book chapters, co-authored books, and published several articles on this topic. Her current focus is working on digital story telling/journaling as a tool for identity formation and post-traumatic growth.

Mavis Osei, PhD, is an art educator who began her career as a lecturer at age 28 in 2009 at the Kwame Nkrumah University of Science and Technology (KNUST) in Kumasi, Ghana. She has a BA in Art (2003) and a PhD in Art Education (2008), both from KNUST. In 2015, she obtained a Fulbright Scholarship to pursue an MA in Clinical Art Therapy at CW Post, NY. She has published several articles and currently lives in Ghana, where she teaches art therapy.

Unnur Ottarsdottir, PhD, ATR, has worked as an art therapist since 1990. Unnur is a practicing researcher at the Reykjavik Academy. She holds a PhD in art therapy from the University of Hertfordshire (UK) and has taught art therapy in a variety of academic institutions. She has written articles and book chapters about art therapy and the methodology of Grounded Theory and has given lectures at conferences and organizations in Iceland and worldwide.

Sojung Park, PhD, LCAT, ATR-BC, is an assistant professor in the department of art therapy education at the Ewha Womans University in Seoul, Korea. She earned her master's degree in art therapy at the School of Visual Arts in New York, and her doctorate in expressive therapies at the Lesley University in Cambridge, MA. Her research interests involve multicultural issues, addiction, self-psychology, and the use of digital media in art therapy.

Jordan S. Potash, PhD, LPCAT (MD), LCAT (NY), ATR-BC, REAT, has worked with clients of all ages in schools, clinics, and community art studios both in the US and in Hong Kong, where he co-founded the Master's of Expressive Art Therapy Program at the University of Hong Kong, the first program of its kind in Asia. He is Assistant Professor in the Art Therapy Program at the George Washington University in Washington DC, Editor of *Art Therapy: Journal of the American Art Therapy Association*, and the former chair of the AATA Ethics Committee.

Sangeeta Prasad, MA, ATR-BC, works as an art therapist with children and adults. She coordinates projects with several non-profit organizations and presents in the US and in India. She is on the Board of Directors of the American Art Therapy Association. Sangeeta authored *Creative Expressions: Say It With Art* and co-edited *Using Art Therapy with Diverse Populations: Crossing Cultures and Abilities* (Jessica Kingsley Publishers, 2013). She continues to paint.

Michael Pretzer, MA, LCPAT, ATR-BC, lives in Washington, DC and works with adolescents. He is a graduate of the Art Therapy Program at George Washington University and holds a master of arts in teaching from the Rhode Island School of Design and degrees in journalism from Northwestern University and the University of Kansas. For more than 30 years prior to becoming an art therapist, Michael worked as a magazine editor and writer.

Pamela Reyes H., MA (in Art Therapy), is Director of the Master of Arts in Health and Art Therapy Program at the Finis Terrae University in Santiago, Chile. From 2004 to 2015, she was Director of the Art Therapy post-graduate program at the University of Chile. Her professional experience has been in community psychology under the paradigm of health promotion, as well as in clinical mental health settings. For the past ten years, she has also worked as an art psychotherapist in private practice. She is a doctoral candidate.

Mary Roberts, EdS, LPC-ACS, ATR-BC, ATCS, is Program Director and Associate Professor in the Graduate Art Therapy and Counseling Program at Eastern Virginia Medical School, Norfolk, VA. She has over 20 years of art therapy experience, providing trauma informed care for adolescents, veterans, and military service members. She facilitated the hiring of art therapists in detention facilities, was responsible for creating seven positions, and developed standards of practice and curricula for art and music therapists.

Mary Ellen Ruff, MS, LPC, ATR-BC, received her MS degree in Art Therapy from Eastern Virginia Medical School in Norfolk, VA in 1996. Her private practice focuses upon adolescents and adults dealing with substance abuse, trauma, and mood and anxiety disorders. She also works with court-involved individuals in the city of Alexandria, VA. She has taught in the Graduate Art Therapy Program at George Washington University since 2007 and regularly creates her own art.

Jane Scott is a pen name under which a Registered Art Therapist (ATR) and Licensed Professional Counselor (LPC) has written her chapter.

Gwendolyn M. Short, MA, LCPAT, ATR-BC, is a native Washingtonian who graduated from the George Washington University with a Master's degree in Art Therapy. Gwendolyn has served on the Art Therapy Credentials Board and the American Art Therapy Association's Board of Directors. She worked for a county health department for 33 years and is now Art Therapy Director at CREATE Arts Center in Silver Spring, MD, where she works with adults living with mental illness. Gwendolyn received AATA's Clinician Award for her work with adults.

Elizabeth Stone, MA, LPC, LCAT, ATR-BC, is a New York State-licensed psychoanalyst and art therapist in private practice in Grenoble, France. She has been a faculty member of the Ecole de Psychologues Praticiens of the Catholic University of Lyon, France; previously, at New York University's Graduate Art Therapy Program. In Europe for 30 years, she has supervised the training of art therapists in Italy, Switzerland, and France, while lecturing and publishing widely on creative expression in art therapy and psychotherapy.

Todd C. Stonnell, MA, LPC, ATR-BC, began his path towards art therapy as a costumed character at an amusement park. Through the process of greeting others as a cartoon figure, he learned how to connect with people without using words. During his art therapy career, Todd has worked with adults living with HIV/AIDS, children at a cancer treatment hospital in India, youth on the Autism spectrum, and adolescents seeking help for various mental health issues.

Sharon Strouse, MA, LCPAT, ATR-BC, is a licensed, board-certified art therapist with 30 years of experience. After her 17-year-old daughter Kristin ended her own life, Sharon immersed herself in a collage practice which became the foundation of her book, *Artful Grief: A Diary of Healing.* She has written chapters in Neimeyer's *Techniques of Grief Therapy: Creative Practices for Counseling the Bereaved* and in Thompson and Neimeyer's *Grief and the Expressive Arts: Practices for Creating Meaning.* She leads national workshops, weekly art therapy sessions, and spiritual development circles for survivors of loss.

Tally Tripp, MA, MSW, LCSW, ATR-BC, is a board-certified art therapist and licensed clinical social worker in the Washington, DC area, specializing in working with trauma-related disorders. Tally is certified in advanced trauma approaches, including Intensive Trauma Therapy, Eye Movement Desensitization and Reprocessing (EMDR), and Sensorimotor Psychotherapy. She is the Director of the Art Therapy Clinic at the George Washington University where she also teaches the Trauma, Group, and International Diversity classes.

Jennifer Vivian, MA, is an art therapist of Inuit and European descent who lives and works in Canada. Jennifer is passionate about art therapy's role in truth-sharing, storytelling, reconciliation, and healing across Turtle Island (North America). She strives to work within an Indigenous framework of art therapy, which is amended as she travels along her path and receives additional teachings.

Diane Waller, OBE, MA (RCA), DPhil, Dip. Psych., FRSA, Emeritus Professor of Art Psychotherapy, Goldsmiths, University of London, Principal Research Fellow, University of Brighton, Honorary President, BAAT. Established the art therapy program at Goldsmiths (1974); headed a team that persuaded the Department of Health to establish a career and salary structure for art therapy in the National Health Service (1982); led negotiations that resulted in the statutory regulation of art, drama, and music therapists (1997). A founding member of Health and Care Professions Council (2002–2013), Diane was awarded the Order of the British Empire in 2007 for Services to Health.

Shirin Yaish, MA in Art Psychotherapy, founded Kaynouna Arab Art Therapy Center in 2012 and has provided thousands of refugees and underprivileged children, youth, and women with art psychotherapy groups and more than 15 NGOs with training. She is considered to be a pioneer in Trauma Informed Art Therapy in the Arab world and internationally. She has presented papers in Hong Kong, Toronto, Amman, and London, and her work has been featured on CNN, Al Jazeera, and other media outlets.

Key to Art Therapy Credentials, Certification Bodies, and Professional Membership Organizations Cited Above

AATA	American Art Therapy Association
ANZATA	Australian and New Zealand Arts Therapy Association
ATCB	Art Therapy Credentials Board (registers and certifies art therapists in the US)
ATCS	Art Therapy Clinical Supervisor (with the ATCB)
ATR	Registered Art Therapist (with the ATCB)
ATR-BC	Registered, Board-certified Art Therapist (with the ATCB)
AThR	Registered Art Therapist (with the ANZATA)
BAAT	British Association of Art Therapists
HCPC	Health and Care Professions Council (registers art therapists in the UK)
HPCSA	Health Professions Council of South Africa (registers art therapists in South Africa)
LCAT	Licensed Clinical Art Therapist
LCPAT	Licensed Clinical Professional Art Therapist
LGPAT	Licensed Graduate Professional Art Therapist
LPAT	Licensed Professional Art Therapist
REAT	Registered Expressive Arts Therapist

FOREWORD

Judith A. Rubin, PhD, ATR-BC, HLM

Audrey Di Maria has assembled a veritable *who's who* of art therapists for this book. Each has considerable experience and expertise, and each has tackled an ethical dilemma that is deeply meaningful and critically important. The reader is therefore in for a thought-provoking exploration of an area sometimes viewed as dry and uninteresting. Rather, ethics in art therapy deals with both the most personal and the most public aspects of our work—from touching a client to showing images of them or their art. After reflection, I decided that the best way to write this foreword was to tell some relevant stories.

Story 1: Touching—an Ethical Hot Potato

Touch is one of the most delicate ethical issues when working closely with someone in therapy. Most art therapists, like other clinicians, strive to create what Winnicott (1960) called "a *holding environment*," a psychological space in which someone would *feel* safely "held."

Actually, art therapy allows for a very special kind of touching that does not violate any physical boundaries. Alice Karamanol describes it beautifully in the film *Art Therapy Has Many Faces* (Rubin, 2004). While drawing a portrait of one of her adolescent students, Alice says: "I love to draw people's faces, and when the students reach like a creative block, I'll say, 'Well, you don't have to work. Let me draw you.' But then I always stop after the pencil part of it, and let them complete it." What follows is one of the most eloquent statements I have ever heard about the uniquely respectful and ethical intimacy possible in art therapy: "The drawing of the picture is a way that *I get to touch them without touching them. It's very intimate attention when you draw someone.*" Drawing someone's portrait is indeed intimate but not intrusive, a fine example of *respect*—the fundamental underpinning of ethical conduct in art therapy as in any interpersonal relationship. If there is sincere respect for the other, ethical guidelines flow naturally.

Story 2: The Editor of this Book—Embodying Ethical Behavior

From her very first communications to her contributors, the editor of this book has behaved with *respect*. It is striking how the *form* (i.e., the way this book has *evolved*) is synchronous with its *content* (i.e., what it is *about*). The way in which Audrey Di Maria has approached her role has been, it seems to me, a beautiful example of ethical behavior. This is not new for her. In fact, I would like to begin by sharing a story of how very thoughtfully she has dealt with me.

In 2012, Audrey was invited to write a chapter for a book that was to be published the following year (Howie, Prasad, & Kristel, 2013). She wanted to include a story I had told her a long time ago about going back to an adolescent therapy group that had terminated to be sure the participants were comfortable with a film the leaders had made about the group. Although the youngsters had signed permissions to be filmed and for us to make a film, we wanted to be certain they felt they had been fairly portrayed, so we invited them to watch the first draft and to sign new releases. Most agreed but some did not, requiring additional editing.

What impressed me as profoundly respectful and thoughtful was that Audrey Di Maria—author of that chapter and editor of this book—wanted to be absolutely certain that I was comfortable with her description of the story. She therefore sent me her written draft along with a consent form, which seemed to me a beautiful example of behavior that, while unnecessary, was profoundly ethical. Checking with me about publishing the story as she had written it in her chapter seems to me to be a clear instance of following not just the *letter*, but the *spirit* of the law.

Showing Images of People and Their Art—Ethical Dilemmas

Showing images of *people* on film, which is even more revealing than showing images of their *art*, is indeed one of the most challenging ethical areas in art therapy. As someone who has been making films and publishing books with photos of people and artwork for over four decades, it is an issue with which I have often wrestled. Since I am convinced that teaching art therapy requires that students see *authentic* examples of the work, the challenge has always been how to do it most respectfully.

To clarify the complexity of the issues involved, I'd like to share two more stories. One is about some blind children who were in the first film I ever made (Rubin, 1972). The other is about an adult whose writing I included in a book (Rubin, 2005). Each has to do with being recognized—one wanting it and the other not wanting it. My conclusion was that both wishes needed to be respected. The issue of showing people's faces in books and films is also discussed in Story 6.

Story 3: "We'll Show You What We're Gonna Do!"

A group of blind children were shown a film about their art therapy program prior to releasing it, to be sure they were comfortable with what had been included. Since they had different degrees of useful vision, some could see it, some could only hear it, but all were engrossed during the screening. Their faces and their artwork as well as some audiotaped excerpts from interviews were included, along with my narration. Several youngsters were upset that I had changed their names in the narration and insisted that they be identified accurately, at which point the others wanted their own names to be used as well. Although their parents had already consented to the film with disguised names, we now needed to get their permission to use actual names, so we showed it to them again. Despite being less comfortable than their children, they were also proud of their youngsters' honesty, so they finally agreed.

The school administrators had a different problem. They were not worried about names, but did have grave concerns about the aggressive impulses expressed by some of the children in the film. However, when we showed it to them with the parents, the latter persuaded them that it was important to show all kinds of feelings. I had led a mothers' group at the school and had trained them to run support groups for other mothers whose children were not involved in the art program, which no doubt facilitated their greater comfort with honest expression.

Story 4: A Woman Gives Permission to Include Her Writing but Not Her Art

Marjorie, a mental health professional who was going through a very difficult time in her life, wrote between sessions and brought her writing in for me to read. She was also doing art at home and bringing that in for us to view together. Having read some of my books, she had said she would be happy for me to include her artwork in one. However, by the time she had finished therapy, she had changed her mind and said that she did *not* want me to reproduce any of her artwork.

What had happened, which was actually quite wonderful, was that painting had become not only a therapeutic relief from stress, but also a valued *avocation*. In fact, because a number of friends had admired her work, she had started to have exhibits in her hometown, and was concerned that even if her *name* were disguised, her *art* would be identifiable to anyone who had seen her paintings. While revoking permission to show her art, however, she did say that it would be all right to share her written reflections (Rubin, 2005). The following excerpt, written during the termination phase of therapy, conveys what the art had come to mean to her:

> As I write about the art, for probably the last time in therapy, feeling the connection with termination. A sense of impending loss, an empty space, where the therapeutic alliance has been. And the art a bridge … And now with Judy, taking the art with me as I prepare to depart, leaving the writing in case it can be of use. Feeling enormously thankful for the therapy, for the art, both having enriched my life in unexpected ways … It has been a fascinating and satisfying artistic journey for me, at a time when my journey in life was filled with pain and turmoil. As Judy has been the midwife for the artistic process for me, I seem to have served as the midwife for the art. Because it really has seemed to have a life of its own from the beginning, needing room to emerge and define itself, to unfold and evolve, resisting my efforts to intervene and transform. The process has seemed much like my life (thinking of my adolescence), trusting my

intuitions, willing to explore uncharted territory, an inherent sense of direction and goodness (or poorness) of fit as things emerged. The process similar in life and in therapy and in art …

Marjorie's art, initiated at first to please me, became an oasis for her, something she was able to keep as her own, along with the therapeutic gains she had accomplished through her hard work. I am grateful for what she taught me, and for her willingness to teach others through giving me permission to share her written reflections.

Story 5: A Man Discovers His Art in a Book 30 Years after Therapy as a Child

The first book I ever published was called *Child Art Therapy* (Rubin, 1978). Because I was no longer seeing the children or families described in it, my supervisor felt it would be unduly intrusive to contact them for permission to print either their images or their art. My publisher in that less litigious era did not require signed permissions, so I never contacted anyone. I *did,* however, change their names to disguise their identities. Thirty years later, I received an email from a young man who had been in a children's art and drama therapy group at the clinic where I worked. It read:

> Hi. Just wanted to pass along something that happened recently. I was getting some books ready for my student aides to reshelf when I noticed one written by you, *Child Art Therapy*. I leafed through it and low and behold stumbled on my own story—I still have the artwork that is shown in the book!!!!!

As you can tell from his message, he had become a librarian, the director in fact of the library at a nearby university which happened to have an art therapy training program. When I received his email, I wrote and asked if he would be interested in getting together to tell me how it felt to see artwork that he had actually saved (so it was therefore clearly important to him) in a book where I had told his story using another name. He responded cautiously: "I think it would be interesting to talk about how seeing my artwork in your book felt. I would be happy to meet with you to discuss it."

When we met in a colleague's office he was candid, saying that when he first saw the images and read his story in the book, he had been angry about not having been asked for permission to have them included. Invited to tell me more about his reaction, he said that, after getting over the shock and surprise of finding his story and his artwork in print, he felt more comfortable, and was relieved that his name had been disguised. It was a vivid reminder to me, as in Marjorie's story, that "*the art is the person,*" something art therapists can too easily forget.

I had asked his permission to include our brief encounter in this Foreword, and he said he would be happy for me to do so. Recently he wrote asking if I had ultimately included anything about our meeting, adding "And I don't remember if I emailed you to tell you how much I enjoyed the time we spent together." I wrote back to let him know not only that I too enjoyed getting together, but also to send him a draft of this part of the chapter. He replied that it was fine and that he got a kick out of being referred to as "a young man." As with Marjorie, I am grateful for his permission to include the rest of his story.

Knowing What You Don't Know—Professional Ethics

The most sophisticated and accomplished individuals I have met during my career have also been the most modest; they are always learning, aware that they will never know it all. That attitude of humility is the most honest and ethical way to proceed, I believe, regardless of how many years of experience one has accumulated. What follows is a story about that issue.

Story 6: A Highly Successful Play Therapist Studies Art Therapy

My favorite example of this kind of professional ethics is the true story of a woman who was already a very well regarded play therapist when she decided she needed to study more because she didn't understand enough about the art of the children she was seeing. Although she had earned an MA in Psychology in 1978 and a PhD in Marital and Family Therapy in 1982, in 1994 she voluntarily undertook a two-year post-doctoral training program in art therapy with stringent requirements: 21 credits consisting of graduate courses, participation in an internship program, completion of a colloquium paper, and 700 hours of clinical supervision. She did all of this work—not required but desired—despite a very busy clinical and teaching schedule.

By the time she started the training, this highly ethical individual had already published seven books for lay and professional audiences, one of which became an instant classic in her field (Gil, 1991). And by the time she finished the training, she had published three more, one of which became a classic on work with families (Gil, 1994). Eliana Gil *knew what she didn't know*, and wanted to know more so that she would be doing an honest, accurate, and therefore *ethical* job of working with children in art. She wanted to understand what children were telling her in their creations, and to do so at a level of sophistication not sought by most play therapists, though all of them offer their clients art media.

Showing the Real Faces of Art Therapy—Another Hot Potato

Earlier in this chapter, I described the potential ethical dilemmas posed by including actual vs. disguised names, as well as by including writing or artwork in books and films. As one who has made teaching films, written articles, chapters, and books with illustrations (some with DVDs included), I have chosen to use actual photos or video-tape of genuine art therapy whenever possible. Why have I made this admittedly controversial decision? Simply put, it is because for me the idea of ethics requires *honesty*. Although there are some art therapy videotapes and films in which students or others appear, rather than actual clients, the films achieve a feeling of *authenticity* only when those volunteers express their own personal concerns. When they do, the tapes or films look and feel as honest as real art therapy sessions. It is my firm belief that if we are to represent what we do—whether to students, other professionals, or the general public—it should be in the most honest (ethical) way possible. There is real human passion in authentic art therapy. It is something to be understood and respected as a vital aspect of what we do. For that reason, I believe that we have a responsibility to represent it in as true a way as possible.

Moreover, if therapy goes well, those who have been served are more than happy to share their experience with others. When I was in private practice, although colleagues often sent patients, the majority of referrals came from "satisfied customers," those who had been helped. I believe that is true for most clinicians, whatever their discipline.

Story 7: A Grateful Client Freely Gives Permission to Use a Video Clip

Almost 20 years ago, when I was making the first version of the film *Art Therapy Has Many Faces* (Rubin, 2004), Dr. Aina Nucho sent me some videotapes she had made of therapy sessions conducted by another colleague, Dr. Mala Betensky. I wanted to include in my film a clip from an art therapy session that appeared on a videotape but, because the tape had been made for teaching purposes, I wanted to make sure that the clients would be comfortable with my doing so. Although Mala had died, with assistance from her colleague and her daughter, I was able to get contact information for the wife of a couple that had appeared on tape.

When I called and explained the reason, the woman readily gave her permission to include the clip, saying she remembered the session well since she and her husband had re-viewed the tape many times. When I asked where I should send a release form for them to sign, she replied with some distress that she was offended. When I asked why, she told me that it would be unnecessary, since her therapy with Dr. Betensky had saved her life and, if I were a friend of Mala's (which I was), she would be honored for the clip of her session to be included in my film.

It had been many years since she had seen Dr. Betensky, but she was clearly delighted that their work together could be helpful to others and found the notion of signing a form to be offensive. Her bond with her therapist had not been on the dotted line; it had been deep and personal and had involved profound trust, a necessary condition for a good therapeutic alliance. She also told me that her son had been in art therapy with Mala off and on throughout his growing up. I asked if he was the one on several videotapes also recorded by Dr. Nucho and she said that he was and that, as with her own experience, the therapy had been vital to him. I wondered about sending him a release form, but she rejected that offer, saying that she would ask him herself and would call me if he were not comfortable being included. She went into some detail, telling me that, although he was developmentally disabled, he had become a happy young adult now living on his own, which she attributed to his therapy with Dr. Betensky. This was a powerful and moving conversation, one I will never forget.

It was a reminder that, while maintaining the privacy of our interactions with patients during and after treatment is essential, it is not unethical to want to share their art, their writings, and even their faces and voices if it can help others as they have been helped. What was most heartening was that this woman's positive experience in art therapy enabled her not only to *allow* her videotape to be used, but to *want* it to be included so that others could be helped as she had been.

I could tell many more stories, but I think I have probably made my point by now. Ethics in art therapy, whether about touching, telling, or showing the art or faces of those you serve, will probably never be reducible to a simple list of do's and don'ts. Rather, it is founded on *sincere respect* for the other and open communication. It is also founded on humility, on *knowing what you don't know,* and on striving to learn whatever is needed in order to do no harm and to help as much as possible.

A Cautionary Note

In regard to *doing no harm,* I should like to conclude with some excerpts from *A Cautionary Note.* I wrote it to end my first book, *Child Art Therapy* (Rubin, 1978), and have often quoted from it in commencement addresses for students graduating from training programs. Because art therapy looks and seems so *simple,* it is especially vital for those practicing it to be aware of how powerful it is—that it has huge potential to help, but equally huge potential to harm. It is thrilling to realize how much we can assist others, but to do so ethically, we need to be aware of art therapy's hazards …

> The procedures described in this book may seem simple, perhaps deceptively so. Art is a powerful tool—one which, like the surgeon's, must be used with care and skill if it is to penetrate safely beneath the surface. Using media with those who are significantly disabled or disturbed (even without analysis of process or product) requires an understanding not only of art, but also of the world of those with whom one is working. The use of art with all kinds of children or families as a symbolic communicative medium is a clinically demanding task, which carries with it both a tremendous potential and an equally great responsibility. Dealing with those who are already vulnerable, or "opening up" others in a way that creates a certain vulnerability, can be either helpful or harmful. One need not be afraid to do many wonderful and meaningful things with children in art, but one must always respect the importance and the uniqueness of a child's emotional life. One also grows to respect, with some awe and humility, the potency of art, especially in the context of those special human relationships promoted in art therapy … The message of this note, therefore, is this: be neither fearful nor fearless, but proceed with open eyes, and with respect for the value of the child as well as the power of art. If you are just beginning, be sure you have someone who understands diagnosis and therapy much better than you do to guide you. If that person also understands art, so much the better. Even "natural clinicians" can add depth of understanding to their intuition. All who undertake the awesome task of helping others, I think, have a responsibility to carry out their work with as much sensitivity and skill as they can possibly develop.
>
> *Rubin, 2005, pp. 387–388*

This foreword ends, and this book begins, therefore, with the hope that those who read it will indeed carry on, but that they will do so with care.

References

Gil, E. (1991). *The healing power of play: Therapy with abused children.* New York: The Guilford Press.

Gil, E. (1994). *Play in family therapy.* New York: The Guilford Press.

Howie, P., Prasad, S., & Kristel, J. (2013). *Using art therapy with diverse populations: Crossing cultures and abilities.* London: Jessica Kingsley.

Rubin, J.A. (1969). Preparing to teach elementary art. *Art Education,* 22(9), 4–11.

Rubin, J.A. (1972). *We'll Show You What We're Gonna Do!* 16 mm film. DVD Revision, 2008. Pittsburgh, PA: Expressive Media.

Rubin, J.A. (1973). A diagnostic art interview. *Art Psychotherapy,* 1, 31–34.

Rubin, J.A. (1978). *Child art therapy* (3rd ed. 2005). New York: John Wiley & Sons.

Rubin, J.A. (2004). *Art therapy has many faces* (Rev. Ed. 2008). Pittsburgh, PA: Expressive Media.

Rubin, J.A. (2005). *Artful therapy.* New York: John Wiley & Sons.

Winnicott, D.W. (1960). The theory of the parent–infant relationship. *International Journal of Psycho-Analysis,* 41: 585–595.

PREFACE

This is not a book about theoretical constructs; it doesn't present a litany of *dos and don'ts* concerning ethical conduct. This is a book that presents real-life ethical dilemmas that art therapists have encountered on the job and describes how they endeavored to resolve them; *endeavored*, because some ethical dilemmas defy solution.

There are many multi-step protocols available to assist mental health professionals in making decisions that are ethical—some are included in these chapters—but the aim of this book is to encourage readers, when facing an ethical dilemma, to look not only at laws and ethics codes, but also at other relevant factors, such as what they might be bringing to the ethical decision-making process.

ACKNOWLEDGEMENTS

My heartfelt appreciation to all those who have contributed—in so very many ways—to the development of this book. Most importantly, to the chapter writers, who have generously shared not only their experience and expertise, but also their uncertainty and their missteps, so that we readers might benefit as we wrestle with the ethical dilemmas that confront us, and to Judith A. Rubin, PhD, ATR-BC, HLM, an art therapist whom I have admired for decades, for her gift of the Foreword.

To Finlay McInally, who created the artwork on the cover of this book, and to all the other art therapists and art therapy students who answered the Call for Art for the cover. To Brenda Barthell, Anne Corson, Bani Malhotra, Kristina Nowak, Jid Shwanpach Ratanapinyopong, Min Kyung Shin, Sarah Vollman, Hannah Wittman, and Amelia Zakour, whose artwork eloquently introduces the sections of this book. The art in art therapy is certainly alive and well!

To all of our clients, students, teachers, mentors, and therapists, who have taught us so much about ethics, clinical work, and life in general. A thank you to my own teachers, Edith Kramer, Hanna Yaxa Kwiatkowska, Mildred Lachman, Bernard Levy, and Elinor Ulman—as well as to my mother, who taught grammar for decades (not only at school, but also at home)!

To Amanda Devine, Elizabeth Graber, and Christopher Teja, my gifted editors, as well as to the wonderfully efficient Jamie Magyar, editorial assistant, at Routledge. To Kris Siosyte, production manager at Taylor & Francis, UK, and to Kelly Winter, project manager, and Hamish Ironside, copy-editor—true professionals, all!

To Dr. Raymond Pasi, whose idea of asking students to interview mental health professionals about ethical issues lit one of the sparks that led to the development of this book.

To Trudy Summers, friend, sounding board, and Wednesday luncheon companion for the past four decades; to my dear friends Wilma Scheuren, Barbara Mandel, Chuck Ludlam, and Paula Hirschoff, fellow members of the Levy Watercolor Group since

1984; and to the amazing women with whom I had the privilege of working at a small psycho-educational facility in DC during the 70s, 80s, and 90s (now shuttered). As Harriet Crawley put it, "We grew up together!" For their sage advice, exemplary models of ethical behavior, and warm friendship, I thank them all.

To Raymond I. Band, M.D., for his wisdom (and patience).

To Christian Gonzalez for his wizardry in organizing the files of the final manuscript.

To Nora Stinley, who first mentioned my name to Routledge, and to Samantha Ahwah, for raising an extremely challenging ethical question.

And, to Ken, whose unstinting support has come in many guises, among them the creation of *a writing room of my own*, the door to which was equipped with a cat flap, through which hot cups of tea and homemade blueberry/cranberry muffins would miraculously appear. Ken's help, perspective, and Aussie sense of humor made this venture possible.

Also gratefully acknowledged are the following copyright holders, for their permission to include quotations:

> From *Advanced Ethics for Addiction Professionals* by Michael J. Taleff (2010), republished with permission of Springer Publishing Co., permission conveyed through Copyright Clearance Center, Inc.
>
> From *Art as Therapy With Children* by Edith Kramer (1971), Schocken Books, an imprint of the Knopf Doubleday Publishing Group, a division of Penguin Random House LLC.
>
> From *Art on Trial* by David E. Gussak (2013), Columbia University Press. Reprinted with permission of the publisher.
>
> From *The Collected Works of W. B. Yeats, Volume I: The Poems*, by W.B. Yeats, edited by Richard J. Finneran. Copyright 1928 by The Macmillan Co., renewed 1956 by Georgie Yeats. Reprinted with permission of Scribner, a division of Simon & Schuster, Inc. All rights reserved.
>
> From *Ethical Issues in Art Therapy* (3rd ed.) by B. L. Moon (2015), courtesy of Charles C. Thomas Publisher, Ltd., Springfield, IL.
>
> From "From China to South Korea: Two perspectives on individual psychology in Asia" by S. Sun and J. B. Bitter. *The Journal of Individual Psychology, 68*(3), Fall 2012. Reprinted with the permission of the University of Texas Press.
>
> From "Help! My Supervisor is Unethical" by Frederic G. Reamer. June, 2013. Reprinted with the permission of *Social Work Today*, Great Valley Publishing Co.
>
> From "Korean Families" by B. C. Kim and E. Ryu. In M. McGoldrick, J. Giordano, & N. Garcia-Preto (Eds.), *Ethnicity and Family Therapy* (3rd ed.) (2005). Copyright Guilford Press. Reprinted with permission of Guilford Press.
>
> From *The Paper Office* (4th ed.) by Edward L. Zuckerman (2008). Copyright Guilford Press. Reprinted with permission of Guilford Press.
>
> From *Trauma and Recovery* by J. Herman (1992). Reprinted by permission of Basic Books, a member of the Perseus Books Club.

PART I
Looking Beneath the Surface

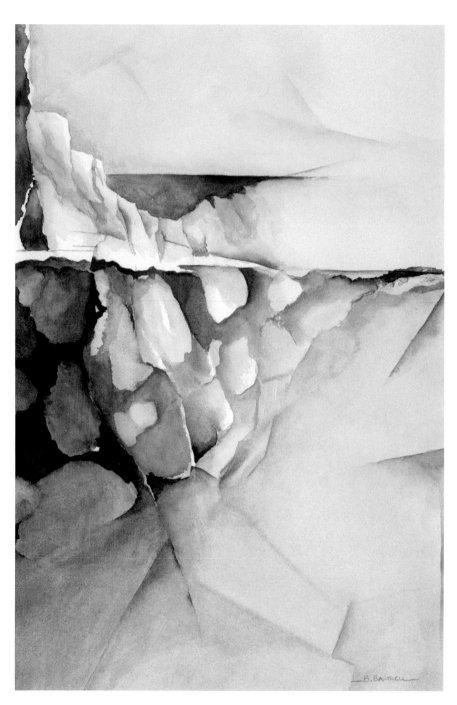

Brenda Barthell *(see color insert)*

1

FACTORS THAT CAN INFLUENCE THE ETHICAL DECISION-MAKING PROCESS

Audrey Di Maria

Rummaging through the attic of my childhood home recently, I pried open a trunk to find a stack of 40-year-old graduate school notebooks. As I flipped through their pages, my mind drifted back to a course I had taken as a first-year student: "Art as Therapy with Children."

All eyes were riveted upon our professor, Edith Kramer, as—her hand slicing the air, her long gray braid bouncing on her back as she moved from one side of the room to the other—she described one of the earliest and most challenging experiences she had had while working at a residential treatment facility for boys who, at that time, were referred to as "disturbed." Ten-year-old Martin—whose relationship with his mother was characterized by provocation (on Martin's part), punishment (by his mother), and reconciliation—was energetically painting an unflattering picture of the school administrators, when suddenly he obliterated the image, destroying his work. Edith told us that the excitement that she had felt while Martin was painting was immediately replaced by a surge of anger toward him. As she explained in the section on transference and counter-transference in her classic book, *Art as Therapy with Children*:

> I had identified with Martin. By painting the caricatures, Martin had expressed for me my own hostility against the school's directors, and on a deeper level he had expressed my childhood rebellion against parental authority. As long as his caricatures were good, he had gratified my aggressive desires in a way that was acceptable to me. I had indulged in more vicarious gratification than is permitted to the therapist and so I was doubly hurt when Martin reverted to raw destructiveness. I was not only attacked in my role as Martin's teacher who had helped him to make the picture, but I was much more deeply hurt because identification with Martin made me experience his regression as my own. Since breakdown of sublimation was to me the most serious menace to my integrity

as an artist, I experienced Martin's attack on his painting as an attack on me, and I reacted with panic, regression, and counterattack.

Kramer 1971, pp. 41–42

In an instant, Edith conveyed to us how easily our own feelings could become intertwined in the work that we would do as art therapists. Her generosity in sharing this experience gave us a glimpse of Edith, *the person* (rather than Edith, the theoretician, Edith, the author, Edith, the artist) as she went about her work. She made it OK to talk about mistakes. In allowing us to see the motivations underlying her action, she challenged us to become more aware of our own.

When confronting ethical dilemmas, we neglect a big part of the picture if we fail to take into consideration what we, as individuals, are bringing to the decision-making process. As much as we might strive to be, we are not objective observers, nor should we be. Our internal responses can inform our understanding of the work, but we must factor our own values, sensitivities, and blind spots into the equation if we are not to be inadvertently led by them.

What, specifically, do we take into consideration when faced with dilemmas that might involve or impact our clients? The informed consent document they signed upon beginning treatment might seem to be a blueprint for treatment, outlining the roles and responsibilities of both parties, but what about aspects of our clients that do not wend their way onto a sheet of paper or into a computer file, such as their belief systems, their cultural traditions, their religious convictions?

The Graphic

The graphic (Figure 1.1) does not present a sequence of steps, but a *mandala* of variables that can (knowingly or unknowingly) influence our ethical decision-making process. At the center of it all is our client. The phrase at the top of each ring (e.g., Laws, Ethics Codes, Policies and Procedures, Job Descriptions, and Professional Training, Experience, and Skills) references material that is easier to codify than that which is represented by the phrase on the bottom of each ring. Even "Professional Training, Experience, and Skills"—which might seem to be less discrete or to have boundaries that are more elastic than, say, the Law—can be embodied by graduate course syllabi and grades, descriptions of jobs held, credentials indicating the meeting of licensure or certification requirements, or Continuing Education certificates confirming the completion of skill-based instruction. Not so with the descriptors at the bottom of the rings and the central circle. Thus, our client's goals, expectations, concerns, values, and culture are inherently more difficult to define or delineate than the terms of the informed consent document that the client has signed. The outermost ring has been left blank in order to accommodate other factors that might affect our own ethical decision-making process, such as our personal traits and tendencies.

Ethical dilemmas can easily arise when there is tension or conflict *between* the rings (e.g., when a therapist's values are in opposition to an administrator's actions) or *within* the rings (e.g., when the norms of a workplace do not reflect that institution's policies and procedures). Even more important are the dilemmas that are generated by friction

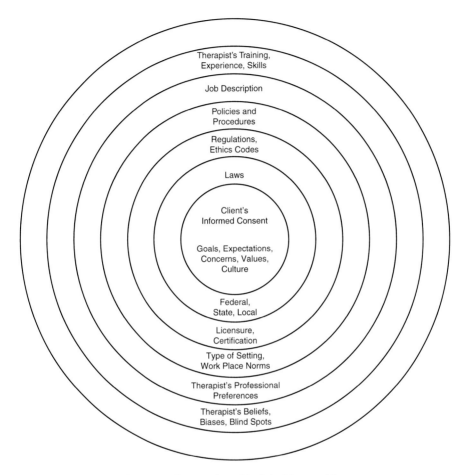

FIGURE 1.1 Factors that can influence the ethical decision-making process.

between factors represented by the concentric circles and the rights, preferences, and needs of the individual who is at the very core of our work (e.g., when our blind spots include an appreciation of the important role played by our client's culture).

Laws, Ethics Codes, and Informed Consent

It is our responsibility to know the laws and the ethical principles that govern our work, but are they as definitive as they appear to be? What happens when international, national, provincial, or municipal laws conflict with one another or with the ethics codes of our profession (Di Maria, 2013a)? How judiciously are laws constructed and how equitably are they applied?

State laws in the US (e.g., regarding the age of consent, the duty to warn, the statute of limitations for prosecuting the sexual abuse of children) vary widely. Those governing the licensure of art therapists are no exception (e.g., with regard to title protection, reimbursement by insurance companies). Some state laws (e.g., regarding the privacy of client records) have stricter provisions than federal laws. Anne Patrick's book, *Liberating Conscience*, (1997) written from the perspective of a Catholic feminist, makes the point that rules can be used to justify behavior that is unethical or immoral. As I write this, the federal government appears to be chipping away at *home rule* here in the District of Columbia (*The Washington Post*, July 24, 2018); our city council's decision to declare Washington a "sanctuary city" might have repercussions in terms of the allocation of federal funds; and District residents are still not represented in Congress by a voting member.

Imagine that you are an art therapist who works in DC, San Francisco, or one of the other sanctuary cities. You have been seeing the child of a parent who is an undocumented immigrant, and one day that child arrives at a session with visible bruises. The child wants to draw, and both the content of that drawing and the comments made by the child regarding the artwork indicate that the bruises might have been inflicted in the home. Art therapists are mandated reporters. Is your course of action clear? Does the context make a difference?

Some of us live in places where there are no regulations governing the practice of art therapy, in particular, or mental health treatment, in general. For guidance, we might turn to the ethics code of a certification body (such as the Art Therapy Credentials Board in the US) or a professional membership organization (such as the American Art Therapy Association). Aspirational values, such as autonomy, nonmaleficence, beneficence, fidelity, and justice (which—along with creativity—are included in the Preamble to AATA's *Ethical Principles for Art Therapists*, 2013) can help to clarify what is at stake when we are confronting situations that are ethically challenging. (Although I refer here to AATA and the ATCB, due to my greater familiarity with the provisions of their codes, many other countries have professional art therapy membership organizations and credentialing bodies, several of which are referenced in the chapters that follow.)

In the absence of an art therapy association, credentialing procedure, or training program, we might turn to the policies and procedures of the agency in which we work or to the cultural norms and traditions of the workplace—as well as the description of the position we hold. Most importantly, there is the agreement that the client and therapist have made with each other; whether it is called an informed consent document or goes by another name, it forms the basis of our contract with the client, outlining what the client has given us permission to do.

The Clientele, the Setting, and the Mode of Treatment

Are some ethical challenges more likely to arise in specific types of settings or when we are working with clients who have particular mental health conditions? How might our response to an ethical issue (such as one involving the use of non-erotic touch, gift giving and/or receiving, self-disclosure, or the creation of artwork with, or alongside, a client) vary in settings as diverse as an early intervention program for preschoolers, an assisted living facility, a detention center for adolescents, a private practice, a community-based studio, an inpatient hospital for members of the armed services, a camp set up for those displaced by a natural disaster? What is the effect upon our decision-making process of our mode of treatment, be it individual or group, couples, family, or community-based work)?

Our Theoretical Orientation, Training, and Experience

How often do we automatically rely upon tenets that we absorbed during art therapy classes or internships? To what extent does our current theoretical orientation reflect that of our training program, our supervisors, our co-workers, our therapists? Whose example do we endeavor to emulate—or did we vow never to replicate? To what extent did these early experiences become professional preferences that might narrow our focus when we're facing ethical dilemmas?

Our Values, Traits, and Tendencies

In an engaging workshop, Catherine M. Iacuzzi, PsyD, MLADC, introduced us to the set of wonderfully provocative questions that comprise Michael Taleff's (2010, p. 30) Ethical Self-Exam:

- Do you live via or through a certain set of ethical (moral) standards?
- If you do, could you easily spell them out if asked, or would you find yourself having trouble coming to an answer?
- If you do have standards, essentially what are they? (Write out a list.)
- Do you assess different ethical situations by the same standards or do you use different standards for different ethical situations?
- If you do assess different situations by different standards, what reasons can you cite for this action?
- Do you ever cheat on your standards? If so, on what particular circumstances do you usually or most often cheat?
- Do you judge others with one set of standards and judge your actions by a different set?
- If so, can you recall the last time you did this, and on what did you cheat?

Might taking this "quiz" highlight areas that could have an undue influence upon us when we are endeavoring to make a decision that is ethical?

On my first day of work as an art therapist, 40 years ago, I was told to report to the office of the chief psychiatrist at the facility, a psychoanalyst, for the customary welcome to new employees. I don't recall what was said, except for his parting words: "Remember, when in doubt, do nothing." Silently, I protested, "That's you, that's not me! When in doubt, I'll do ... something."

And I did. I cringe to think about it. It took both work and life experience, good supervision, consultation, and my own therapy (psychoanalysis) to recognize—among many other things—that thinking is, indeed, doing something (I can hear my analyst asking, "Are you thinking, Audrey, or ruminating?") and that figuring out why "taking action" was so important to me was time well spent. Why do I share this? Because, in analyzing the possible courses of action (so to speak) open to us when we face an ethical dilemma, it is important to be aware of our well-worn paths; the preconceptions, biases, and blind spots through which our thoughts are being filtered—often, without our knowledge.

In a writing class he had attended, my 89-year-old Uncle Waddie was given an assignment to write a "one-word biography" of each of his siblings; the one that he chose for my mother was "principled." I ask students in the Ethics course I teach, "If you had to describe yourself in one word, what would it be?" I then ask them to create artwork that illustrates how that quality might affect their ethical decision-making process. A student who had been in the military services came up with the word "protective" and illustrated ways in which this characteristic might affect his decision-making process in ways intended and unintended.

How would you respond to the following questions? Am I inclined:

- To look before I leap, just leap, or look and look and look?
- To rely upon my instincts?
- To question authority?
- To shy away from conflict?
- To take a stand?
- To side with the majority?
- To allow loyalty to play a role in my decision-making process?
- To make excuses? For whom?
- To identify with some clients? What do they have in common?
- To worry about alienating people as a result of my actions? Whom?
- To become defensive? About what?
- To ask for help?
- To become incensed by particular situations? What are they?
- To acknowledge my mistakes?
- To respond thoughtfully to criticism?
- To refrain from questioning the motivations or actions of certain people? Name these people. How did they become part of this group?

Might aspects of our decision-making process reflect our response to any of these questions?

How might our familial and personal experiences inform our decision making? Growing up in a home with one parent, my sister and I did not witness the "sandpapering of ideas" (a phrase coined by Bernie Levy) that can occur when consensus is reached as a result of the thrashing out of divergent points of view. In our home, it was more of a "the buck stops here" approach, as one parent stepped up to make whatever decisions had to be made. And, although I didn't yet know the term, the often confusing nature of multiple relationships was felt early on, as, in our small town, my Aunt Barb was also my sixth grade teacher—and my mother was my seventh and eighth grade teacher! Indeed, my journey through each grade was travelled the following year by my cousin Jeff, the next year by my sister Gail, and the year after that, by my cousin Vaughan.

Not long after a member of my family committed suicide, I recall participating in a treatment team meeting in which I speculated that the client being discussed seemed to be exhibiting signs of depression. When our consulting psychiatrist said, "Oh, Audrey, you always think that people are depressed," I responded, "Well, aren't they?" (I knew I was—and I wasn't taking chances with anyone else.)

Deciphering and Challenging our Biases and Blind Spots

The ATCB *Code of Ethics, Conduct, and Disciplinary Procedures* (2018) states that:

> Art therapists will not discriminate against, or refuse professional services to individuals or groups based on age, gender, gender identity, gender expression, sexual orientation, ethnicity, race, national origin, culture, marital/partnership status, citizenship or immigration status, ability, religion/spirituality, or any other bias.
>
> *Standard 1.1.2*

When we read the phrase, "or any other bias," what comes to mind--political party affiliation, mode of dress, body size? An exercise that may illuminate implicit biases is Harvard University's "Implicit Bias Test" (1990). "See No Bias," by Shankar Vedantam (2005), explores the process further. Personally, I have found Charles Ridley's *Overcoming Unintentional Racism in Counseling and Therapy: A Practitioner's Guide to Intentional Intervention* (1995) to be very helpful (Di Maria, 2013b).

As therapists, it might be eye-opening to look through the *Diagnostic and Statistical Manual of Mental Disorders* (5th ed.) (American Psychiatric Association, 2013) and rank order the categories by the ease which we would feel in working with clients who have been diagnosed as having the conditions listed. (Could we be biased against people who have certain mental health conditions?)

As art therapists, we might want to examine the potential influence of the degree or type of artistic skill shown by our clients. And let's not forget the tools of our trade, the art materials. Each of the chapters that follow includes "Reflective Art Experiences" (thank you to Mary Roberts for suggesting that term) and "Discussion Questions" that are geared toward the professional development of the reader (rather than being directives for use with clients). Let's try a couple of Reflective Art Experiences to do with art materials …

REFLECTIVE ART EXPERIENCES

1. Create artwork using your favorite art materials; the ones you use most often when creating your own artwork. Afterward, consider the extent to which the materials you favor either deliberately or inadvertently influences the choice of materials (a) you are inclined to present to your clients; (b) you are apt to make most readily available (i.e., within easy reach) in the art therapy space; or (c) you tend to order for your art therapy practice.

2. Choosing art materials that you like the least, create a second piece of artwork. Next, jot down some of your reactions to the piece, the process of

creating it, and the qualities of the materials, themselves. Then, think about ways in which your own feelings about the use of these particular materials might indirectly be conveyed to your clients. Consider what might have been gained or lost by your clients as a result. What aspirational values might have been impacted by your decision?

On those occasions when we wish that we had made a decision other than the one we made, Welfel offers a helpful "Three-Step Model of Recovery," within a section on "Self-Monitoring: Taking Responsibility in the Absence of a Complaint" in her book entitled *Ethics in Counseling and Psychotherapy: Standards, Research, and Emerging Issues* (2016). I have found Welfel's book to be a useful textbook—along with Bruce Moon's ground-breaking, *Ethical Issues in Art Therapy*, 3rd ed. (2015).

I could go on, but I recall Elinor Ulman admonishing us to "Say what you have to say, then sit down," as well as to "Leave them wanting to hear *more*—not *less!*" So, I'll leave you with the following.

Films Fraught with Ethical Dilemmas

When teaching Ethics, the first assignment I give is the viewing of one of these films, to be discussed during the following class. It always generates hearty (at times, heated) debates about how the dilemmas raised in the films could or should have been resolved, as well as cogent reflections upon the ethical decision-making models exhibited by the characters (Fletcher, as cited in Moon, 2015). My thanks to Reverend Brendan Whittaker for recommending the film *Gone Baby Gone* (US, 2007), which became the first on an ever-lengthening list of thought-provoking films, dutifully researched (popcorn in hand). Some of my favorites are:

A Fantastic Woman (Chile, 2017)
Against the Current (US, 2009)
Crash (US, 2004)
Eye in the Sky (UK, 2015)
Far From the Tree (US, 2017)
Gett: The Trial of Viviane Amsalem (Israel and France, 2014)
Graduation (Romania, 2017)
Land of Mine (Denmark, 2015)
Last Men in Aleppo (Syria, 2017)
Proof (Australia, 1991)
Snowden (US, 2016)
Spotlight (US, 2015)
The Darkest Hour (UK and US, 2017)
The Innocents (France, 2016)
Weiner (US, 2016)

And, since watching the films listed above can be disquieting, I'll end the list with:

What About Bob? (US, 1991)

References

American Art Therapy Association (2013). *Ethical principles for art therapists.* Alexandria, VA: Author.

American Psychiatric Association (2013). *The diagnostic and statistical manual of mental disorders* (5th ed.). Washington, DC: Author.

Art Therapy Credentials Board (2018). *Code of ethics, conduct, and disciplinary procedures.* Greensboro, NC: Author.

Di Maria Nankervis, A. (2013a). Ethics in art therapy. In P. Howie, S. Prasad, & J. Kristel (Eds.), *Using art therapy with diverse populations: Crossing cultures and abilities* (pp. 56–64). London: Jessica Kingsley.

Di Maria Nankervis, A. (2013b). Working cross-culturally with children at risk. In P. Howie, S. Prasad, & J. Kristel (Eds.), *Using art therapy with diverse populations: Crossing cultures and abilities* (pp. 134–142). London: Jessica Kingsley.

Editorial: "Here we go again" (2018, July 24). The Washington Post, p. A16.

Harvard University (1990). The implicit bias test. Retrieved from www.implicit.harvard.edu

Kramer, E. (1971). *Art as therapy with children.* New York: Schocken Books.

Moon, B.L. (2015). *Ethical issues in art therapy* (3rd ed.). Springfield, IL: Charles C. Thomas.

Patrick, A.E. (1997). *Liberating conscience: Feminist explorations in Catholic moral theology.* New York: Continuum.

Ridley, C.R. (1995). *Overcoming unintentional racism in counseling and therapy: A practitioner's guide to intentional intervention.* Thousand Oaks, CA: Sage.

Taleff, M.J. (2010). *Advanced ethics for addiction professionals.* New York: Springer.

Vedantam, S. (January 23, 2005). See no bias. Retrieved from www.washingtonpost.com/wp-dyn/content/article/2005/01/23/AR2005040314622

Welfel, E.R. (2016). *Ethics in counseling and psychotherapy: Standards, research, and emerging issues.* Boston, MA: Cengage Learning.

2

INFORMED CONSENT AND MORE

Positioning the Private Practice Contract at the Crossroads of the Art Therapist's Ethical, Clinical, Financial, and Legal Responsibilities

Anne Mills

> Thus there are four aspects of the psychotherapy practice: the therapeutic, the ethical, the legal, and the financial. These four dimensions interact, intertwine, and may compete with one another.
>
> *Zuckerman, 2008, p. 10*

This chapter consists of the contract I use in my private practice (see Appendix A), my commentary about various sections of the contract (with reference to the line numbers as shown in the appendix), and vignettes that illustrate the relevant ethical issues. Each comment or vignette is introduced by the number of the line on the contract to which it corresponds. The reader will derive the most benefit from this chapter by—after reading each comment or vignette—turning to the contract to read the line to which that comment corresponds.

A Cautionary Note

Readers are welcome to use all, or to adapt any part, of my contract. However, readers should also be warned that it is their responsibility—and theirs alone—to adapt the contract in accordance with the laws, regulations, and ethics codes to which they are subject at the time that they make use of this document, and to have it reviewed and revised by a lawyer specializing in mental health law.

I write as the sole proprietor of an unincorporated business in an American city. I am the only therapist in the practice. I offer art therapy and other mental health services to children and adults, as well as supervision and consultation to mental health professionals. To whatever extent this description does not match you or your practice, your policies and, thus, your contract may differ substantially. Preferences and solutions that work for my business may not be appropriate for yours.

Many forms of giving information (e.g., privacy policies that comply with the Health Insurance Portability and Accountability Act [HIPAA]) and seeking consent (e.g., permission to treat) occur in private practice, and many of them are enfolded within this contract. Many physicians prefer to present us with numerous single pages of notifications, asking us to sign each one. I find it simpler to present most notifications and consents within one document, calling for one signature. It is a matter of personal preference and what your lawyer recommends. My contract does not address all situations under which a clinician gives information and seeks proof of informed consent. Others include: client intake forms, including emergency contact information; coverage by another therapist during vacations; a professional will; permission to photograph client artwork; and consent to use hypnosis. However, the contract is an attempt to anticipate areas of risk and to manage them proactively.

In a sense, a contract is a statement of where and how the clinician and the client are setting boundaries *around the therapy* in order to protect therapy. As society, ethics codes, and laws change, clarifications must be made and new issues addressed. For that reason, I update my contract three times a year.

Presenting the Contract

The style in which I work is a little unusual. During our first contact, potential clients are told that I offer an initial evaluation during which time they are asked to evaluate me, to see if they could perhaps develop a good working relationship with me. I tell them that I will be seeing if my skills are a good match for what they seem to need. I explain that they will draw pictures during the initial evaluation because that is the best way I have to get to know someone quickly. I expect both of us to think about how the meeting has gone and then to talk on the telephone a day later to compare notes. If either of us feels that it is not a good fit, I aim to give three referrals which are clinically, financially, and geographically appropriate.

During the initial evaluation I give the potential client a copy of my contract, asking him or her to read it later, as it provides information about me and how I work. If we mutually agree to work together, the contract is reviewed aloud thoroughly and signed in the next meeting, which is the first session.

Because many of the people with whom I work have attachment disorders and attachment avoidance, they tend to be highly anxious when contemplating beginning a new therapeutic relationship. Some attempt to cope with their anxiety by truncating the process—that is, rushing to a quick decision. I view the decision to work together as a serious commitment that we both must undertake thoughtfully, which is why I instituted this particular approach. Some clinicians move into evaluation and commitment to treat in the first meeting; others extend both processes over three sessions. Each clinician must find what works for his or her particular situation therapeutically, ethically, financially, and legally.

Since part of my practice is long-term work with survivors of severe early trauma, reviewing the contracting process after some years of working together ensures that the conditions under which we are working will be the same as those of newer clients and provides a reminder of the boundaries inherent in the contract.

Ethical, Clinical, Legal, and Financial Considerations

Each line of my contact has been included for a specific reason. The comments and the vignettes I provide in this chapter indicate why particular lines were deemed necessary. Although my contract covers many topics, I will focus upon a few, for spatial considerations and to avoid repeating subjects (e.g., telehealth, termination) that are covered in detail in other chapters. (My contract can be found in Appendix A, page 389.)

Contract Line 22: *Credentials*

Although I was licensed as an LCAT in New York State, since the license is now Inactive, I do not include it in my professional materials. Inactive licenses, and degrees that do not pertain to the services being offered, should not be listed among our credentials or appear on our signature line.

Contract Line 25: *Telehealth*

Although regulations governing telehealth and telemedicine are continually shifting, requirements (at the time I am writing) include that one be licensed in both the state where he or she practices and the state where the potential client is situated. Since I offer distance psychotherapy but have not completed specialized training in distance psychotherapy (this training is not required in all jurisdictions), it is ethically necessary for me to state this unequivocally. For our own legal protection, it can be advantageous to state the limitations of our practice in writing. Of course, we do not work beyond our areas of competence.

Contract Line 41: *Collaboration*

When I began in private practice, I was aware that some people who sought art therapy did not yet perceive it as *real therapy*. Some sought it as an expression of discomfort with the status of their verbal psychotherapy. Certainly, I witnessed the intense immediate positive transference to the art materials, as well as the idealization of the art therapist, who was imagined to be more fun or permissive or to have fewer boundaries than the primary therapist. As a new private practitioner, I did not want to take on cases whose demands exceeded my abilities, nor did I wish to be misperceived as a therapist who would steal others' clients. I was wary of people who added an art therapist to their treatment team and then fired their primary therapists without the art therapist's involvement or awareness. The way I dealt with this in an early version of the contract was to state, "If the client chooses to terminate with the primary therapist, I would need to terminate as well, unless the client immediately selects a new primary therapist," which encouraged discussion of the issue. However, the day came when it was not in the best interest of the client for me to terminate with that individual when he or she wished to stop working with the primary therapist.

In addition to asking potential clients who has referred them, I ask if they already are in therapy with someone, if they have discussed their interest in art therapy with their primary therapist, and if their therapist approves of adding art therapy to their treatment (Mills, 2011). When a potential client is already seeing another therapist, the client comes to me as a "package deal." If I am uncomfortable with the other professional or their treatment approach, it is unfair to all parties for me to accept work with this client. This is a very delicate situation which may require a frank, thorough conversation with the other therapist and tact in referring the patient onward. In these cases, I request a release of information in the evaluation session and more time than the usual 24 hours for the potential client and me to arrive at a decision about whether to work together. I contact the primary therapist to verify the situation and learn about the client and the treatment from that therapist's perspective.

I tell all collaborating psychotherapists that I need: (a) to have a way to leave detailed information for you about my work with the client, asynchronously (e.g., via a confidential HIPAA-compliant voice mail that allows an extended recording time); (b) to hear regularly from you about how treatment is going on your side; and (c) to know that the client is seeing you regularly. If the primary therapist and I agree that we will work together, we also exchange information about coverage and vacations.

I was trained always to request information from, and to follow up on information provided by, prior therapists. I regard it as a courtesy to the client and the prior therapist to ensure that clinical wisdom is carried forward from past treatment; it may also reduce the number of times that the client has to tell his or her story. However, I have found that relatively few other mental health professionals engage in this practice. In my many years in private practice, no prior clinician has offered to send me a written discharge summary, and requests for information often seem to be misinterpreted as requests for clinical assistance. I cannot emphasize too strongly the importance of collaboration. In one case, I did not know that another mental health professional was seeing my client until the cost of the sessions was revealed by the public agency tasked with paying for the child's psychotherapy. Although all parties (including the other therapist) knew of my ongoing involvement, none had informed me or collaborated with me, resulting in an incomplete, uncoordinated treatment plan and a clinical situation that could have caused my client much confusion, if not harm.

Contract Line 44: *Release Forms for Collaborators*

My experience with the case discussed in the following ethical dilemma led to the wording of lines 44–49.

MY ETHICAL DILEMMA

Conflicting priorities

A high-functioning client was very concerned about privacy. He paid in cash for sessions and made it clear to me (his primary therapist) and his psychiatrist (previously his primary therapist) that he did not want any paper trail (including email) about his treatment. He did sign a standard release allowing me to communicate with his psychiatrist. The client, who lived alone, had a chronic, progressive, debilitating, and life-threatening illness that was treated by a number of medical specialists. He was deeply depressed by this illness and had been medically hospitalized briefly a year before when he had been physiologically unstable.

Due to his depression and lack of energy because of his medical condition, the client became irregular in making appointments with me and cancelled most of them at the last minute because he could not muster the energy to come. I contacted him weekly to set up sessions, providing some supportive therapy by phone, and although he said that he wanted to attend, nine weeks elapsed since our last appointment. At about this time, the psychiatrist copied me in an unencrypted emailed collaboration with the client's many medical specialists. It was helpful to receive the information about the client's health and to know that he was meeting regularly with the medical professionals.

My dilemma was three-fold: (a) Should I continue to provide services? (b) Should I clarify or renegotiate the status of the therapeutic relationship? (c) Should I seek the patient's written permission to participate in the email collaboration of my client's other providers, so that I might share germane information such as the fact that the client had not attended sessions for several weeks?

How would you respond?

For the writer's response, see Appendix B.

Contract Line 65: *Document Retention*

All private practitioners should have a document retention policy that states our policy on encryption, code names for clients' names in phones or appointment books, emails, texts, files of original art, digital images art, sensitive information such as clients' social security numbers or credit card numbers, insurance/client payment files, Records of Consultation (clinical notes, progress notes), and Notes (personal notes, psychotherapy notes). It should include when material will be scanned or shredded and how all the material is kept secure.

Contract Line 69: *Risks of Unsecured Email*

The HIPAA Omnibus Final Rule (2013) specifies that if a health care provider informs the client of the risks of sending protected health information by unsecured email, and the client still wants to receive the information by email, he or she can give consent to receive normal, unsecured emails from their psychotherapist (Huggins, 2013). This means that stating my preference that email be used only for scheduling might not be necessary. Specifying "encrypted email" and "normal, unsecured email" might be a good idea. How would you re-write this section?

As a federal statute, HIPAA would normally be more powerful than a state law, but if a state law about health professionals communicating with the public sets a higher standard of protection for the public than HIPAA, the art therapist must follow the state law. Art therapists in private practice need to know local laws regarding communication using various forms of technology. At times, federal law might seem less restrictive than our own moral code or common sense. Imagine a client whose concerns include being subjected to violence by an intimate partner. HIPAA may allow us to get permission from a client to send emails that refer to treatment, but could those emails put the client in danger if seen by an abusive partner? We choose the right path when we consider the client's safety before our expediency.

Contract Line 93: *Talking About Fees*

MY ETHICAL DILEMMA

"I'm only asking."

Example 1: I created a budget for my new private practice based upon business expenses and projected income. Deciding upon a fee, I advertised it with confidence and felt empowered to explain it should the fee be questioned or disputed by clients. A former supervisee, now a practicing art therapist in a distant state, was paying me for distance consultation on setting up a private practice. When he said, "I think I'll set my fees at the same level as you, to start out," I wasn't sure how to respond.

Example 2: I received an email from a psychologist who had just moved to the area. This person, who did not seem to have art therapy credentials, asked what the average fees charged locally by art therapists were, saying that, "as an art therapist and psychologist," he planned to charge 25% more.

How would you respond?

For the writer's response, see Appendix B.

Contract Line 99: *Paying On Time*

MY ETHICAL DILEMMA

"It's my money—isn't it?"

A client attended weekly sessions, but paid about every other week. When I reminded her verbally of the outstanding payments, she gave reasons for not paying the debt in full on the spot.

How would you respond?

For the writer's response, see Appendix B.

Contract Line 102: *Late Cancellation Policy*

Self-examination around late cancellation policies abounds in therapists' discussions with one another, as the ethical, therapeutic, and financial dimensions of the policy can all lead to dilemmas. It is emotionally loaded, and perhaps the most common area for acting out or enactments by both client and therapist. Some clients readily accept the therapist's late cancellation policy, volunteering the late payment fee without hesitation, while other clients persist in "forgetting" the fee even after the therapist and client have talked through one late cancellation.

While the therapist has a choice about how firm or flexible to be in administering the late cancellation policy, it is important to understand that applying, or failing to apply, a late cancellation policy can affect the therapy negatively (e.g., leading to premature termination) or positively (e.g., deepening the sense of safety and trustworthiness). Some therapists are flexible on cancellations when a client has a cold, so they won't be exposed to germs. Some charge for late cancellations only if they become customary or only after the reasons behind a client not showing up for therapy have been explored in session. Others charge for late cancellation fees except in emergencies.

MY ETHICAL DILEMMA

What constitutes an emergency?

A client called shortly before her session, saying that she didn't know why but she had to pull over to vomit by the side of the highway on the way to the session. She had not missed any prior session.

How would you respond?

For the writer's response, see Appendix B.

With particularly complex issues such as this, it can be helpful to print—in the margin of the contract, beside the section describing how that issue is addressed in therapy—a horizontal line on which the client may place his or her initials, indicating understanding and acceptance of that section of the contract. Ensuring that the policy is stated clearly also offers the opportunity for the therapist to say confidently why this is important and fair, and for the client to state if it is not acceptable or affordable. If the therapist's and client's needs or expectations diverge widely, it may be best to refer the client to a different therapist (Mikel, 2013). Interestingly, it is rare for a therapist to have a policy that penalizes *the therapist* for cancelling a session with less than 24 hours' notice—which raises another ethical issue!

Contract Line 112: *Payment*

If a client offers to pay you "if I can first present receipts to my insurance company and get the reimbursement," what is being proposed is fraudulent. All paperwork (dates of service, diagnoses, costs) must be accurate. To knowingly do otherwise would be health care or insurance fraud—crimes that may constitute a felony.

Contract Line 142: *Termination*

It is important to know that psychotherapists have much narrower grounds for unilateral termination than physicians (The Doctors Company, 2015).

Contract Line 173: *Location Tracking*

An example that illustrates the rationale for this inclusion is that of a client who might be in danger from an abusive spouse who is able to identify the pattern of the client's movements.

Contract Line 179: *Referrals*

Once Client A has referred someone to me (someone who might become Client B), I cannot discuss the matter; I can neither confirm nor deny to either client that the other is or is not a client.

Contract Line 185: *HIPAA*

HIPAA was established to raise the standards of confidentiality within healthcare and research in the United States (USHHS, 1996). Because of the need to maintain the confidentiality of protected health information, HIPAA affects private practice contracts.

HIPAA-covered entities may also be affected by sections of the Health Information Technology for Economic and Clinical Health (HITECH) Act (2009).

Contract Line 186: *Release of Information*

May a third party receive information about the fees a client pays, the client's medications or prognosis, or the client's history of hospitalization? It depends upon which third party is requesting the information, the details of the consent form signed by the client, and the state in which you practice (Jaffee-Redmond, 1996). Local laws may regulate the information we may disclose, even if our client has given written permission. Sometimes federal security clearances or law enforcement mental health background checks are pursued with such vigor that the mental health professional may lose sight of this. It is important to know the statutes that apply to the site of your practice and re-read them when information is requested. For instance, the District of Columbia Mental Health Information Act of 1978 provides clear limits and outlines civil damages and criminal penalties for violations of the limits of disclosure by clinicians or clients in group sessions. The Act protects clinicians by giving us the authority to limit authorized disclosures, and protects our personal notes. Because of this, I have found it acceptable to respond to these requests by writing:

> The enclosed request for client information and treatment plan asks for information that would be illegal for me to disclose under District of Columbia law. I have enclosed a copy of the relevant DC statutes. The information that I am allowed to reveal is …

In closing, I have written:

> If you have questions about this information, or require further information, please feel free to contact me. If the information is within the bounds acceptable by law and [client's name] consents to the information being revealed, I will be happy to help.

Check with your lawyer about this issue, however.

Concluding Thoughts

When I give talks on ethics and private practice, I ask the audience, "What do you wish you'd known before embarking on private practice?" One respondent said that private practice is all consuming, requiring high stakes decisions that can have life-or-death consequences.

Decades ago, the American Art Therapy Association's Standards of Practice specified that one had to be in practice a minimum of two years after achieving registration (the ATR) before one could work in private practice, as I recollect. My recent survey of licensure laws and ethics documents revealed when a person is legally able to *practice,* but did not specify when that individual is qualified to embark upon a *private practice.* Consequently, relatively recent graduates of art therapy training programs sometimes consider starting private practices with limited clinical experience, merely because they are licensed or license-ready. I encourage readers to consider that one cannot begin private practice ethically until there is a healthful intertwining of their understanding of themselves and their developmental level as a psychotherapist, their financial well-being, and their legal and business preparedness. There is too much at stake—not only for the private practitioner, but also (and more importantly) for that practitioner's clients.

REFLECTIVE ART EXPERIENCES & DISCUSSION QUESTIONS

1. Create artwork that reflects a time when you applied a particular policy either firmly or leniently, only to find that doing so had an unsatisfactory outcome.
2. How did the choice you made (above) impact later decisions with that client? What about with other clients?
3. Create artwork that juxtaposes your concerns about your client's financial difficulties with your concerns about your own.
4. How would you respond to a client's request that she have a phone session in lieu of a late cancellation, "So I'll get something for my money"?

References

The Doctors Company. (2015). Terminating patient relationships. Retrieved from www.thedoctors.com/KnowledgeCenter/PatientSafety/articles/CON_ID_000326

Huggins, R. (2013). Clients have the right to receive unencrypted emails under HIPAA. Retrieved from https://personcenteredtech.com/2013/10/clients-have-the-right-to-receive-unencrypted-emails-under-hipaa/

Jaffee-Redmond. (1996). The federal psychotherapist-patient privilege (Jaffee vs. Redmond, 518 US 1): History, documents, and opinions. Retrieved from http://jaffee-redmond.org

Mikel, E.H. (2013). *The art of business: A guide for creative arts therapists starting on a path to self-employment.* London: Jessica Kingsley.

Mills, A. (2011). Therapist's page: Adjunctive therapy. Retrieved from http://many voicespress.org/backissues-pdf/2011_04.pdf

United States Department of Health and Human Services. (1996). Health Insurance Portability and Accountability Act of 1996. USDHHS Office for the Assistant Secretary for Planning and Evaluation. Retrieved from https://aspe.hhs.gov/report/health-insurance-portability-and-accountability-act-1996

Zuckerman, E.L. (2008). *The paper office. Forms, guidelines, and resources to make your practice work ethically, legally, and profitably.* New York: Guilford Press.

PART II
The Ethical Dilemmas

Although the chapters have been grouped within seven categories of ethical issues, since many of the chapters address multiple ethical issues, they could easily fall within a number of those categories. While some chapters deal with dilemmas that may be unique to the practice of *art* therapy, others deal with dilemmas that art therapists share with other mental health professionals.

Each chapter presents from one to several ethical dilemmas, asking the reader, "How would you respond?" Readers will get the most out of the chapters by taking a moment to reflect upon (in words or in images) how they think they might respond to each dilemma, before turning to Appendix B to discover how the chapter writer endeavored to resolve the dilemma. Reflective Art Experiences (a thank you to Mary Roberts for suggesting this term) and Discussion Questions—geared toward the professional development of the reader, rather than for use with clients—appear at the end of each chapter. The most valuable aspect of these exercises may well be the thoughts and discussions that they generate.

In writing these chapters, each of us has pledged to abide by the standards of the ethics codes to which we are bound, specifically with regard to the presentation of clinical material. The case examples that are included are de-identified and/or composites of experiences with clients, staff, and others. No reference to any (living) person is intended or should be inferred. The resolutions to ethical dilemmas described herein are not meant to be prescriptive in nature, but to exemplify various ethical decision-making processes. No responsibility for loss caused to any individual or organization acting upon or refraining from action as a result of the material in this publication can be accepted by Routledge/Taylor & Francis or the Editor.

Assumptions, Discrimination, Exclusion

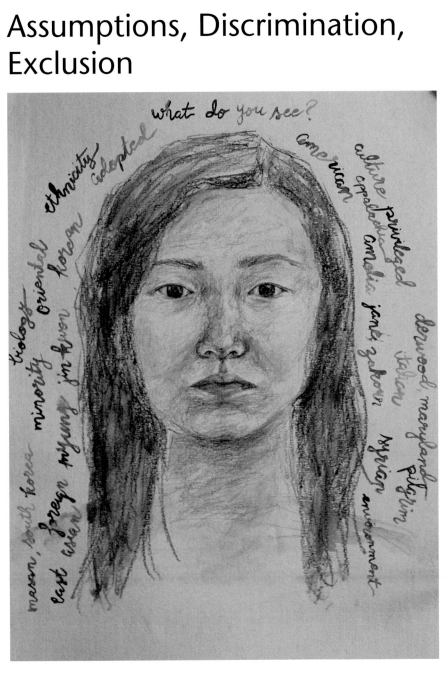

Amelia Zakour

3

AFTER THE TYPHOON

We Brought Art Materials, They Wanted Coffee

Maria Regina A. Alfonso

On November 8, 2013, the most powerful recorded typhoon to hit land, Super-Typhoon Yolanda (known internationally as Typhoon Haiyan), killed at least 6,300 people and left 11 million homeless in the Philippines (BBC News, 2013). As a Filipina myself, who witnessed the wrath of the storm, I wanted to do something to help. As an art therapist and expressive arts therapist, I thought that art-making might have a place in the long-term recovery process of the survivors.

Laying a Foundation

Four years prior to Typhoon Yolanda, members of the Cartwheel Foundation, an education-focused non-profit organization for indigenous peoples that I founded in 1999, were invited by the community and church leaders of the town of Culion in the province of Palawan to collaborate with the elders of three island communities. Our aim was to build schools for the approximately 100 families residing there as they had no access to formal education. These isolated islands are inhabited by the Tagbanua, one of the oldest of 110 indigenous or ethno-linguistic groups in the country. They subsist on income from harvesting and selling seaweed and have limited access to basic services (running water, education, health care). Socio-culturally, the Tagbanua remain partially isolated from the mainstream and have a long history of feeling excluded. The original settlers of Culion, they were displaced in 1904 to make way for a leprosarium established under the American Commonwealth of the Philippines.

Though gravely affected by the typhoon, Palawan was getting very little attention from the media, so my colleagues from Cartwheel and I thought it would be good to focus our efforts there, among families we knew personally. Beyond offering our presence and support, our hope was to offer a space where art making might invite a gentle shift from the pervading sense of helplessness among survivors to an awakened sense of their inherent self-agency. We believed that the act of "making" or "creating" would help them to regain their internal locus of control and their ability to re-imagine a future beyond tragedy. We were also aware that the resilience and strength of the survivors would teach us as much, if not more, than we could ever offer them.

Location of the Work

The Philippines is an archipelago of 7,107 islands, approximately 2,000 of which are inhabited. Palawan is the largest island classified as one province. To get to the affected islands off its shore, one must travel an hour by plane from Manila, the capital, then 40 minutes by bus, and an hour by boat. Including transfers, waiting time, and weather delays, this trip can take up to two days.

Context of the Work

Typhoon Yolanda struck the communities in the dead of night. As their bamboo homes were blown away into the sea, families struggled to find each other, swimming blindly to stay alive. When the winds and rains stopped, they found none of their homes, boats, or belongings on the shore where they live. The only structure that was left partially standing was the preschool classroom we had built together for their children; the only half concrete-walled structure on the islands, it had sheltered families from the ocean at the height of the storm.

After the typhoon, collaborative efforts made possible the provision of basic necessities such as food, clothing, and supplies to rebuild homes and boats. Beyond the immediate emergency response, however, the psychological well-being of the Tagbanua was of serious concern. Three months after the typhoon hit, we initiated Project RISE (Re-Igniting Community Strength through Education), a community, strength-based, rehabilitative and preventive program to support the islands (Cartwheel Foundation, 2016). Its scope included the provision of technical assistance to a local team of psychosocial support workers, the training of teachers to use resilience-strengthening, arts-based activities to transform their classrooms into healing spaces, and longer-term engagement with community elders and local government to ensure their continued access to health care and ways to make their livelihood.

The process began with an island visit or *kamustahan*, which gave us an idea of the community's socio-emotional needs (*Kamusta ka* is "how are you" in Filipino). Then a five-day workshop was held for Culion-based volunteers of various ages and backgrounds, including the volunteer-teachers of Cartwheel in the community pre-school, local government and Department of Education staff, as well as church catechists. Since the volunteers had also felt the wrath of the storm, time was devoted to express, through art making, and process what they had experienced. Within a circle of trust, surrounded by artwork that told their stories, the volunteers expressed concern and support for each other. In succeeding days, their commitment to help their neighboring islands grew, as did their confidence. They learned psychological first aid and psychosocial support approaches using art, music and dance, as well as mind/body-based activities such as breathing, tapping, massage, and yoga, all of which they would soon share with the affected families.

A form of deep listening and attuning with reverence, known in Australia as the indigenous healing practice of *dadirri*, seemed to cradle the process of sharing and learning during the workshop. This creation of space for deep contemplative, heart-based listening built strength among the volunteers (Davis, 2015). Stories of trauma and pain were shared and witnessed with loving acceptance. Similarly, the shared Filipino value, *pakikipagkapwa-damdamin*, the mutual holding of hearts and feelings, seemed to drive the generosity of the volunteers, allowing each one to experience being accompanied with genuine empathy and compassion by another (Carandang & Nisperos, 1996). During their visits to the islands in the year following the typhoon, the volunteers aimed to recreate these spaces by providing informal workshops in which people of all ages could play, make art, and relax their anxious minds and bodies.

We Don't Have Coffee

After the five-day psychosocial workshop in Culion, the volunteer psychosocial team was divided into groups to visit the three islands affected. As I had met the preschoolers and teachers in Cartwheel's early childhood and adult literacy programs on one of the islands, I accompanied the team there. As our boat docked ashore, where we were met by smiling children and their mothers, I was shocked to see the extent of the devastation. All of their homes had been destroyed.

First, we needed to pay respects to the chieftain and request permission to visit the families on the island. After he officially welcomed us, we were granted permission to visit with each family. We had carefully crafted our questions before the visits began, to avoid sounding pushy and making direct references to the storm. As I walked along the shoreline, I saw four women near their half-rebuilt bamboo homes. I approached and squatted side-by-side with them, sitting with them first in silence and then, at the appropriate time, inquiring:

Me: *Kamusta po kayo?* — [How are you?]

Mother 1: *Ganito pa din…* — [The same as usual …]

Me: *Napadalaw lang po ako dahil gusto po naming malaman kung kamusta na po kayo … Ano po ang mga pinagkaka-abalahan niyo ngayon?* — [We are visiting to check in with you. What is keeping you busy these days?]

Mother 1: *Pareho pa din.* — [The same.]

Mother 2: *Ngayong mga araw, malungkot kami.* — [These days, we are sad.]

Me: *Bakit po?* — [May I ask why?]

Mother 2: *Kasi walang kape; walang pang gastos pumunta sa bayan at bumili ng kape sa Culion.* — [Because we don't have coffee. We don't have money to buy coffee in Culion.]

A memory from a previous visit there surfaced. I had met a mother cradling her child and was alarmed by the black blotches around the baby's mouth. She said it was coffee. Due to the scarcity of food, some children, only months old, are fed ground coffee.

Lady: *Basta may kape, ok kami.*
[As long as there's coffee, we're OK.]

Me: *Ngayon na ilang buwan na nakalipas ang bagyo, papaano po kayo nakakaraos?*
[Now that it's been a few months since the storm, how are you coping?]

Grandma: *Minsan nararamdaman pa di ang takot, pagmalakas ang hangin … Sumisikip ang dibdib …*
[Sometimes we still feel afraid, when the winds are strong … our chests tighten …]

Mother 1: *Ang mga bata, pag-gabi na at may hangin, nanginginig at umiiyak pag minsan.*
[In the evenings, when the winds are strong, the children sometimes shiver and cry.]

Grandma: *Ang iba sa amin, may mga panaginip tungkol sa nangyari. Awa ng Diyos, wala namang. Namatay kahit nawala ang lahat …*
[Some of us still have dreams about what happened. With God's mercy, no one perished, even if we lost everything …]

Me: *Napakapositibo po ng pagtingin ninyo sa nangyari. Nguni't mukha pong may natitira pa ding takot … at naiintindihan ko po ito dahil wala pang isang taong nakalipas ang nangyari.*
[You have a very positive attitude about what happened. But there is still sadness … and I understand this; it hasn't even been one year.]

Mother 2: *Ang mga bata, wala pa ring damit at nakapaa pa din …*
[The children still don't have clothes and are barefoot …]

Lady: *Kami naman walang kape …*
[And we don't have coffee …]

Me: *Ano po ang nakakatulong sa mga panahon na ito?*
[What is helpful to you during these times?]

Mother 2: (smiling) *Kape.*
[Coffee.]

This expressed need for coffee (which they said helped them to cope daily with the devastation they faced) seemed to offer a simple and concrete solution for concerned citizens who wanted to support their recovery. For my companions and I, who had art (rather than coffee) in mind, the situation was more complex. It called for deeper reflection about expressed and perceived needs, and what accompanying others and *pakikipagkapwa* really mean. It also strengthened my belief that answers to ethical dilemmas are usually not black or white.

The "Suring"

When I asked the women what else helps, Grandma told me that it was the *suring*, which she described as their Saturday night dance. Pointing toward a flattened area on a nearby hill, she relayed that the entire community gathers every Saturday there to dance together. "It helps us forget our fears, sadness, and hardship." Suddenly, the female elder sprung up to show me a most graceful rendition of the *suring*, her face radiant, her frail body glowing with energy, her gray hair flowing in the wind. Her enthusiasm was magnetic; I watched, mesmerized, from my squatting position, and suddenly found myself dancing with her. This moment ended with conversation about their native attire and other matters related to the dance; then it was time to say goodbye, for the time being.

Did the Tagbanua Families Actually Need Our Help?

I clearly remember the thoughts that flooded my mind while waving at the community from the boat as we made the journey back to Culion. While I was aware that the visit was a small part of our long-term engagement with the community, I could not help but wonder if we were doing the right thing by coming in as outsiders or so-called "trained psychosocial workers using expressive arts-based approaches." The Tagbanua, who have existed for centuries without help from the mainstream, are models of resilience. Yet, they had told me, "Before we had nothing. Now we still have nothing." While I was saddened and taken aback by this perspective, I recalled contrasting images of Tagbanua children chuckling as they busied themselves trading plastic food wrappers that washed ashore after the typhoon. It made me think about how children, often without trying, stumble into making something out of "nothing." Perhaps our role was to accompany them as they paved the way for their elders. Maybe through play and "making," they would lead their community to a deeper awareness of their inner resources, reserves, and gifts, which were already evident to us, typhoon or no typhoon.

As I envisioned one such treasure, the traditional Tagbanua courtship dance called the "*suring*," I saw that the expressive arts are at the very heart of this community's cultural tradition! I could not help but think about the importance that van der Kolk (2014) places upon body-based approaches in trauma treatment. If the Tagbanua already have this capacity for self-healing, did we even have a role to play at this stage? And yet, the statement about having "nothing" lingered in my thoughts. Interestingly, "*suring*" is a word from the Tagbanua dialect which, when translated to Filipino, means "to test" or *pagsuri*. I wondered if it might allude to some kind of "test" for us, as "caregivers." Despite our best intentions, it was critical that we think through the ethical implications of our work. Thoughtfully evaluating them would ensure that we stayed true to the United Nations General Assembly's Inter-Agency Standing Committee Guidelines to "do no harm" (UNICEF, 2007).

MY ETHICAL DILEMMA

When there is a power dynamic between a psychosocial support team and the survivors of a disaster, should it be addressed? If so, how?

One thing I became increasingly aware of as we visited the typhoon-affected islands was the distinction made between "mainlanders" and "natives" by residents of Culion. This non-inclusive perspective has deep socio-political and cultural roots. Unfortunately, all members of the volunteer psychosocial support team had not fully shed their view of the Tagbanua as the "disempowered." They seemed unaware that this viewpoint perpetuated the greater collective impression of indigenous peoples as the "have-nots" in society. As this attitude became more apparent, we facilitators wondered whether this needed to be addressed. We asked ourselves: What would the possible repercussions of this attitude be upon the community? How could a gentle shift in perspective among the team-in-training be encouraged? Could we lead future workshops in a way that would ensure that volunteers used a strength-based approach and took extra care to safeguard the emotional safety of the families? Our ultimate dilemma was whether to introduce the arts-based workshops and gatherings in the communities, given this fundamental issue and its potential impact upon the work.

How would you respond?

For the writer's response, see Appendix B, page 396.

MY ETHICAL DILEMMA

Is it ethical to introduce mainstream arts-based approaches into an indigenous community that has its own cultural heritage and practices? Is this yet another power dynamic? If the decision is made to engage, how does one proceed?

After my visit with the women on the island, I began to question the advisability of introducing more mainstream art-based approaches. Particularly after hearing about the "*suring*," I asked myself how sharing the art-based approaches I had learned as an art therapist would impact their recovery. If we introduced new ways of art-making, could this be perceived as dismissive of their resilience and contribute to the further extinction of Filipino pre-colonial cultural traditions? Was it possible to introduce additional methods of dealing with anxiety, fear, and loss that would complement or build upon the existing practices of the Tagbanua?

How would you respond?

For the writer's response, see Appendix B, page 397.

MY ETHICAL DILEMMA

Would it benefit a community to take part in a post-disaster psychosocial support program that does not have a long-term plan for sustainability?

While most humanitarian aid providers and organizations are very well intentioned, the short-term nature of their engagement can negatively affect intended recipients of psychosocial support. Sometimes, assistance is provided to survivors by non-local professionals who leave after the prescribed life of the project, without training a local support team. If sustained funding for a project is uncertain, would a short-term intervention be better (or worse) than nothing? If, as in our case, this concern is resolved and the decision is made to engage, how do we ensure the accessibility of the support, given the island community's distance from the mainland? The use and consequent depletion of already exhausted community resources to gain access to support had to be considered.

How would you respond?

For the writer's response, see Appendix B, page 397.

MY ETHICAL DILEMMA

If the community has expressed a need for coffee, why bring art supplies?

What would bringing art supplies instead of the coffee requested communicate? Would it indicate that we weren't listening deeply enough? If we did bring coffee, how would that be helpful in the long-term? Does the long-term even matter in a case such as this, where the community has expressed that they have "nothing"?

How would you respond?

For the writer's response, see Appendix B, page 397.

Conclusion

At the heart of this experience of "dancing" to the life ways of the Tagbanua was the enchanting discovery of an "ethics of listening" in "intercultural art making" that has begun to impact our own personal lives and our understanding of the use of the arts for healing (Macneill, 2014). This "ethics of listening," practiced among other indigenous groups around the world, is extremely relevant to the process of offering psychosocial support and navigating ethical dilemmas that arise as we strive to attune ourselves to community needs, expressed and otherwise.

We came with art supplies. We learned their dances first. We struggled with the issue of coffee. Our experience continues to teach us that reflecting upon ethical issues offers a critical space for the ongoing re-evaluation of standard ways of working that may seem second nature to most art therapists. It keeps us alert to the importance of putting the community's welfare and safety first. Perhaps, in the end, wanting to be ethical is the best caring we can offer. Through it, trust is built and, somehow, we find ourselves—like the women by the shore or the children at play—dancing the *suring* and stumbling into unassuming but heroic stories of resilience and healing.

REFLECTIVE ART EXPERIENCES & DISCUSSION QUESTIONS

1. Create art in response to the art form of an indigenous community as a way of deepening your connection with that community.
2. Create an art piece that would reflect a shared space in which you and the leaders/teachers of an indigenous community might meet to connect, exchange stories, and learn from each other. What would this space look like? What values and guidelines would ensure that this space is inclusive and emotionally and physically safe for all?
3. With sensitivity to the natural power dynamic that may occur when an "outside" group engages with an indigenous community, what are other ways in which you could initiate contact and engage with the community? What questions would you ask to establish a connection? What stories about your own life would you share to make it a learning exchange and not an "interview"?
4. What local materials could you encourage the members of an indigenous community to use for continued art making if the art supplies that art therapists usually use (e.g., paints, paper) were not readily available?

References

BBC News (2013, November 14). Typhoon Haiyan: Aid in numbers. Retrieved from www.bbc. com/news/world-asia-pacific-24899006

Carandang, L., & Nisperos, M. (1996). *Pakikipagkapwa-damdamin: Accompanying survivors of disasters*. Manila: Bookmark.

Cartwheel Foundation (2016). Strength within: Harnessing Tagbanua resiliency. Retrieved from http://cartwheelfoundation.org

Davis, J. (2015). An indigenous approach to healing trauma. Retrieved from http://upliftconnect.com/indigenous-approach-to-healing-trauma/

Macneill, P. (Ed.). (2014). *Ethics and the arts*. New York: Springer.

UNICEF (2007). Inter-agency standing committee guidelines on mental health and psychosocial support in emergency settings. Retrieved from www.unicef.org/protection/guidelines_iasc_mental_health_psychosocial_june_2007.pdf

van der Kolk, B. (2014). *The body keeps the score: Brain, mind and body in the healing of trauma*. New York: Penguin Group.

4

ART THERAPIST? YES. MINISTER? THAT, TOO!

Ethical Issues That May Arise When One Has Dual Roles

Martina E. Martin

The Harm in Making Assumptions

As an African American cisgender woman from Pittsburgh with a name like Martina Estella Martin, I have absorbed more than my fair share of other people's assumptions about my name, race, and cultural identity over the years. My name has Latin, German, and Italian roots, and I have learned to embrace its cultural ambiguity and the curiosity it fosters in others. Once, I applied for, and was offered, a job as an administrative assistant after successfully completing a phone interview with a hiring manager. I felt confident after the interview and believed that we had genuinely connected. On my first day, I arrived on-site and waited patiently in the lobby for my new supervisor to escort me to my office.

While waiting, I noticed a tall, African American woman standing in the lobby, closely examining each new face that passed by. After about 10 minutes of waiting impatiently, she called out in exasperation, "Martina E. Martin?" Somewhat confused as to why it took her so long to call my name, I stood up and stepped forward as her jaw dropped. "You're Martina E. Martin?" she asked. "Yes," I responded. "I thought you were going to be Latina," she exclaimed. "I wasn't expecting a black woman with locs!" After laughing it off uncomfortably, I accompanied her to the office where I later learned from my colleagues that the hiring manager, who was white, was looking to diversify the branch and therefore did not want to hire any more African Americans because the majority of the staff was African American already. A few weeks later, when I finally had a chance to meet the hiring manager and thank him face-to-face for giving me the opportunity, I noticed that he, too, was in shock, as he asked in disbelief, "You're Martina Martin?" "Yes," I responded. In that moment, he must have realized his own folly. He had made the assumption that my name, and perhaps even my qualifications, could not possibly be attributed to a person of African descent. He was wrong.

Henry Winkler quipped that "assumptions are the termites of relationships." This is true, also, of the therapeutic relationship. Whether assumptions emerge from clients' distortions or from therapists' inability to clearly define their role(s), they can corrode the alliance between client and clinician and undermine the positive benefits to be reaped from their work together. Although the American Art Therapy Association's (AATA's) *Ethical Principles for Art Therapists* (2013) and the Art Therapy Credentials Board's (ATCB's) *Code of Ethics, Conduct, and Disciplinary Procedures* (2018) both assert that art therapists are responsible for avoiding ambiguity and ensuring that clients are clear about the different roles that exist within the relationship, helping clients understand this delineation can be difficult. This is particularly true when clinicians find themselves functioning in more than one role within a given treatment setting.

When the Art Therapist is a Minister

As a Board Certified Art Therapist and Licensed Professional Counselor, I work at a non-profit community-based health center that specializes in meeting the needs of youth and adults living with complex physical and mental health conditions. Our organization places a particular emphasis upon providing high quality HIV/AIDS and LGBTQ+ competent care. My work with gender nonconforming, gender fluid, and trans individuals has made me sensitive to the importance of using each client's preferred pronouns.

In my work, I frequently encounter individuals who are in the midst of existential and spiritual crises. My primary responsibility as a mental health clinician is to provide them with a safe, non-judgmental space within which to explore and work through their thoughts, feelings, and ideas. Whether they are concerned about being punished for prior wrongs or are angry with God, religion, or a particular faith community, I am called upon to assist these individuals in communicating their thoughts and feelings in a meaningful way through the art therapy and counseling services I provide.

The Unintended Consequences of Self-disclosure

Having a Master of Divinity degree and a background in pastoral care makes me particularly sensitive to the ways in which a client's physical or mental health challenges might be negatively impacted by their spirituality or religion and vice versa. I have encountered clients who felt as though their diagnosis of certain chronic illnesses such as HIV/AIDS or cancer was a direct result of some sin they had committed. For example, one client ended our work together because I would not collude with his own internalized homophobia. "Don't you think I should go to hell for having romantic thoughts about men?" he asked. "No," I countered, "but what I think is irrelevant. Why do you believe you should go to hell for having such thoughts?" I asked.

Infuriated by my response, the client stated that he did not understand how a person with a Master of Divinity would not condemn him to hell for being a gay man and having romantic thoughts about other men. Given the important role spirituality played in his life, and the nature of his beliefs, it is likely that, over the years, he had encountered a number of ministers who had willingly colluded with him in the belief that his sexuality marked him for condemnation. When I refused to hop on the fire and brimstone bandwagon and defied his assumptions about how a minister should respond, it seemed to push him headlong into a state of cognitive dissonance that could not be overcome in our initial session together. Working through the inherent conflict between his spiritual beliefs and feelings would require his willingness to go there and, at this point, he was unwilling and did not return to therapy.

When I reflect upon the ethical decision I made to answer his question directly (disclosing my personal opinion), I remain conflicted. While the ethics codes of AATA and ATCB forbid discrimination on the basis of religion or sexual orientation, neither offers much guidance on how best to respond my client's question. If I had refused to answer his question at all or had relied upon the boilerplate response, "Why do you ask that question?" would it have prolonged our time together or would it have made me appear more standoffish and unapproachable? If, in an effort to appease the client, I had answered the question in the affirmative, I would have compromised the very ethical principles I am required by law and conscience to uphold. Perhaps terminating in this way enabled the client to consider that alternative viewpoints on the topic of condemnation and faith do exist.

Hearing clients use words such as "sin," "judgment," and "condemnation" sets off alarm bells, tuning me in to how my clients conceptualize their maladies in relation to their faith. It also helps me to understand whether their spiritual beliefs and/or religious practices appear to be helpful or harmful to their recovery process. Once this is known, I can then work with the client to determine which of these beliefs and practices, if any, can serve as viable coping strategies. If it appears that their beliefs and practices may be incongruent with their recovery goals, we can work together to see if a healthier balance can be struck by reframing their situation or examining the etiology of these beliefs and practices.

When the Minister is an Art Therapist

As a Provisional Deacon in the United Methodist Church, I feel not only called to live out my faith through my profession as an art therapist and counselor to marginalized populations, but also concerned about the mental health of our congregations and society at large. For several years, I have facilitated expressive arts workshops in a variety of congregational settings on topics ranging from grief and loss to self-care and rejuvenation. Working in the field of mental health has made me more sensitive to the needs of fellow parishioners who appear to be suffering in silence with issues that cannot be solved by prayer and fasting alone. For example, in the African American community, many feel overwhelmed and traumatized by the repeated incidences of racial profiling and police brutality that have resulted in the senseless deaths of individuals such as Tamir Rice, Michael Brown, Eric Garner, Sandra Bland, Philando Castile, and Alton Sterling. After a grand jury failed to indict police officer Darren Wilson for any crimes related to the death of the unarmed teenager Michael Brown, I noticed a distinct undercurrent of anger and helplessness among the members of my church, most of whom are African American. Although some members had been actively involved in the Civil Rights Movement of the 1950s and 1960s, many lamented that they were too old now to march. In an effort to provide them with an opportunity to express their outrage at what many perceived to be a gross miscarriage of justice, another art therapist, Brittney Washington, and I held an impromptu "art break" during which they could create protest postcards to voice their feelings of anger and frustration in a constructive and cathartic way. Before they were mailed off to the Department of Justice, the postcards were strung together and stretched across the altar to unite the congregation in intercessory prayer during the season of Advent.

As an art therapist, I utilize art-making as a means of helping people process those things for which they can't find words. Whether they have experienced the sudden death of a loved one, survived a personal tragedy, or weathered a natural or human-made disaster, we labor together to "make sense" out of the seemingly senseless. My role as a minister provides me with an opportunity to participate directly in this process of intercession with my faith community, through the facilitation of expressive arts workshops. While I am not functioning as a therapist or counselor in these settings, my background and training enable me to advocate for, and to speak responsibly on, issues related to the mental and emotional well-being of those I serve in ministry. I also create my own art, as shown in this mixed-media story cloth (Figure 4.1).

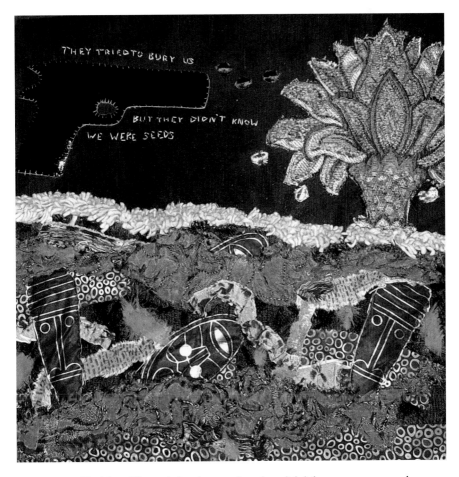

FIGURE 4.1 Uprising: They tried to bury us but they didn't know we were seeds *(see color insert).*

MY ETHICAL DILEMMA

How do I hold the therapeutic frame while experiencing strong counter-transference?

I encountered a particularly challenging ethical dilemma when I worked as an art therapist and activities coordinator at a day treatment program. The mission of the program was to enhance the quality of life for individuals living with HIV/AIDS through the provision of comprehensive day treatment services that were offered in a safe, home-like, community setting. Not long after I assumed this role, I met a client who was fairly new to the program. In addition to being HIV positive, he had recently received a terminal cancer diagnosis which had exacerbated his already complex mental health profile. At times pleasant and cordial, the client's mood could shift rapidly, making him angry, demeaning, and overly critical. When confronted about his behavior by staff, the client would become defiant and oppositional before ultimately becoming tearful and remorseful. Given the unpredictability of his mood, it was not surprising that many of the other clients in the program limited their interactions with him.

One day, when the client was in a particularly good mood, he pointed toward the name placard on my door and asked, "What do the letters M-D-I-V after your name stand for?" I told him that, in addition to going to school for art therapy, I had also attended Divinity School. Genuinely interested, the client bombarded me with difficult questions about life, death, and God, in an effort to understand the basics of theodicy. "Why do bad things happen to good people?" he would often ask, and "Why do good things happen to bad people?" Knowing how precarious his health was, I understood that his constant questioning was an attempt to make sense out of the seemingly senseless. As time went on, our conversations led to even more curiosity on his part. However, knowing that any attempt at proselytization was in direct violation of the ethical principles of my profession, I took care that our conversations remained general in nature.

When volunteers from a local church came to lead a Spirituality group, my client would often use the time as an opportunity to ask them the questions that I refrained from answering and to interrogate them about their faith. "What kind of God goes around killing people?" he would ask and then quickly interject, "That don't sound like no God I want to serve!" "How can you come in here sharing what is supposedly 'good news' about that kind of God? That don't sound like good news to me," he would boom. Often, his questions overwhelmed and derailed the group and at times I wrestled with the idea of having him removed from the group, so that he would not interfere with the experience of others. However, as time went on and his prognosis got worse, the desperation in his arguments became more palpable. I came to understand that he didn't want to know why God parted the Red Sea and smote Pharaoh and his army, he wanted to know why God was smiting him with an inoperable form of cancer!

After receiving discouraging news from his doctor, the client returned to the program distraught and enraged. His anger toward me was so unbridled that I actually feared for my personal safety. "You're just like my ex-wife," he screamed as he charged toward me, backing me into a corner. "You think you're so holy and righteous! You think you're better than me, don't you?" Totally undone by his negative transference toward me, I didn't know how to respond. As soon as I could, I took refuge in my office, shut the door behind me, and sobbed, feeling like a powerless child. I contemplated my future as a therapist as I wondered, "At what point can I wash my hands of this case? He is just too much to deal with!"

How would you respond?

For the writer's response, see Appendix B, page 418.

Concluding Thoughts

Even though I never cross the line into full-fledged ministry with my clients, I try to provide them with unconditional positive regard, empathy, and genuine concern. Whenever I take extra measures to ensure that my clients feel cared for and respected, regardless of their mental, physical, or emotional challenges, I am not only providing good care as a mental health clinician, but also fulfilling my calling to "the least of these" among us.

In this instance, my client made a lot of assumptions about my role as an art therapist and my role as a minister. In addition to transferring onto me some of his own negative experiences with his ex-wife and religion, he seemed to assume that my personal beliefs were the litmus test by which I judged him and his worth. He was wrong. What was unclear to me at the time, but is abundantly apparent to me now is that, in addition to his complex medical profile, my client probably should have been diagnosed with a personality disorder. When I view his interactions with other clients and staff in the light of this possibility, it is easy for me to see why allowing him to stay in the Spirituality group (even though I secretly wanted to put him out) was so healing and therapeutic for him in the long run. While I certainly regret how my experience of counter-transference unfolded, there is a lesson for me in it, and I am grateful that I was able to hold the therapeutic frame long enough to allow him to resolve his existential concerns in his own time.

REFLECTIVE ART EXPERIENCES & DISCUSSION QUESTIONS

1. Create artwork about a time when you experienced such strong counter-transference (negative or positive) toward a client that you considered terminating your work with the client. Describe that experience.
2. Think about a dual role that you have tried to fulfill and illustrate (through drawing, painting, collage, or clay modeling) how those two roles impacted each other.
3. How do you ensure that preferred pronouns are respected with your clients?
4. Does the topic of spirituality play a role in your therapeutic work? If so, in what way? If not, why not?

References

American Art Therapy Association (2013). *Ethical principles for art therapists.* Alexandria, VA: AATA.

Art Therapy Credentials Board (2018). *Code of ethics, conduct, and disciplinary procedures.* Greensboro, NC: ATCB.

5

CAN BIASES EVER BE RIGHT?

The Ethics of Working Internationally as an Art Therapist, a Trainer, and a Professor

Heidi Bardot

Having grown up overseas, I view working internationally—be it conducting clinical work, providing training, or designing educational immersion programs—not as an interaction with "*the other*" from which we can then return home, but as an extension of the idea of *home*, as we open up ourselves to the opportunities for growth, reciprocal learning, and connection that the world offers. Adopting this approach, however, comes with the responsibility of questioning our goals and intentions, exploring our biases and expectations, and approaching every situation with our ethical guidelines and boundaries firmly in place.

Questioning Intent: Now, *Why* Do I Want to Do This?

One of the most difficult steps in preparing to work internationally is questioning why we want to do the work. Oftentimes, it is due to the misguided *Savior Complex*—a desire to *save* disadvantaged people by introducing them to the magic of art therapy. While we all came into this profession wanting to assist and support others, the idea that only *we* can do this, only *we* have the answers, reflects a dangerous colonial viewpoint (Potash, Bardot, Moon, Napoli, Lyonsmith, & Hamilton, 2017). One of the joys of working in other communities is the reciprocal learning that takes place. However, this, too, can become twisted when interactions become less about learning from each other and more about what we can get out of this experience, add to our resumes, or post on Facebook. The "Art Therapy International Work Assessment" (ATIWA) (Hillinga-Haas, Bardot, Anand, & Prasad, 2015) is a self-assessment tool designed to encourage therapists to ask themselves questions such as:

- What are the top three obstacles confronting those living in the area in which you intend to work?

- What is the role of art in the culture of the country in which you intend to work? What kind of artwork is typically done in the country where you plan to work?
- Have you faced dangerous and/or threatening life situations before? Are you prepared to for these types of situations?
- Are you prepared to have your expectations and ideas challenged?
- How willing are you to abide by the cultural norms of the areas in which you will work (e.g., will you wear skirts that are no shorter than below the knee or refrain from using your left hand to eat with)?

Hillinga-Haas et al., 2015pp. 1–4

By focusing upon the emotional, physical, and spiritual challenges that a therapist should consider before working overseas, the ATIWA (2015) can help one to prepare him- or herself for the "realistic and non-romantic aspects" (p. 1) of international work.

Awareness of Biases and Boundaries: When to Step, Jump, or Stomp All Over Them

As therapists, we all realize the importance of recognizing and being aware of our personal biases—those inherent beliefs we have due to past experiences and/or the influence of others.

These cultural, racial, gender, sexual, spiritual, or age-based beliefs can inform our interactions, behaviors, hopes, and fears. In international work, these biases can easily sneak into our expectations (e.g., assuming that one culture will welcome art therapy while another will resist it)—with both positive and negative results. Healthful boundaries are one sign of an experienced and well-adjusted therapist. Having strong boundaries allows one to loosen, or step over, them when the culture, or a situation, demands it.

From the Perspective of a Clinician: Letting Go of Expectations

Internationally, I have worked in refugee camps, prisons, safe houses, youth programs, psychiatric centers, and schools. I always tell my students that, in order to do international work, you need to examine everything that you already know, discard most of it, and create something new that responds to the specific situation, culture, or client you are encountering. Traditionally, in India, children are taught in art classes to create or copy beautiful images, so that they can feel proud of the final result. When we asked them to scribble and express their feelings, stating that it was okay to create "ugly" pictures and that it was the process of creating that was important, we were met with distress by the children and redirection by their teachers. Learning the cultural expectations of art activity enabled us not only to clarify the difference between art therapy and fine art, but also to alter our projects in ways that would result in a positive finished product.

In the Middle East, I conducted art therapy groups in a mountain prison notorious for riots and overcrowding; built to accommodate 3,000 inmates, it houses nearly twice that number. I worked with 20 men in the mental health ward, all of whom had committed murder. Ranging in age from early 20s to mid-80s, many have lived there for more than 30 years, as their families refused to take them back after they had served their sentences. I quickly discovered that my usual approach to conducting art therapy sessions had to change, due to cultural expectations. In my previous work in psychiatric facilities, I was accustomed to sitting with my back to the door, for easy egress in case of an emergency. On this ward, I was shown to a chair in the corner of the room, far away from the only exit, where I was offered Arabic coffee and a peeled tangerine. I had split seconds to evaluate and respond to the situation. I knew that these men had committed murder and I knew that I could become ill from their offerings (the coffee having been made from—and the tangerine having been washed with—untreated water). I was also aware of the culture of giving and the open nature of these men; in effect, *I was being invited into their home as their guest.* I assessed the potential danger, listened to my instincts, and decided to bend my rules. I accepted the chair, the coffee, and the fruit they offered me. The result was an open and honest therapy session during which we discussed strengths, hopes, and spiritual beliefs within a relaxed environment of gained trust.

I would not always make this decision. Not long afterward, we were turned away from the life-sentence ward, as a riot was in progress—overpopulation and deplorable living conditions leading to frustration and anger. Having worked in many facilities in different countries, nothing much shocks me anymore; however, I actually lost my breath when I saw this prison, as it looked like the set of a post-apocalyptic movie. Barbed wire was strung over the whole building; towels, blankets, and clothing hung out of every window and crevice, drying in the hot sun. The ground was strewn with trash. Arms and hands protruded from every opening. The noise from the men pounding on the walls, stomping on the floors, and yelling and screaming was so intense that the bars on the windows were actually shaking. As we stood outside the prison, waiting to see if it would be calm enough to enter, I questioned my limits. I felt lucky that the riot did not break out after we had already entered the ward; in the past, the prisoners had taken visitors hostage. If I were struggling with fear and feeling unsafe, would it be possible to function effectively as a therapist? All of us must determine our own limits, deciding when, where, and why we are willing to step over the boundaries we have learned. It is our duty to protect not only our clients, but also ourselves. We never made it onto this ward, as the riots continued throughout my stay.

From the Perspective of a Trainer: Is it Ethical to Train Others in Art Therapy Techniques?

Some suggest that training non-art therapists in art therapy techniques undermines the intensive training that students pursue in order to become art therapists; others say that, since people are already using the arts in counseling, classrooms, and community centers, why not train them to use it properly? In my international work, I have met many people who are art therapy pioneers in their own countries; individuals who have the inherent intuition to use the arts effectively and are seeking ways to approach the arts ethically and usefully as they recognize the power behind it. Therefore, when I train non-art therapists or provide workshops, I am focusing upon the school teacher who wants to look at art from a deeper perspective and have her students talk about their work thoughtfully … the relief worker who sees trauma on the front lines in her work with refugees but does not know how to respond to their art in a positive and supportive manner … the counselor who would love to be trained in art therapy but is unable to do so because of financial, visa, or family issues. I am also looking at how the trainees can better inform me about their specific needs, concerns, challenges, and cultural influences, so that together we can create an approach that works for them.

I was about to present a week-long introduction to art therapy techniques to drama therapists, counselors, educators, and relief workers in Lebanon. Having taught similar courses before, I knew that I might have to adjust the format and structure, depending upon cultural needs; what I did not realize was how much I had to change. I began by asking each of the 38 participants to choose a small magazine picture that would introduce him- or herself to the group, a process that generally takes a minute or two; in this group, however, it took 5–10 minutes per person. Each individual spoke with such lyrical beauty about the shapes, colors, content, and connection of the image to his or her own life—a lovely cultural piece that I wanted to honor and a process that they taught me was important. Therefore, the next day the introductory ritual was done in small groups, so that each person would have the time to share deeply. I am continuously learning and adjusting.

When introducing an idea to people of another country, we must always think about sustainability, so as not to offer a service that is ripped away when we leave that country. Sustainability should, and often does, require training locals to continue the work. When we started a summer abroad program in South Africa, the work that we initiated in a youth center was continued by a local social worker whom we trained to use the arts.

From the Perspective of a Professor: How to Support Students and Clients While Remaining Culturally Sensitive

Recognizing the need to train students who will become culturally sensitive art therapists who are able to work with an increasingly diverse population, in 2007 I developed the Art Therapy International Social and Cultural Diversity Course, a three-week summer session that has taken students to France, India, South Africa, the United Arab Emirates, and Croatia. The initial idea for the course was to place students in a situation where they did not know the language, might feel uncomfortable with the customs, and could internalize some of the stress and vulnerability that minorities often experience as clients. These experiences were then paired with the Cultural Diversity course, which was designed to increase self-awareness, knowledge, and skills, enabling students to bridge the "theory to practice" gap (Ruddock & Turner, 2007; Pedersen, 2009; Sue & Sue, 2008). Often, students assume that psychological theory and practice are enough to interact effectively with people from other cultures; they do not take into account that they are coming to that interaction from a Western,

European point of view (Campbell, Liebmann, Brooks, Jones, & Ward, 1999; Cattaneo, 1994; Hiscox & Calish, 1998; Moon, 2015; Pederson, 1994; Sue & Sue, 2008).

When I take students overseas, I must provide them with a safe and mentally stimulating learning environment and ensure that they process what they are experiencing and learning in a positive and supportive manner. Because students in this exciting, but vulnerable situation experience a variety of emotional reactions—from anxiety and the questioning of beliefs (and even identity) to growth and awareness—the journey must be a thoughtful endeavor, planned with great care (Bardot, 2011). Our internship sites are chosen with both opportunities and risks in mind, allowing students to stretch themselves and their boundaries (e.g., by determining how to deal with touch when a client has lice; with their discomfort with the cultural practice of removing one's shoes, even in hospitals). To support the students, I created an evening ritual whereby they would process each day's experiences by journaling and creating artwork and then share with the group, recognizing commonalities and discussing differences. Many students have found this ritual to be their favorite—and most effective—learning tool.

MY ETHICAL DILEMMA

Can biases ever be right?

The first time that we took a group of art therapy students to India, two students who had been placed at one of the internship sites—a psychiatric facility for children and young adults—expressed great distress at having seen teachers hit children with sticks and tie them to chairs, in an effort to control them, then leave them isolated for hours. That evening, the interns shared these concerns with the group and received their support. During the discussion, we explored the extent to which we were being influenced by our western biases, since, in the psychiatric facilities in which we had worked, staff were bound by strict rules of conduct, as well as child endangerment laws. The two interns were determined to return to the site the next day to promote change in the system by asking staff about the reasons for their approach and suggesting other options. However, during supervision and our processing ritual the following evening, the students reported that their efforts to talk with the teachers were met with angry comments that this was the only way to control the children: *"If they act like animals, they need to be treated like animals."* This response seemed to go against what we had seen and heard about the Hindu religious belief that all creatures (human and animal) had to be treated with respect and care. Our students again reported witnessing staff chasing and hitting the children on their backs and heads with sticks and seeing the same boy in isolation, tied to a chair. Sobbing, they expressed both the helplessness they experienced and the anger they felt towards the staff. Despite feeling guilty about abandoning the children, they decided that they could not return to the facility and watch what they could not change.

The evening's ritual focused upon the tension inherent in forcing a change, the powerlessness of feeling that one could do nothing, and the strength of the fabric of culture. The group wondered, "Can biases ever be right?" Students questioned the definition of bias as a prejudice for or against something, usually considered unfair (Merriam-Webster, n.d.). Was it a bias to disagree with people mistreating others, even in situations in which corporal punishment is considered culturally acceptable? Was this a human rights issue? When should we be culturally sensitive and when should we object and fight for what we believe is *right*? Can a bias ever be right?

How would you respond?

For the writer's response, see Appendix B, page 399.

Conclusion: Broadening Awareness, Boundaries, and Biases—Oh My!

With increased interest by students and professionals in working abroad, we have to explore even more deeply our motivations, our inherent biases, and our expectations of the people, our interactions, and the experience, itself. We have to recognize when caring and empathy take precedence over skill, self-awareness, and boundaries. And when we are inevitably tested, it is essential that we look within and seek support from without. It is then that we can hope to respond ethically in a therapeutic and culturally aware manner, viewing each instance as a growth experience.

REFLECTIVE ART EXPERIENCES & DISCUSSION QUESTIONS

1. Create a list of your own personal biases. Try to be as honest as possible, without censorship. Choose one of these biases and explore where the origination point of this bias might be. (The origination point is usually a personal or family experience that, over time, has broadened to include all interactions of that kind, rather than remaining relegated to that one particular interaction). Discuss.
2. Create an image of an imagined positive encounter with the subject of your bias. Discuss.

References

Bardot, H. (2011, July). Out of the darkness comes understanding and awareness: Students' process during an international course. Paper presented at the meeting of the American Art Therapy Association's 42nd Annual Conference, Washington, DC.

Campbell, J., Liebmann, M., Brooks, F., Jones, J., & Ward, C. (Eds.) (1999). *Art therapy, race and culture*. London: Jessica Kingsley.

Cattaneo, M. (1994). Addressing culture and values in the training of art therapists. *Art Therapy: Journal of the American Art Therapy Association*, 11(3), 184–186.

Hillinga-Haas, H., Bardot, H., Anand, S. & Prasad, S. (2015, July). Art Therapy International Work Assessment (ATIWA). Paper presented at the meeting of the American Art Therapy Association's 46th Annual Conference, Minneapolis, MN.

Hiscox, A.R. & Calish, C.A. (Eds.) (1998). *Tapestry of cultural issues in art therapy*. Philadelphia, PA: Jessica Kingsley.

Merriam-Webster (n.d.). Bias. Retrieved from www.merriam-webster.com/dictionary/bias

Moon, B. (2015). Multicultural and diversity issues in art therapy. In B. Moon, *Ethical issues in art therapy* (3rd ed.). Springfield, IL: Charles Thomas.

Pedersen, P. (2009). Teaching towards an ethnorelative worldview through psychology study abroad. *International Education*, 20(1), 73–86.

Pederson, P.B. (1994). *A handbook for developing multicultural awareness* (2nd ed). Alexandria, VA: American Counseling Association.

Potash, J., Bardot, H., Moon, C., Napoli, M., Lyonsmith, A., & Hamilton, M. (2017). Ethical implications of cross-cultural international art therapy. *The Arts in Psychotherapy, 56,* 74–82.

Ruddock, H. & Turner, D.S. (2007). Developing cultural sensitivity: Nursing students' experiences of a study abroad programme. *Journal of Advanced Nursing,* 59(4), 361–369.

Sue, D.W. & Sue, D. (2008). *Counseling the culturally diverse: Theory and practice* (6th ed.). Hoboken, NJ: John Wiley & Sons.

6

CULTURALLY ADAPTIVE ART THERAPY PRACTICE

Is it Ethical?

Mercedes Ballbé ter Maat

Nearly 40 years ago, I left my native country of Argentina to arrive in the United States of America (US) as a legal immigrant under the status of "permanent resident." I knew what that meant … I could stay in the US for as long as I wanted and could return to Argentina as often as I wanted. So I did, not because I did not like the US, but because I missed Argentina terribly. And 40 years later, I still do, so much so that now I spend half of my time in the US and half of my time in Argentina.

The fact that I was educated in US-based universities—receiving a bachelor's degree, master's degrees in Art Therapy and in Counseling, and a doctorate in Counseling—meant that my formal training and practice in the mental health field took on an Anglo-American perspective. All the classes I took but one were taught by white professors; the clinical case studies they presented were primarily about white clients. In effect, I learned techniques that would work with clients from mainstream America. There was no mention of how to work with individuals who were from different cultures (e.g., Black or Hispanic clients); we worked under the assumption that the treatment of individuals was all the same. I knew it was not, because I knew that I was different from white America. Not better or worse, just different.

Whiteness, as I call it, permeated all aspects of my life. I did not come across other Hispanics in high school, college, or graduate school, so I quickly began to incorporate whiteness as my norm for communicating, relating, and behaving. For instance, I stopped kissing people when I saw them for the first time that day or when I would leave a gathering. (Welcoming people by kissing them on one cheek is a customary greeting for Argentinians.) This personal boundary became rudely clear as white America seemed horrified by my attempts to kiss them, stepping back as I approached them. Another example of the differences in personal boundaries was seen in the way we "hanged." Hispanics tend to be collectivistic, often hanging in groups, eating, laughing, and talking loud. It is not uncommon to see large Latin families composed of multi-generational members living under one roof and spending meal time together.

As an immigrant, all but my immediate family were in Argentina. And, soon upon our arrival in the US, my siblings and I sought educational opportunities in different parts of the country, separating us even further. My same-aged single friends and relatives in Argentina were still living with their parents in intact families. This was seen as "enmeshment" by white professional standards and "weird" by my friends. In the US, I lived either with one roommate or alone as a student and young professional, until I married and had a family of my own.

Whiteness also permeated the way I practiced psychotherapy. The theories and techniques, as well as the ethical principles and standards of conduct, were designed for working with white clients and did not take into consideration that similarities and differences may exist when working with those who have different backgrounds, cultures, values, world views, and life experiences. I trained as an art therapist in two prestigious private hospitals in the District of Columbia that seemed to cater only to white people. My exposure to working with African Americans did not start until I changed jobs in 1988 to work at St. Elizabeths Hospital, a DC government-run institution that, incidentally, was the first publicly funded mental hospital in the country. It wasn't until ten years later that I began to work with immigrant children and families.

By then, I had suspended my Hispanic ways of relating, to adopt white macro-culture ways of being and doing psychotherapy. That is, I was abiding by a set of rules dictated by the psychology and art therapy communities that governed my professional behavior. I was trained in the early 1980s by two significant forces: a university program with a psychoanalytic orientation and a dear uncle who was a psychiatrist and psychoanalyst in Buenos Aires, Argentina. And so, I greeted clients with a handshake or a verbal hello; I abided by strict time limits (i.e., the 50-minute hour) and starting/ending times. I thrived on transference and counter-transference; eating or drinking during sessions was not permitted; clients could not join groups if they had arrived after the group had started; and self-disclosure was non-existent as I kept a working distance from my clients. I did not accept or give gifts; I did not drive clients in my car nor would I ride in a client's car; and the list went on—until I started working overseas, and with immigrant clients within the US.

MY ETHICAL DILEMMA

To work effectively with immigrant families, must I unlearn what I've been taught about conducting art therapy and psychotherapy?

I considered myself a solid professional, an ethical clinician who hardly thought about ethics, until I was hired by Arlington County (Virginia) Public School System in 1997 to use art therapy with recently arrived Latin American immigrant students and families—a community that shared my culture and often challenged my professional rules and demeanor. I began to struggle with questions such as, "Is anything that I learned about conducting therapy applicable to this job?" and "Do the art therapy guidelines regarding ethical conduct apply here?" I told myself that there must be a way of working with immigrant students and families that remains true to counseling and art therapy without violating ethical and legal standards. There must be a way that I can reciprocate my clients' greeting (with a kiss on the check) without worrying about crossing a boundary or being accused of physical or sexual harassment. There must be a way of giving and accepting gifts without strings attached. There must be a way of appropriately disclosing my immigration experiences without the fear of inappropriate counter-transference. And there was. For me, it started with a graduate-level course at the University of Virginia taught by Dr. Courtland Lee, entitled "Multicultural Counseling." Multicultural counseling became my way of counseling and conducting art therapy, and awakened my passion for working with those who, like me, did not quite fit into whiteness.

I began to do a few things that seemed unconventional in the world of ethics and psychotherapy at that time. I started to speak Spanish with the children and parents, contrary to what some school personnel were prescribing: "We are in the US, speak English," and "Speaking English is the only way children are going to learn English." Although these statements hold truth, speaking the families' native language enabled me to build rapport and convey my warmth and acceptance. I also encouraged parents to come to the school whenever it was convenient for them, without an appointment. I would mention a day of the week when I was more available but not a specific time, allowing parents to come when they could. I understood that, since most held multiple jobs, coming to school for a meeting at a particular time might not be possible. They understood that, if I were busy at the time they arrived, they would need to wait a bit. This flexible schedule drastically decreased the number of parent-meeting cancelations.

I also understood that, in order for immigrant students and families to enhance the quality of their lives in the US, they needed to reproduce what they had left behind: a sense of community and *familiarismo*. I organized monthly family nights during which families could join each other for a light dinner, followed by an educational discussion. We kissed each other on the cheek as they came in. Students would participate in art therapy groups while parents would join the speaker, who would discuss topics that kept parents coming back, such as parenting issues, helping their children to succeed in school, communicating with teachers, navigating their children's educational system, finding a job, understanding and adapting to US culture, feeling safe in the community, blending and/or reuniting families, and exploring immigration and legal status issues. It was remarkable to see how these evening events supported the collectivistic nature of this cultural group. Parents began to get to know each other, share similarities, develop trust in each other, generate friendships, and foster a sense of community—all aspects of the life they'd left behind. They saw me as their friend and ally; I saw myself as their advocate and cultural broker. This was 1997. Was what I was doing ethical?

How would you respond?

For the writer's response, see Appendix B, page 398.

MY ETHICAL DILEMMA

Could I lead an effective art therapy group, given the current group's cultural norms and social psychology orientation?

Another unconventional event that questioned the ethical principles that I not only had learned and practiced, but also was teaching to students at the master's level, arose in 2013 when I traveled to Argentina to offer art therapy services to those affected by a huge flood in my hometown of La Plata. One would think that whiteness would not have been an issue, as I was returning to my native country. But it was.

Upon arriving in Argentina, I met with two social psychologists who invited me to join them at the newly founded, private community center where they practiced. Participants were adults affected by domestic violence who had been displaced by the flood. Group therapy was offered during week-day afternoons and individual therapy was provided by a clinical psychologist. I assisted the social psychologists with group sessions, first by observing and then by leading a 12-session art therapy group.

As I observed the groups, I kept saying to myself, "Go with the flow and observe," and "This is not your group, these are not your clients, you are a guest here." The gatherings seemed more like friendly, casual get-togethers than therapeutic encounters. Participants arrived at different times and proceeded to the kitchen area where others had gathered. (The practice was located in what used to be a small row-house; the kitchen was the only large space that could host the group.) As participants came in, they sat around the kitchen table to drink tea, coffee, or *mate*—a traditional drink made of yerba leaves and hot water, passed around for everyone to sip through a metal straw. The refrigerator held snacks and *masitas* (small pastries) brought by the participants or the psychologists. The conversations were led by the social psychologists, who typically addressed one or two participants per group while the rest (usually 8–12 members) would observe and occasionally chime in. There was no structure, theme, or time limit; groups could last from two to four hours and participants would come and go as they pleased. The sessions seemed like individual therapy taking place within a group setting. Yet, as they sat in the kitchen, sharing experiences of the flood and domestic unrest, there was a true feeling of respect and camaraderie among the participants—males, females, mothers and daughters, victims and (unrelated) abusers. We greeted each other with a kiss as we entered the center; we kissed as we said goodbye. Smoking, eating, and drinking were allowed during group. After group, participants would share car rides to the center of town to catch the bus to go home.

I struggled with how to behave, as I saw myself stretching ethical boundaries and establishing dual relationships—something I had not done before. I passed judgment as to what I thought was *right* and *wrong*, *ethical* and *unethical*. I questioned whether my "whiteness"—a value system that I did not think existed in me—was getting in the way of understanding, assimilating, adapting to, and accepting the cultural norms before me, norms that were part of my own culture and upbringing. Should I share my way of doing psychotherapy or try to adapt to theirs? Social psychology brought people together as a community, to rely upon one another for help. My ethical dilemma was whether to alter the structure of this group in order to facilitate art therapy in the way I had been practicing it for years in the US or to negotiate, compromise, or expand ethical boundaries to maintain the current group culture. Would a culturally adaptive art therapy group be ethical?

How would you respond?

For the writer's response, see Appendix B, page 398.

Concluding Thoughts

In my work with Latin American immigrant families in the US and with adults in my native Argentina, I learned to incorporate culturally specific ways of behaving, in an effort to enhance a structured, supportive, and productive therapeutic environment. I learned that one could relax about time schedules, kissing, food, gifts, and self-disclosure and that expanding one's personal boundaries does not necessarily result in a loss of professionalism or effectiveness. In summary, I learned that there is no one way of conducting art therapy sessions and that following my heart, to be true to the culture I share with my clients, is not unethical.

REFLECTIVE ART EXPERIENCES & DISCUSSION QUESTIONS

1. Think back to when you were young—as early as you can remember. Think about something that happened when you were with your family, perhaps not your entire family, but at least one family member. If you were to play the whole memory as a movie and then to stop it at one frame, what would be happening? Create artwork representing what is happening in that frame.
2. Memories from early childhood are typically associated with deeply rooted cultural norms. What does the memory that you drew illustrate about your cultural upbringing and make-up? What feelings are expressed? Why do you think you remembered this particular event? What was it trying to convey?
3. Think of a time when, as an art therapist, you worked with an individual or a group of individuals who did not share your cultural views and moral values. Visualize your reaction, thoughts, feelings, and body sensations at the moment when you were presented with this ethical challenge and represent them on paper, using lines and colors.
4. What do the lines and colors in your artwork convey? What steps did you take to resolve this cultural and ethical dilemma?

7

DO NO MORE HARM

The Ethical Practice of Art Therapy with Hospitalized Adults Who Have Severe and Persistent Mental Illness

Deirdre M. Cogan

Some of America's most marginalized and misunderstood individuals reside within the walls of long-term psychiatric hospitals and residential facilities. These individuals struggle not only with the debilitating effects of severe and persistent mental illness; their day-to-day realities are lived within the confines of institutional settings. Progressive legislation, spirited ethical debates, and consumer advocacy groups have dramatically changed the face of mental health treatment over last few decades. However, the stigma associated with mental illness persists. It follows that the ethical practice of art therapy with individuals who have severe and persistent mental illness (SPMI) requires not only sensitivity to this cultural stigma, but also an understanding of the complex and variable nature of SPMI.

A Changing Context

When I began my tenure as an art therapist treating individuals at a state psychiatric facility, I was initially overwhelmed by the nature of their illness. Clinical presentations took on myriad forms, ranging from intrusive symptoms such as hallucinations and bizarre, repetitious behavior, to negative symptoms such as apathy, lack of volition, and poverty of speech. Most individuals suffered from one or more severe psychiatric conditions that caused significant functional impairment for an indefinite period; they struggled with intractable conditions which permitted relief only during periods of partial remission. Length of stay varied from several months to several decades.

Within my first year at the hospital, momentous changes took place. Like so many state hospitals around the country responding to the push toward community living, the institution which once housed several thousand individuals now provided care to a few hundred, within a new facility. Sadly, many patients resisted this change; some felt safer in the hospital than in the community. Periods of institutionalization had fostered dependency and acute sensitivity to stress. I viewed art therapy as an antidote to their resistance. "The arts therapies draw on the healthier dimensions of the personality and celebrate aspects of feeling and thought that transcend the more problem-oriented tasks sometimes occupying the traditional verbal therapies" (Blatener, 1992, p. 406). The facilitation of authentic feeling and restoration of personal agency are central to our modality.

Clinicians and their clients were called to embark on a road to recovery which was dotted with potholes. When working with individuals who have SPMI, often there are many forces at play. For instance, art therapists have a duty to "do no harm," yet it is equally important to offer clients opportunities for autonomy, despite the fact that these opportunities might introduce risk. Equal access to art therapy services is crucial, yet, because the nature of their pathology might preclude their participation (especially if they pose a danger to others), not all individuals who would like to participate in group art therapy can do so. One must constantly assess the situation and the context, while reconciling opposing ethical obligations.

Ethical Values

The values set forth in the Preamble of the American Art Therapy Association's Ethical Principles for Art Therapists (AATA, 2013) proved to be enormously useful in navigating this unchartered territory. Before describing how, I will discuss an issue that is especially germane to working with individuals with SPMI: therapeutic boundaries.

Boundaries

While respect for clinical boundaries is fundamental to creating meaningful alliances with individuals who have SPMI, deviations from standard practice can be supportive of treatment. I recall working with a husky man who towered over me. In group, he would reach out and forcefully touch my arm. Over time, I learned that this action served an important function for him. Due to his florid symptoms, he was unable to distinguish me from his hallucinations. Eventually, a prosocial "fist bump" provided him with a sensory pathway that enabled him to make this differentiation.

In another instance, I encountered a frantic woman pacing the hallways of the admissions unit. At second glance, I realized she was someone with whom I had worked—a lively, deep-voiced individual who loved to recite poetry. She inquired, "Do you hear them talking?" When I reassured her that I heard only the two of us talking with one another, she sighed with relief, saying "Thank you, I was not sure." Following that candid interaction, we developed a strong therapeutic relationship.

While clinician transparency can be a powerful tool to forge a positive alliance, it can also have adverse consequences. Judgments must be contextual and they vary greatly on a case-by-case basis, depending upon the nature of the individual's mental illness. During a lively session of an empowerment group, one group member, a former educator who experienced chronic bouts of depression, inquired whether I had ever been depressed. I pondered the ethical implications of self-disclosure. While I thought that my self-disclosure might reduce the stigma and sense of isolation that she could be experiencing, I wondered if this type of disclosure might be alarming to her and awaken latent issues of over-identification. I chose to acknowledge that I, too, had experienced periods of depression. After my candid disclosure, she shared that her perception of me had immediately changed from that of a powerful woman to someone who did not possess the strength to help her. In this case, perhaps less transparency would have been more beneficial.

Autonomy

Respecting the clients' right to choose is especially important in a residential setting. Therefore, given the availability of other treatment options, if an individual decides not to participate in or to continue with art therapy groups, I believe that that person should have the option to do so. This is especially true of long-term hospitalized patients who are of legal age to make critical life decisions, yet, due to the nature of their illness, are surrounded by others who continually make decisions for them.

I began to fully value the principle of autonomy through my therapeutic alliance with a cognitively impaired man who was considered to be "hard to reach." When he joined my group, he had been in the hospital for three decades. He had a waif-like appearance and a gentle manner and he quickly became engrossed in the multisensory activities, often creating intricate, textured collages. He was proud of his creations, often beaming when he shared them with peers. Thus, I was surprised when one day he announced that he wanted to leave the group. When questioned about the reasons for his request, he informed me that he wanted to experience similar successes in other groups. This posed an ethical dilemma for me. I was emotionally conflicted, feeling torn between encouraging him to remain in a group which seemed to be so beneficial for him and respecting his decision to leave it. I also became aware of my own counter-transference; I enjoyed having him in the group and I liked to think that I was helping him. After reviewing his history, I was able to glean the importance of his decision. As a young child, he had gone from placement to placement; his childhood experiences seemed to have been built on shifting sand. While in the hospital, he had avoided therapeutic relationships. In short, it seemed as though he had never established a stable base from which he could separate. Understanding this dynamic, I fully endorsed his decision.

The client periodically stopped by my office to tell me how he was doing in his new groups and I told him that I was delighted to hear about his progress. Eventually, he was placed in the community. Supporting his autonomy had two-fold benefit: first, he practiced his ability to assert himself and communicate effectively; second, he created object constancy by checking back in with me. He seemed to regard me as a trusted ally who would not infringe upon his rights. I would like to think that, as a result of the collaborative alliance we developed, I played some small part in helping him prepare to become more independent.

Beneficence

The promotion of the clients' sense of well-being is a central aim of our profession. Individuals with SPMI appear to be exquisitely sensitive to psychological intrusion and to being questioned, assessed, and re-assessed. Anticipating the fact that delusions and paranoia might foster a sense of distrust, one can create interventions that will minimize the level of suspiciousness by shifting the focus of activities to self-efficacy. Even when individuals are struggling with debilitating symptoms, there are areas of strength that can be built upon, thereby helping clients to develop self-confidence and an increased level of comfort in the group. Key is to ensure that the art therapy room is a space that can be experienced as a safe haven away from the commotion of day-to-day life in a hospital. The goal is to cultivate a space where participants do not associate groups with harsh judgment or with adverse stimuli that they wish to avoid.

Fidelity

Clinicians often share stories with one another as a means of debriefing and exploring meaning. Although working with adults with mental illness does provide interesting stories and anecdotes, it is crucial to remember that individuals with SPMI are not only legally, but also professionally, entitled to their dignity as well as their privacy. We must make certain that discussions take place in a clinical setting and adhere to the provisions of confidentiality. People with SPMI are extremely sensitive to perceived slights and degradation; breaches of privacy can undermine the ethical integrity and level of professionalism of an entire program.

Justice

Though a commitment to fairness and equal access to services is important, there is a delicate balance between justice and safety. Fairness must be measured against the potential for harm. Depending upon the individual and the circumstance, the behavior of clients can be unpredictable. In order to maintain a safe milieu, individuals are held accountable for their conduct during groups. Demonstrating empathy does not require one to collude with pathology. Empathy requires one to listen and respond to the individual's emotions and perceptions. It does not require unconditional acceptance of unacceptable behavior. If group participants are unable to accept this responsibility, they may need to be temporarily, or permanently, suspended from the group.

I once worked with a man who experienced paranoid ideas of reference. His thought disturbance led him to interpret the actions of others as hostile. Once, he aggressively struck a group member (i.e., a perceived antagonist) who had smiled at him. When he vehemently protested his prompt removal from the group, I made it very clear that I was not questioning his perception; however, I was prohibiting his aggression. Later, he was able to acknowledge that his conduct had been unacceptable. While his persecutory thoughts persisted, he refrained from further destructive action. In the long run, his removal from the group seemed to increase his sense of ownership of his mental health. He was able to apply this self-awareness not just within, but outside, the group.

When Values Collide

Autonomy versus Beneficence

One year, the patients were invited to exhibit their work outside of the hospital, in government buildings and in juried exhibitions within galleries. From a legal perspective, the process seemed relatively cut and dry: a release form would be created and, once it was signed, the client's artwork could become part of an exhibit. Since many of the patients with SPMI were not competent to sign the release forms, an additional signature by their *guardian ad litem* would be required.

Since there is a difference between legal and ethical obligations, resolving the former does not absolve the clinician from the latter. While I wanted the patients to benefit from the boost to their sense of self-esteem and competence (in effect, their sense of autonomy) that exhibiting their artwork might provide, I was concerned about how some of my patients would react to seeing their artwork exhibited in a public forum. And, although I could agree with administrators who felt that the patients could benefit, emotionally, from the reinforcement they would derive from seeing that other people valued their work enough to buy it, I believed that—in addition to all the other possible negative consequences of a sale of client artwork (e.g., the feelings of patients whose work did not sell)—I believed that involving myself in any financial transactions violated my ethical obligation to my patients.

My concerns seem to have been well-founded. A talented client who experienced magnificent delusions of grandeur had been lucid when the release form was signed. Later, he developed a delusion that the gallery had sold his artwork for millions of dollars and then had withheld the funds from him. By placing myself outside the process of dealing with his artwork as a commodity, I was not experienced as a person who had participated in what he experienced as exploitation. Luckily, our therapeutic alliance was protected from this perception.

Justice versus Nonmaleficence

At one point, the facility decided to implement a trauma protocol which had proven to be effective with women on forensic units. Being among the first clinicians in the hospital to implement the initiative, initially I was steadfast in my fidelity to the modules, only to learn rather quickly that modifications would be necessary.

The need for this was revealed when an actively psychotic woman was referred to the trauma group. The group seemed to provide her with an outlet for feelings pent-up during years of abuse; however, an increase in the acuity of her illness was quickly observed. In one session, she complained of tactile sensations such as feeling insects crawling around inside her. In the next, she stated that the therapist was reading her mind. I began to question whether our interventions were antithetical to her treatment goals. While creative arts therapies can give voice to emotional experience, traumatic memories can awaken overwhelming feelings of helplessness, fear, and unbearable physical sensations. While potentially destabilizing for any individual, this can be debilitating for a vulnerable individual with SPMI. Sadly, little had been written about trauma intervention with people with SPMI.

In her seminal book, *Trauma and Recovery*, psychiatrist Judith Herman refers to trauma as a disease of disconnection, stating that "Survivors feel unsafe in their bodies. Their emotion and thinking feel out of control. They also feel unsafe in relation to other people" (Herman, 1992, p. 160). Using Herman's model of establishing safety as a priority, we were able to modify the modules in order to tailor them to meet the needs of our patients. Art therapy was used in a variety of applications to promote positive connections between individuals—and, thus, opportunities to give and receive validation and compassion—while avoiding triggering flashbacks and tactile memories.

MY ETHICAL DILEMMA

How can I best serve both the Hospital Review Board and my patients?

The Hospital Review Board reviews and votes on the treatment team's recommendations for individuals who have involvement in the criminal justice system. A comprehensive clinical and administrative review is scheduled after the unit administrator submits a report detailing the individual's diagnosis, responsiveness to current goals and objectives, and current functioning. After reading the report and listening to the treatment team's presentation, the Board discusses the case and votes on the treatment team's recommendations.

While I was never a permanent member of the Board, as a department supervisor, I served as an alternate for my supervisor in her absence. There were times when this led to friction between my administrative goals and my clinical goals. For example, I was once asked to assess and vote on a client's readiness to participate in a day treatment program. The individual had been in one of my groups for several years and I had established a strong attachment to him. Although initially guarded, he was compassionate towards others and had shared childhood memories of having been torn from his mother's care and placed in foster care. I now see that I had developed a maternal transference towards him and delighted in his remarkable progress.

During the review, it was revealed that he had become assaultive towards another individual shortly after the report was submitted. I was deeply conflicted regarding my clinical obligations and my duty to the Board. My client had made steady progress over the course of several years, but it was apparent that he could be unpredictable and dangerous. Should I recommend that he be moved into day treatment or remain in the hospital?

How would you respond?

For the writer's response, see Appendix B, page 401.

Concluding Thoughts

The trend toward deinstitutionalization that I mentioned at the beginning of this chapter has continued, unabated, and a focal point of treatment for persons with SPMI has been to find alternatives to long-term hospitalization. While many individuals with

SPMI are responsive to community-based treatment, it can be challenging for those whose symptoms wax and wane. Decompensation can occur when there is lack of attunement between what the individual values—and can tolerate—and the mission mandated by the institution.

It is incumbent upon art therapists to modify interventions to support community readiness goals. For instance, an individual who goes on community outings might be asked to create drawings or collages in response to being in the natural setting or at events outside the hospital. Imagery frequently generates lively conversations and can reveal barriers to community readiness. When processing their artwork, individuals often identify situations that make them fearful or environmental stimuli that exacerbate their symptoms. Together, the art therapist and the individual can engage in shared decision making about how to manage the distress associated with these situations. Using art to support psychosocial rehabilitation has two benefits: imagery can give voice to perceptions that clients may not be able, or willing, to verbalize and it can help them diffuse anxiety by bringing clarity and form to confusing experiences and feelings.

REFLECTIVE ART EXPERIENCES & DISCUSSION QUESTIONS

1. Imagine you are living in an environment where you are familiar with the routine and know everyone around you; draw yourself there. Suddenly, you are asked to leave that place—to go somewhere that those in charge believe is better for you.

   a. Draw how you might feel.
   b. Draw what you might need in order to make that transition.

2. Describe an occasion when you wondered whether programmatic initiatives were unsupportive of, or detrimental to, your client's treatment goals.
3. Describe a time when self-disclosure did not have the result that you intended.

References

American Art Therapy Association. (2013). *Ethical principles for art therapists.* Alexandria, VA: AATA.

Blatener, A. (1992). Theoretical principles underlying creative arts therapies. *The Arts in Psychotherapy,* 18(5), 405–409.

Herman, J. (1992). *Trauma and recovery.* New York: Basic Books.

8

NOT JUST ANOTHER OLD PERSON

Art Therapy with Those Who Strive for Autonomy and Respect within a Culture of Invisibility

Emery Hurst Mikel

Picture an old woman on the street, carrying her groceries home. What do you see? Wrinkles? Slow movement? A stooped posture? Do you worry about the person tripping or falling down? What if you learned more about the woman walking past you? What if it turns out that she has been married 64 years? What if you then find out that this woman is a Holocaust survivor? This isn't just another old person. This is Rose, a woman in her 90s who loves her little apartment in Brooklyn, where she and her husband have lived very full and rewarding lives. She has children and grandchildren. She has stories to tell you and eventually you'll realize that a gleam comes into her eyes and a flush rises in her cheeks when she talks about some of the adventures she has had. Every time you leave, she takes your hand and tells you, "Don't do anything I wouldn't do!" before chuckling and sending you on your way.

No one is just another old person. I will generalize throughout the rest of this chapter for the sake of time and space, so please keep this in mind as you continue to read.

What is so Scary about Older People?

Well, for starters, they make us face our own aging, mortality, and fear of waking up one day to a life unlived. When we see an "old" person, many professionals and lay people alike see deterioration, inability, frailty, fear, and the great unknown. Is this a misconception? Not exactly, but it is only a very small part of the much bigger picture that is the immense value of each person's life, painted in unfathomable depth and color. The problem is that many people—including clinicians—approach this age group with a sense of trepidation; few are brave enough to acknowledge, let alone challenge, their preconceptions in order to find out who the person beyond those fabricated barriers really is.

Ethical Issues

Respect and autonomy seem to be at the root of most of the ethical dilemmas I have witnessed. The first time I meet with my art therapy interns, I talk about boundaries, because some of the choices they will need to consider in their interactions with older adults appear to be in direct conflict with what they are learning, for good reason, in school.

Touching a Client

Half the time that I sit with a person in hospice care, we are holding hands. Touch is also an important way to communicate with those who have dementia. As an art therapist, I often use the hand-over-hand approach to assist some clients as they begin their work. Since touch is more likely to occur with older adults, it is crucial to learn how to use it in a professional and respectful way. One option is to ask the person's permission before touching. When there is no chance to ask or the client does not have the ability to answer, I often place my hand close enough for the client to reach. I may slowly and softly place my hand on the client's hand. If I touch someone and the person moves away—even after many positive responses in the past—I immediately remove my hand and sit back in my chair, giving the client more space. I will also apologize. It is important to respect where someone is at the moment, and not base our actions upon what has happened before.

One day, I was so concerned when a client pulled away from me that I consulted a nurse after the session. It turned out that he had just had his flu shot and his entire arm was extremely sensitive. The next time I arrived, I got a hearty handshake.

Disclosing Personal Information to a Client

Fletch is an 82-year-old man who has been on hospice care for three months. In a nursing home and confined to bed, he can still sit up to create art. Fletch really enjoys making art together, so Julia, the art therapist, often draws alongside him or introduces interventions where they work on the same sheet of paper. Last week, Fletch talked about his late wife and the wonderful life they had shared together. When he asked Julia if she was married, she said that she was engaged. Fletch suggested that she bring her fiancée in sometime. Julia smiled and said she thought that would be fun, but that her partner's work schedule made it unlikely.

Consider how Julia handled the situation. When working with other populations, we don't share much personal information because it doesn't serve our client or the relationship we are building. With older adults, it may seem disrespectful not to converse in a sociable manner during a session. I usually respond to personal questions with two or three sentences about myself and then return the focus to the client. That way, I don't share too much or monopolize the client's time. In the vignette above, Julia felt fine sharing that she was engaged, but when asked to bring her fiancée in to meet Fletch, she set a boundary. Perhaps she was maintaining confidentiality, avoiding the creation of a dual relationship, or feeling uncomfortable.

Giving and Receiving Gifts

After Julia told Fletch that her partner's work schedule would make it unlikely that he would stop by, Fletch asked Julia to get a pocket watch out of his dresser drawer. She did so and handed it to him. "This is a wedding gift for you and your new husband. Every young couple should have a pocket watch!"

What are your thoughts? Many ethics codes state that we should not accept gifts from our patients. Setting this boundary shows respect for the family (who might expect to inherit that watch), the client (whom we are already being paid to see), and the therapist (who would be creating a dual relationship and, possibly, generating misunderstandings or accusations if the client forgot that he gave you a present). Sometimes cultural and other factors make this difficult. The practice I have adopted is to thank genuinely, refuse politely, and suggest that the client and I each create and exchange a piece of artwork during the session. This process is in line with our agreed-upon relationship, the intention of the art making is clear, and role confusion is avoided.

Making Art With, or in the Presence of, a Client

The question of whether to make art with, or in the presence of, a client always raises an ethical dilemma for me. I try to resolve it by asking myself: Why am I considering doing this right now? What are the benefits and risks? Whose needs would be met by doing this—the client's or mine? In other words, would this be respectful of my client's space, abilities, and autonomy or would it serve to quell my own anxiety and do away with the need to devise an approach that would better serve my client?

Many of the older adults with whom I have worked felt uncomfortable if I just sat with them while they made art, so I often set up materials for myself, but then would wait to see if I needed to make art in order for them to feel more at ease. There are many ways to make art with clients. I have made art with people watching or directing me. I have had clients gain control, choice, and independence through showing me how to paint. I try to involve my clients in these decisions as often as possible, so they can let me know what they feel comfortable with and why.

Confidentiality

Colleagues who have taken over the leadership of groups that I had run at assisted living facilities have sometimes called to let me know how everyone is doing. I appreciated the updates and the calls felt normal until a peer questioned the advisability of the exchange in relation to confidentiality. Suddenly, I realized that I was no longer privileged to receive any information pertaining to those clients. My time with them was over. The same would be true of going back to visit clients at a facility where I no longer work.

The Health Insurance Portability and Accountability Act of 1996 (HIPAA) provides guidelines regarding confidentiality, but those lines can look blurry when working in programs for older adults. The social atmosphere can even throw off other professionals.

Nurses may ask us about a current client while we are passing in the hallway. It feels as if we should be able to discuss such things while within the nursing home—until we think about all the other people around who might overhear us.

Ensuring Respect and Autonomy in the Presence of Ageism

When should individuals no longer be involved in the decision-making process about their own health, well-being, and care?

Carol is 70 and diagnosed with early stage dementia. She knows that she gets confused and that it will get worse, but is happy to live at home with her husband George. She likes Dr. Ross and is used to visiting him. As usual, Dr. Ross asks her the date and the day of the week and asks her to remember several words while they chat. Then he turns to George and says, "Carol is doing well, but I see some changes, so let's set up an appointment with the neurologist. Have you noticed changes at home?"

Consider this exchange from Carol's point of view. This process certainly saves time for the doctor and George may figure that he might as well get used to making decisions for Carol—even if he does not yet have her power of attorney— because eventually his wife won't be able to make them. Speaking about her as though she were not in the room is disrespectful, however, and takes away her independence and choice. Caregivers, medical personnel, spouses, and grown children often talk to me in front of clients, as if they are not there and cannot comprehend what is being discussed. Luckily, people can be made aware of and change their behavior. We need to give our clients a chance to maintain their dignity, respect, and independence in whatever way they can.

When should individuals no longer be involved in the decision-making process about their own health, well-being, and care? *"Never!"* We can always try to find a way to involve the client.

Obtaining Informed Consent When Clients Have Dementia

I want to include client artwork and stories in a book I am writing. I know I need to get art release forms and informed consent paperwork signed. Some of my clients, however, have dementia. What should I do?

My approach is based upon my ethical responsibilities, including my need to respect my clients' right to choose regardless of diagnosis. On several occasions over a three-week period, I bring up my book project, ask clients what they think of it, and ask whether they would like their art to be included. For clients who say "no" the majority of the time, the process goes no further. If I still really want the artwork of those clients in my book, I have to admit that to myself and then not put it in the book. Someone once asked me, "Can't we just use it? They won't remember." No!

If certain clients answer "yes" most of the time, I then consider how their participation would serve them versus me. If I am still uncertain what fits best for them, I may turn to their family members—not to ask whether I should include the art, but whether they believe that the client would have wanted the art included. If the answer is yes, I approach the person who has the client's power of attorney. Sometimes clients will want to sign the form themselves, even if they are no longer deemed legally competent to make those decisions. I am okay with that, as it offers them a sense of autonomy. I then approach the person with power of attorney, to get the form officially signed.

Elder Abuse

One day I was working with residents of a small group home for people with dementia, creating paper collage trees and discussing seasons, when a relatively new aide walked over to Mary and, without warning, lifted her out of her chair and began walking her out of the room. Mary yelped in surprise, flailed a bit, almost tripped over a chair, and then kept asking, "Where are you taking me?" The aide just smiled and said, "Don't worry." No other staff seemed to notice what was happening.

I was a new art therapist at the time and stood there dumbfounded, trying to figure out what to do for Mary, why this scene bothered me so much, and if I had a right to say something. No one else responded, so I felt unsettled as well as upset about Mary's anxiety and confusion. I did nothing that day, but after discussing it in ATR supervision, gave the manager of the facility, who had hired me, a call. I described what I had witnessed and she thanked me; after that, the aide seemed to change her behavior. It can be a struggle to make a decision like that when it is not just theoretical, but finding the support to make that phone call or bring awareness to a situation that could result in someone being harmed is a duty we have to our clients both ethically and legally.

Elder abuse is a very sad reality. We tend to think of extreme cases, but small incidents take place every day. As mandated reporters, we are legally obligated to report not only observed, but also suspected, abuse and neglect.

The National Research Council (2003) explains that mistreatment occurs when a caregiver, or other person in a relationship of trust with a vulnerable adult, takes an intentional action that causes harm or creates a serious risk of harm. It does not matter whether or not the harm, itself, was intentional and can include failure, by the caregiver, to provide for the adult's basic needs or to protect the person from harm. Types of mistreatment range from physical and emotional to financial and healthcare fraud. Robinson et al. (2015) give a comprehensive list of signs to look for—whether they be unexplained bruises or a caregiver yelling at, belittling, or threatening an older adult or allowing that adult to go unwashed or wear soiled clothing.

MY ETHICAL DILEMMA

How do I maintain confidentiality on a home visit?

I was riding up an elevator to make a home visit with a hospice patient whose condition had seriously deteriorated. I made sure my identification badge was facing forward so my client could see it and remember my name. As I exited the elevator, a neighbor of hers, Sara, stood there with her dog and said, "Oh, you're from hospice! We met when you last visited Mrs. Goodrich. How is she doing?"

How would you respond?

For the writer's response, see Appendix B, page 419.

Concluding Thoughts

Older adults have lived full lives, been through wars, fought for the rights we have today, and done other remarkable things. Even when their words no longer make sense, so much can be learned from, and communicated by, people who have dementia. If we are lucky, one day all of us—and all those whom we love—will be older adults. How will we want them, and ourselves, to be treated?

REFLECTIVE ART EXPERIENCES & DISCUSSION QUESTIONS

1. Think of an older adult in your life whom you cherish. Draw an image that represents your connection and relationship. Afterward, consider all the things that make that person important to you and all the ways that he or she is an amazing, unique individual. On the back of the paper, write a brief letter to a future caregiver who will meet this person when he or she is no longer verbal. What is important for that caregiver to know and to understand?
2. What brings joy and meaning to your life and makes you uniquely you? If your ability to care for yourself were taken away, what would be important for a caregiver or therapist to know in order to sustain/improve your quality of life?
3. Think of a moment when you felt that a client was being mistreated in some way. Use art materials to explore how you felt as a witness, how the client might have felt, and how the instigator might have been feeling.
4. How do you handle a situation in which a client is being mistreated? Does your response differ when there is clear abuse rather than something more subtle? What about when your client is subjected to something even less tangible, such as ageism?

References

The Health Insurance Portability and Accountability Act of 1996 (HIPAA) P.L. No. 104–191, 110 Stat. 1938 (1996).

National Research Council (2003). Concepts, definitions, and guidelines for measurement. In R.J. Bonnie and R.B. Wallace (Eds.), *Elder mistreatment: Abuse, neglect and exploitation in an aging America*. Washington, DC: The National Academies Press.

Robinson, L., Saisan, J., & Segal, J. (2015). Elder abuse and neglect: Warning signs, risk factors, prevention, and reporting abuse. Retrieved from www.helpguide.org/articles/abuse/elder-abuse-and-neglect.htm

9

REDRESSING SOCIAL INJUSTICE

Transcending and Transforming the Borders of Art Therapy Training in South Africa

Hayley Berman

My white privilege pervaded my upbringing in an apartheid South Africa. The majority of the population did not have the right to vote, did not have access to a decent education, and had very little access to tertiary education. I always knew that something was fundamentally wrong. Being subjected to the unequal power relations of the medical sphere after a spate of surgeries during adolescence heightened my sensitivity to the need for inter-subjective, democratic modes of engagement. Making sense of my experiences through image making was critical to my emotional survival and I was determined to enable others to do the same. The luxury of being able to obtain my Master's degree in Art Therapy in the United Kingdom, away from an environment subsumed by discrimination and racism, was liberating and emotionally expansive. Within group training, the theoretical framework of psychodynamic thinking, and my own psychoanalytic journey, I could imagine a future of inclusivity. It was in those moments that a seed was planted "to liberate the life-force in a traumatised South Africa," which became the title of my PhD dissertation (Berman, 2012).

Within the South African context of historically restricted access to tertiary education, based upon divisive racist apartheid structures, many could not hope to attain the undergraduate degree that is prerequisite to pursuing training as an art therapist—let alone go abroad to obtain the graduate degree that is considered entry level to the profession. The redress of undemocratic structures in society presupposes a new model of practice—in this case, one that challenges the ethics of the implicit exclusivity and elite premise upon which the training of art therapists rests. My intention was to address this schism by creating access to art therapy training programs—and the profession—through subverting hierarchies with an ethics characterized by reciprocity, transformation, and sustainability.

In 1994, I founded the Art Therapy Centre in Johannesburg, now known as Lefika La Phodiso, Africa's first psychoanalytically informed Community Art Counselling and Training Institute.

Lefika La Phodiso

Lefika La Phodiso ("The Rock of Holding") is situated on the second floor of the Children's Memorial Institute in Johannesburg, which is home to more than 30 child-based non-governmental organizations that provide a multitude of complementary services. Located on the border of Hillbrow, opposite the Constitutional Court, and within walking distance of Wits University, its position exemplifies the richness and complexity of residing on the margins of society, at the periphery of academia, in proximity to the bastion of constitutional rights and social justice. Hillbrow has been rated the worst crime precinct in the province of Gauteng (in which Johannesburg is located), with the highest murder rate, the highest rate of robbery with assault, and the second to highest rate of assault with intent to cause grievous bodily harm (Falanga, 2016).

From the moment one comes up the stairs, art leads him or her into the haven of Lefika. A mural of the Hillbrow skyline, made up of fragments of colorful discarded images created within the Open Studio spaces, welcomes all who enter (see Figure 9.1). I have arrived to find a three-year-old who had navigated her way alone through the busy and often violent streets of Hillbrow to get to Lefika, a place she knows she'll find a nutritious meal and reliable adults who can contain her. Indeed, the assumption we bring to our work at Lefika is that the children who attend our programs have a sense of agency and resilience. Like the three-year-old child, they are self-referred and display a resistance to their current circumstances by seeking out and recognizing a creative safe space, with adults who can enhance their sense of self-worth. I regard the children's responses as a form of positive protest, an unconscious activism

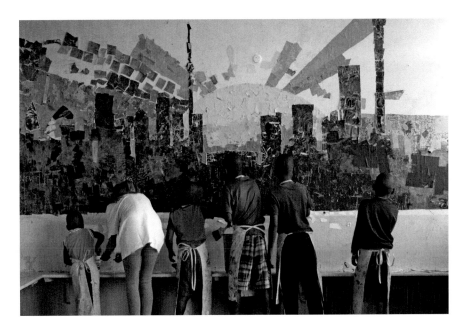

FIGURE 9.1 Children creating a mural of the Hillbrow skyline *(see color insert)*.

in investing in spaces that build social cohesion, ego strength, and empathic relating. This philosophy mirrors all of Lefika's services and training, which build upon existing resources, strengths, and passions.

MY ETHICAL DILEMMA

Informed consent and children's services

What is our ethical responsibility (in terms of informed consent) to children who show up for services on their own?

How would you respond?

For the writer's response, see Appendix B, page 400.

The Overriding Ethical Dilemma

How do we meet the mental health needs of children and adults in a country where resources are scarce and needs are great? In the following pages, I describe how I have endeavored to address that dilemma, by creating non-exclusionary training, developing sustainable services, and ensuring ethical practice.

In South Africa, the hardcore psychosocial reality is that there is a deficit of parental figures in a parentless nation with minimal mental health resources and limitless mental health needs. Lefika's response has been to focus upon building the parental, adult ego function in society by training community workers to provide an internalized model of healthy relationships. Fonagy and Higgitt (2007) comment, "it is the internal working model of attachment relationships that predicts mortality rather than the physical presence of supportive individuals" (p. 19). We see our role as one of enhancing, supplementing, and supporting the parents who are struggling, not replacing them.

Training Community Art Counsellors

In addressing the deficit of mental health resources in South Africa, I have worked collaboratively to build therapeutic capacity within under–resourced communities (Berman, 2011). Over the past 25 years, Lefika has trained over 250 students and reached over 160,000 beneficiaries. Lefika has developed a new professional category, "Community Art Counsellor" (CAC), which has been accredited by the Health and Welfare Sector and Training Authority, and recognized within the South African Arts Therapies profession as an initiative for psychosocial transformation.

Training takes place over an 18-month period within the context of an experiential therapy group in which image making and psychoanalytic thinking are interwoven.

The training is tiered in the way the master's degree program in Art Therapy at my alma mater, Hertfordshire University, UK is structured: to include experiential, theoretical, and practice-based learning. Students include community workers and allied professionals from multi-racial, multi-cultural groups of diverse incomes. Students who can pay for training help to subsidize those who cannot afford to pay. Government and corporate funding also helps to defray expenses.

Criteria for admission includes a history of empathic community engagement, a practice of engaging in one's own image making process, and a capacity for self reflection. Each student has a passion for psychosocial change and a commitment to starting a community project in the area in which he or she lives and works or in an area identified as being in need of a CAC resource. Trainees engage, relate, create, free associate, and participate in eight training modules, each of which includes assessment criteria and procedures. The modules are: Counselling within the South African Context, The Counselling Process, Psychoanalytic Approaches and Theories, Group Work, Trauma, Social Action and Visual Research, Social Entrepreneurship and Creative Leadership, and Bereavement, Loss, and Endings.

Students and CAC graduates must adhere to the codes of ethics of the South African National Arts Therapists Organisation, the South African Psychoanalytic Confederation, the British Association of Art Therapists, and the American Association of Art Therapists. An important element of assuring the ethical practice and implementation of services is that Community Art Counsellors always work in groups, where possible facilitating in pairs, symbolizing the parental couple, and the work takes place within institutions, community-based organizations, or arts centers that focus upon social cohesion and social justice. This results in the building of therapeutic capacity—personally, institutionally, and geographically—and the creation of sustainable, replicable services in under-resourced areas, including those impacted by violence and trauma. This differs from the scope of practice of registered Art Therapists, who can work individually and privately.

Shifting the Psychoanalytic Couch Out of the Consulting Room and into the Community: Holding and Containing

At Lefika, our hope is that providing consistency in terms of time, space, task (group), (art) materials, and adult support (the CACs) will allow for the establishment of what Winnicott (1965) called a *good enough* internal environment. The process of creating in the presence of *the other* (in group work, *others*) facilitates the opportunity to revisit the early negotiations of self in relation to other. Interactions within the group facilitate the development of an internalized capacity to hold, while the creation and use of images lend another dimension to what it means to hold and be held by relationships and *objects* (Winnicott, 1965). Becoming the *developmentally needed object* sometimes requires the breaching of therapeutic ethical norms, for example, by choosing to feed the children before their group begins. Our ethical responsibility to engage actively in repair and redress does not mean abiding by rigid professional boundaries that preclude humanitarian responses.

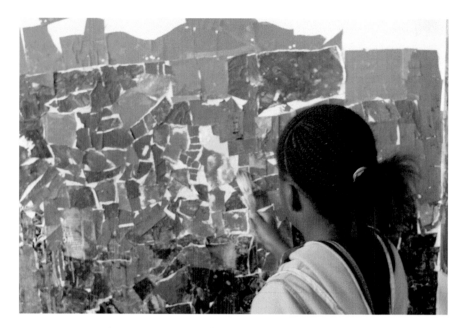

FIGURE 9.2 Transformative potential of material.

Essentially, Community Art Counsellors are trained to provide the transitional space, the holding environment, in which empathic relating and healthy attachment can occur. This expands the "safe spaces" that children are able both to experience in the present and to draw upon as adolescents and adults. In this way, we seek to multiply the function of the *good enough* parent (Winnicott, 1965). The modeling of psychoanalytic concepts such as these becomes internalized and replicated in practice, such as in Open Studio Spaces for children, mural-making projects in schools, trauma debriefing sessions for school children and teachers who have witnessed death, and workshops for students and staff following violent protests (Berman, 2016). Imagine these kinds of experiences—led by psychoanalytically minded adults in studios with an enormous range of evocative objects and materials and consistent boundaries of time and space—in every town, every province, every country. (See Figure 9.2.)

Accreditation

The Health Professions Council of South Africa provisionally accepted Lefika's Art Therapy curriculum in 2005; however, only within the context of a tertiary educational structure. This was a tautological bind, as most of the students did not have undergraduate degrees, due to past educational inequality, and would, therefore, not be allowed entry to a university. Alternative methods of accreditation and recognition were sought. In 1998, the South African government introduced the Sector and Training Authority (SETA) and the Skills Development Act to redress inequality of opportunity as a result of the policy of apartheid. In 2000, the Lefika Training Programme was amended to comply with the SETA requirements and lodged for accreditation. The foreignness of the content and the challenges of presenting course-work that straddled arts and health sectors resulted in the submission being rejected, lost, and resubmitted over many years at great cost. In 2017, accreditation was granted by the Health and Welfare SETA as an NQF 5 (post Grade 12) qualification within an existing category: the "Certificate in Methods of Counselling," granting Lefika the status of an accredited training institution. Alumni have the opportunity to fulfill the assessment criteria to gain accreditation through recognition of prior learning.

Professional Recognition

Lefika has paved the way to create a new mid-level registration category for Community Arts Counsellors with a submission made to the Health Professions Council of South Africa. A task team, composed of representatives of all the Arts Therapies modalities, has been established. The goal is to expand and adapt the CAC training modules to all the Arts Therapies, thereby creating appropriate, accessible arts-based therapeutic resources in under-resourced areas throughout South Africa. There appears to be both a proactive momentum in the country with regard to recognizing the massive shortage of mental health professionals available to meet the population's mental health needs and a consensus among professionals regarding the importance of empowering people to use art interventions within the community settings where they are needed.

Because of the prohibitive cost of training overseas, there are only a small number of qualified Arts Therapists in South Africa. The only Master's-level programs are in Music Therapy, at the University of Pretoria, and Drama Therapy, at Wits University. Initiatives are currently underway to implement an Art Therapy training program in South Africa.

Addressing Sustainability

The inclusion of social entrepreneurial and social action training modules ensures the promotion of an active citizenship, empowering students with proposal writing skills and research methods so that they may develop visions and missions that move away from personal gain to "constructing a future through innovation and action" (Ludema & Fry, 2008, p. 295). This also enables students and CACs to create their own sustainable employment opportunities. In an effort to make this training accessible beyond the immediate vicinity of Johannesburg, Lefika has decentralized its organization through "training the trainers." The trainers comprise a group of 15 senior Community Art Counsellors with extensive experience and an intensive training process to train future CACs, continuing this work within and outside of Lefika. Some of these trainers have been with Lefika for nearly two decades, as facilitators and employees.

Significantly, one of the pioneer CACs has succeeded me as Executive Director of Lefika. In a very tangible way, hierarchies have dissipated and new leadership has emerged.

Supervision

On an organizational level, Lefika is supported by an active board of directors, business mentors, and advisors; on a clinical level, support is provided by psychotherapists and psychoanalysts from the South African Psychoanalytic Confederation and the Institute of Psychoanalytic Child Psychotherapy. Ongoing experiential and academic learning opportunities are essential to engaging with the complexities of this work, including addressing a host of defenses, such as projection, as well as the enactment of transferential and counter-transferential dynamics.

Concluding Thoughts

In attempting to do challenging work, the capacity to contain the uncontainable is imperative, so as to be able to sustain the creation of a safe enough place for reflection. In that space, unprocessed, unconscious material emanating from self and other can be engaged with, in an effort to make sense of it. This work is fraught with paradox, as when things become expansive, they can cease to be containing. There are some things that can't and won't be contained, whether in words or images, or in relationships or systems. However, the space to keep thinking ethically about the complexities remains. As Bollas (2009) says, it may not all be "beautiful," but it is all "important."

Engagement has often struggled with disillusionment as I have endeavored, in my own way, to help make South Africa a more supportive, life-enhancing place in which children can grow up. The process becomes particularly difficult when socio-political structures do not share the same visions and values. My primary struggle has been that of persuading "the powers that be" of the need for more mental health services in South Africa and of the viability of Community Art Counsellors to provide some of those services. The process in which I've been engaged has historically been scrutinized by art therapy colleagues who (like I) have had the luxury of training at international institutions and who work primarily in private practice. How could I make this precious, expensive professional identity available to others, when so many art therapists invested such vast amounts of time and money in their own training? Comments included that I was "bastardizing the profession."

> ...I would argue that we do need to keep talking and we do need to keep finding new ways of enabling more people to talk, and we need to do this because otherwise the divisions within us will overwhelm us. Our world is more pluralistic and it is more hegemonized; to stand a chance of fighting the latter we have to find forms of creative connection across the boundaries of race, class, gender, culture and other differences.
>
> *Hoggett, 2006, p. 14*

Was I breaching my ethical responsibility as a newly trained professional? What do you think?

REFLECTIVE ART EXPERIENCES & DISCUSSION QUESTIONS

1. Create an image (or choose an existing image/object) that represents a time when you felt you belonged. Create a parallel image (or choose an existing image/object) that represents a time when you felt excluded. Share your thoughts about these experiences with someone or journal about them.
2. Facilitate the creation of a mural within the context in which you are working, involving the beneficiaries in determining what they would like to communicate, to whom, and how.
3. What are some of the risks and the benefits of inclusivity within the Art Therapy profession?
4. How can you expand your practice, ethically, to address some of the social and economic injustices in your community?

References

Berman, H. (2011). The development and practice of art therapy as "community art counseling" in South Africa. *ATOL: Art Therapy Online*, 1(3).

Berman, H. (2012). To liberate the life-force in a traumatised South Africa. Unpublished doctoral dissertation. The University of Western England, Bristol, UK.

Berman, H. (2016). *Body of work*. Working Body of Knowledge Series, vol. 1. Johannesburg, South Africa: Lefika Publications.

Bollas, C. (2009). *The infinite question*. London: Routledge.

Falanga, G. (2016, September 5). Hillbrow has highest murder rate in Gauteng, stats show. Retrieved from www.security.co.za/news/33356

Fonagy, P., & Higgitt, A. (2007). The early social and emotional determinants of inequalities in health. In G. Baruch, P. Fonagy, & D. Robins (Eds.), *Reaching the hard to reach* (pp. 3–34). Chichester: John Wiley & Sons.

Hoggett, P. (2006). Connecting, arguing, fighting. *Psychoanalysis, Culture & Society*, 11, 1–16.

Ludema, J.D., & Fry, R.E. (2008). The practice of appreciative inquiry. In H. Bradbury & P. Reason (Eds.), *Sage handbook of action research, participative inquiry, and practice* (pp. 280–296). London: Sage.

Winnicott, D.W. (1965). *The maturational processes and the facilitating environment*. London: Hogarth Press.

10

TRANSLATION OF THE THERAPEUTIC LANGUAGE

Can One Teach or Practice Art Therapy Ethically Without Considering Culture?

Sojung Park

Ethical choices in our practice are based upon the principles, values, cultures, and interests of those involved. When these domains conflict, due to their diverse nature, ethical dilemmas arise. Culture—with its beliefs, customs, and loyalties—is inseparable from ethical practice because one's perspectives and decisions are based upon the way one lives in the world, as shaped by the society to which one belongs. However, society is not a fixed organism, but fluid and changeable. Accordingly, the context of our culture can shift, depending upon the ground on which we are stepping, and this affects the ethical decision-making process.

I experienced a cultural shift when I returned to Korea from the United States. Despite being a native Korean, I soon realized that the decade I'd spent training, practicing, and lecturing as an art therapist in the US had colored the cultural perspectives I had when I left Korea. Teaching at a graduate program in arts psychotherapy in Seoul has challenged me to bridge the cultures of East and West through the application of art therapy. Based upon this experience, I will present some of the important concepts that one should be aware of when either implementing art psychotherapy in Korea or teaching art therapy to students from Korea. I will also share ethical dilemmas that are frequently raised by my students due, primarily, to viewing therapy from a cultural perspective that is grounded in Confucianism and collectivism and to concepts of emotion that I regard as being uniquely Korean.

Confucianism and Collectivism: The Cultural Fundamentals of Korea

While the term individualism is often used to describe the culture of the US, Confucianism and collectivism characterize the culture of Korea; similar perspectives are shared by other East Asian countries such as China and Japan. Although Confucianism might no longer be practiced actively in Korea, its core values of loyalty (to the king) and filial piety still characterize its culture. A key component is a hierarchical structure often governed by age or position, with the person on a lower level expected to show respect to those on higher levels. This dynamic applies to virtually any relationship, including that of student and instructor.

One of the questions I frequently receive from my fellow art therapists who teach at a graduate program in the US is, "I have a Korean student in my class and she won't speak! Is there something wrong with her?" From a Western perspective, the student may, indeed, seem distant or reserved, and teachers often look for a reason behind the quietness. Yet, this is a classic example of how both Confucianism and collectivism shape one's demeanor in a group setting such as a classroom. Barring the existence of a language barrier, the quietness should be considered, first, as a way of showing respect to the teacher. A book that might interest readers in this regard is Cain's *Quiet: The Power of Introverts in a World That Can't Stop Talking* (2012). Furthermore, drawing attention to oneself by expressing one's own thoughts is also contrary to the values of Korea's collectivist culture, which prioritizes the group's harmony over individual needs.

Cultural differences underlie some of the difficulties experienced by the students from Korea, as well. For instance, the students often feel hesitant to call teachers by their first names or to raise their hands during class, as it is against their cultural practice. Since the teacher–student relationship in Korea is formal and fairly vertical, the relatively horizontal relationship in Western culture can be foreign to the students; from their perspective, asking questions of, or expressing opinions to, the teacher could be interpreted as "disrespectful" or as challenging the authority of the teacher. Accordingly, a common phenomenon with a group of Korean students is the lack of questions or interaction in class. Even if they have specific questions on their minds, students are likely to stay silent during class, choosing instead to approach the instructor individually, after class, as a way of showing respect.

This cultural presence may also be reflected in the art-making process. Traditionally, nature and its surroundings were the main features of Korean art (as seen in *sumukhwa* or folk paintings), rather than the artist's direct representation of self or expression of personal feelings. Accordingly, the frequent encouragement (and, usually, requirement) to create art about oneself during class may be unfamiliar to Korean students, in comparison with students from the West. However, I have found that the opportunity to make art about oneself is a wonderful way for Korean students to learn and to practice the different view of the self in the West, though the transition may take time and require understanding on the part of their teachers.

The relationship between teacher and students can certainly parallel that between therapist and clients in Korea. As the dynamics in the classroom show, Koreans often feel uncomfortable addressing individual goals and desires in groups, due to their cultural values. Accordingly, students or clients with a similar Eastern background must be approached differently from students or clients who have a Western perspective. Without this awareness, a Western-trained teacher or therapist might prematurely regard the individual or group as repressed or even resistive. Understanding the cultural context within which an individual lives is, therefore, crucial for any teaching or therapy to be effective; not to do so would not just be uninformed practice, it would be unethical practice.

Concepts That Are Unique to Koreans and Impact Their Sense of Boundaries

In order to understand the cultural contexts of Koreans, one must understand some Korean emotional concepts that cannot be translated into English, such as *jeong, jip-an, and chae-myun*. Sun and Bitter (2012) regard them as key to understanding how to apply psychotherapeutic concepts within the context of Korean culture; in fact, they maintain that, without grasping these important Korean concepts, conducting Western-based therapy with Korean clients would be likely to fail. Implementing the concepts can be quite challenging, however, creating ethical dilemmas for therapists, due to the collectivistic nature of the concepts. The tension between these Korean cultural concepts and the Western concepts of individual boundaries and the therapeutic boundary are explored using questions frequently raised by the students.

Jeong (**"care for others"**). The concept of *jeong* can be summarized as "a heart to care for others." *Jeong* is deeply rooted in collectivism and supports the cultural perspective of "*we*, rather than *I*." Korean society encourages one to extend *jeong* to others, and an individual with *jeong* is usually considered positively, as a person with a warm heart. This cultural practice is naturally reflected in the sense of group boundary that Koreans share. When Korean students in art therapy classes confront the importance placed upon therapeutic boundaries, ethical dilemmas arise for them, as drawing a line between therapist and client seems to contradict the concept of *jeong*. As shown in the following example, the conflict is heightened by the fact that Korean art therapy students often consider themselves to be persons with a lot of *jeong*, due to the nurturing nature of the field.

> **Why can't I feed my young clients when they come to the session hungry?**
> *I run art therapy groups in the afternoon, and my young, elementary school clients have to come to the sessions directly after school, so they are hungry by the time they arrive. I provide snacks for them, so they can eat something before the session. Isn't it better to feed them, so they can focus during the session?*

This type of question is quite common when discussing ethical issues in class. Tension is certainly present between the concept of *jeong*, as expressed in the student wanting to feed a hungry client, and the traditional approach to the drawing of therapeutic boundaries. This illustrates the confusion that arises when a professional sense of boundary becomes intertwined with the cultural emotion of *jeong*; "ignoring" a hungry child is not an act of *jeong*. Learning the importance of therapeutic boundaries can take time and practice for all developing therapists, but, due to this important facet of their cultural background, Korean students often face an extra challenge in this process: to find a balance between their professional identity and maintaining *jeong* as Koreans.

What interests me is that the students often mistake the setting up of a therapeutic boundary for giving up *jeong* in the sessions. Therefore, the most crucial part of addressing this ethical dilemma for Korean students is to acknowledge their fear of losing *jeong* if they draw a therapeutic line. This fear is usually much greater than someone from a Western culture might think, as setting up a therapeutic boundary is frequently followed by guilt, as it can be felt as a refusal to take care of the clients. Moreover, the idea of a therapist who doesn't have *jeong* contradicts the students' very perception of a therapist because, from a Korean perspective, a person who helps others must have *jeong*. Thus, the students may feel even more perplexed about their professional identity and their roles as therapists.

I usually begin to address this complex issue by acknowledging the importance of *jeong* in Korean society and by emphasizing that, in fact, *jeong* is present in therapy in Korea—but from a therapeutic perspective. I assure the students that setting up a therapeutic boundary is not dismissing *jeong* from the session, but including it more therapeutically. Teaching the students to develop the ability to see *jeong* in the session is crucial and I do so by elaborating upon the impact of *jeong* in therapy. With regard to the anecdote, above, I remind them that it is the responsibility of the parent or guardian to feed the child, so that the child doesn't come to the session with an empty stomach. Therefore, if the students continue to do the parent's job because they feel bad for the child, they are taking away from the parents the opportunity to take care of their own child. In many cases, the therapy for the children can begin by educating the parents of their responsibility to the child, in order to have the child fully participate in the session. Moreover, the young clients also need to have a clear understanding of the therapeutic space, as well as the role of a therapist, so as not to confuse the therapist with their main caregiver, who feeds, houses, and clothes them. Clarifying the role of a therapist and helping students to think, from a therapeutic perspective, about the consequences of physically nurturing the children has been helpful in defining the position of *jeong* within the professional boundary of therapy.

Jip-an ("within the house") and Chae-myun ("face-saving"). The Korean word, *jip-an,* which literally means "within the house," draws a clear boundary around the blood-related family. *Chae-myun,* which can be translated as "face saving," has to do with the shame experienced by Koreans when their problems are known outside of their group. Accordingly, *jip-an* aims to keep private matters within the household, in order to maintain *chae-myun.* Kim and Ryu (2005, p. 352) explain:

> Korean families have a clear boundary as to who is "in" and who is "out"… [The term *jip-an*] identifies both family memberships, values, and traditions practiced within a particular family…this boundary also determines what information needs to be kept *jip-an* and what can be shared…Koreans attach shame to such a wide range of problems that they are highly selective about what is revealed.

Notwithstanding, the psychological concept of *jip-an* can extend to the various groups to which one belongs in modern society, such as friends, coworkers, and fellow students, enabling Koreans to select the group with whom they wish to share which of their private issues. Because of this, many Koreans are reluctant to see a professional therapist, which creates another ethical issue for therapists in Korea.

Why can't I accept a friend's child as a client?

My friend has a son who seems to have Attention Deficit Hyperactivity Disorder. She doesn't want to take him to a psychiatrist since she doesn't want a rumor to go around, so asked me to give him art therapy, instead. If I say no to her, she will get upset and probably won't get him treated at all. Isn't it better for me to see him than to not have him receive any treatment?

Issues regarding dual relationships are also common among students in Korea. Though the students may be aware of the danger of dual relationships in therapy, it is challenging to draw a therapeutic boundary that would exclude someone within their psychological circle of *jip-an,* such as close friends, as in this case. Furthermore, the concept of *jip-an* also defines the groups of people whom an individual is required to treat with *jeong.* As in other East Asian countries, people are discouraged from discussing their problems with those who are outside their household—especially strangers, even if they are professional therapists. Instead, people often choose someone with whom they are connected to talk with, since they would rather keep their issues "in the house" and share them only with those whom they consider to be, in a sense, part of their extended family. Because of the culture of *jeong,* Koreans usually expect their friends to take care of their children. Likewise, it is not easy for Korean therapists to turn down a friend who is having an issue with his or her child.

Whenever a similar question arises in class, I encourage students to consider what saying "no" would mean to them and to their friend; usually, this would be regarded as a rejection of those who need help, or *jeong.* I then ask the students to explore the meaning of the therapeutic boundary and to question the consequences of its absence; this usually leads to a discussion of one's professional identity as a therapist. I further add that it is also our job to educate the public (starting with the people in our own groups) about the issue of dual relationships and, in this case, to offer to refer the child to a legitimate therapist who would have a more objective perspective.

MY ETHICAL DILEMMA

Does a gift policy also need translation according to culture?

One day, a client brought me a small amount of food that she had made at home. When I was in the US, I had practiced a "no gifts" policy, with some reasonable exceptions such as an appropriate present at termination. Understanding that it is common for Koreans to share their food with others as a way of sharing their *jeong,* I wondered whether this would constitute a "reasonable exception."

How would you respond?

For the writer's response, see Appendix B, page 427.

Translation of the Therapeutic Language

In regard to the Korean culture, Sun and Bitter (2012) advise that "there is no therapy that can effectively proceed without *jeong*, and any therapy that fails to protect against a loss of *chae-myun* is doomed" (p. 242). What this guidance implies is that a therapist must enter the culture of a client for therapy to be effective. How therapeutic can our work be if we don't include ourselves within the cultural norms of our clients, but insist upon forcing our own cultural perspectives upon our clients, including the cultural norms of therapy?

One of the biggest challenges about my adjustment to Korea as a professional art therapist was to translate the therapeutic language—which was based upon a Western perspective—into a language that would reflect the Korean value system and thinking pattern. Ultimately, the process of translating the therapeutic language was to change my attitude from the concept of *I* to the concept of *we* in therapy and to ensure that the lens through which I viewed my clients in Korea reflected the appropriate perspective. After all, how communicative can we be if we speak a language that is different from that of the client?

The importance of maintaining one's professional identity is crucial in making this transition. Consequently, the real challenge in this process is to find a balance between one's professional identity and one's cultural flexibility. This task certainly cannot be achieved without having a solid foundation in the field, since the ethical principles of the profession and a clear understanding of the art therapist's role become the guidelines within which to integrate multicultural issues in therapy. Therefore, when encountering multicultural ethical dilemmas, our first step may be rather simple—to return to the core values and beliefs of the field of art therapy and to clarify our position as art therapists within the context of the culture of our clients.

REFLECTIVE ART EXPERIENCES & DISCUSSION QUESTIONS

1. Create a symbolic image of collectivism and a symbolic image of individualism. How are they different and what do they have in common?
2. Create an image of your culture. (Keep in mind that the image will be reconstructed to form your next piece of artwork.) Once finished, take a photo of the art. Next, cut the completed artwork into pieces and create a collage that has a new (perhaps abstract) shape, using any additional art materials you choose. Share your experience in translating the image into another piece of artwork (e.g., determining what to keep, what to let go of, what to negotiate) and discuss how you can relate this process to the cultural translation of the therapeutic language.
3. What are the characteristics of your cultural background and how do they impact your ethical standards as a therapist?
4. What tips would you give a therapist from another country who will be working with a client of your culture?

References

Cain, S. (2012). *Quiet: The power of introverts in a world that can't stop talking.* New York: Broadway Paperbacks.

Kim, B.C., & Ryu, E. (2005). Korean families. In M. McGoldrick, J. Giordano, & N. Garcia-Preto (Eds.), *Ethnicity and family therapy* (3rd ed.) (pp. 349–362). New York: Guilford.

Sun, S., & Bitter, J.B. (2012). From China to South Korea: Two perspectives on individual psychology in Asia. *The Journal of Individual Psychology*, 68(3), 233–248.

11

WALKING A NEW PATH

Ethical Considerations in Indigenizing Art Therapy in Canada

Jennifer Vivian

I am an Inuk art therapist who lives and works in Canada. It took me a long time to be able to say that, to get comfortable identifying myself as Inuk, with my blue eyes and blonde hair. My grandmother was Inuk from Labrador. Like many Indigenous people in Canada, she lost her status in the eyes of the Canadian government as soon as she left the reserve. The loss of status meant the loss of treaty rights and benefits. My father fought for over a decade to have his status, and that of his daughters, recognized. Given my appearance and the fact that I grew up outside of my ancestral territory, describing myself as Inuk can open up a wide variety of dialogues, depending upon whom I am talking with and what we are discussing. This is true in my art therapy practice, as well. I am very aware of the privilege that comes with having fair skin and I am cognizant of the fact that I did not grow up with the oppression and systemic racism that affect many, if not all, Indigenous peoples, including members of my family.

After much deliberation, I have come to the realization that I need to be mindful of identifying as an Inuk person in all areas of my life—independent of what may be gained, or lost, as a result. The privilege of deciding who gets to know that I am Inuk does not mean that I feel that I have to disclose my status to every person I meet. However, it does mean that I feel a duty to speak up up when I see evidence of discrimination towards Indigenous peoples. Due to my appearance, I am privy to comments made by non-Indigenous workers when they think that no Indigenous person is around. When this occurs, I feel an ethical responsibility to challenge these kinds of statements and, whenever possible, to educate. My identification as an Inuk practitioner does not make me an authority on working with the more than 600 recognized Indigenous Nations in Canada. Being Inuk is simply part of who I am and influences how I practice. It is important for me to have shared this with you as I describe some of the ethical dilemmas that I have encountered so far in my work with Indigenous people.

Starting to Search: Ethical Issues in Research

For the final project of my Master's degree in Art Therapy, I wanted to honor traditional Indigenous teachings. I longed to create a new model of art therapy based upon Indigenous healing philosophies, but I was filled with questions. Was I *allowed* to write about this? Who was *I* to be taking this on? How could I gain access to this material? How could a paper that required Western research "validity" honor oral traditions and lessons? How would I ensure that I was not attempting to present myself as an expert on the subject? How would my research be different, and honor, rather than exploit, Indigenous people?

To satisfy graduate school requirements, I needed to base my paper upon published texts, but the research process also became a first step in excavating the knowledge and awareness of Indigenous history that would shape who I am, as well as how I approach to art therapy. I read as much as I could to educate myself about the legacy of residential schools upon Indigenous communities. I tried to honor Indigenous ways of knowing. I acknowledged the paper's limited scope (e.g., that it did not include adequate information about oral traditions and customs; that the model I presented was offered as a point of departure for further research). The result was *Full Circle: Toward an Aboriginal Model of Art Therapy* (Vivian, 2013), which I'll discuss later.

Seeking to Serve: Ethical Considerations in the Job Search

After I completed my graduate degree, I had a strong sense of wanting to give back to the Indigenous community. My choices presented an exercise in ethical decision making. If I sought employment within an Indigenous community in Northern Canada, I would have to consider what that would mean. How long was I prepared to work up North? Who was asking me to come (who was the employer)? Would I be going only for personal and professional gain? What could I offer the community? Did the community want and/or need what I was offering? Who was *I* to offer to "help" that community? If I were truly going to truly commit myself to offering my services to an Indigenous community, it would have to be at the invitation of the community, itself, and for the long term. Since I was not in a position to work for more than a year up North, instead I applied to work at a shelter for Indigenous women in a Canadian city. I have heard fellow Indigenous practitioners say that their communities should not be approached by non-Indigenous practitioners. Currently, non-Indigenous people are going into communities whether they are invited or not. I believe that it is the responsibility of these individuals to ensure that they have had training in cultural competency specific to the community in which they will live and work and to continuously seek out knowledge about, and honor the traditions of, that specific community.

When I settled near the Indigenous community which I live close to now, I knew that I wanted to get involved and to offer my services as an art therapist, but how would I approach the community in a way that was respectful and would not be self-serving? What was my intent in wanting to work there? What were my biases and presumptions? When I decided to prepare a proposal for an art therapy program at the local Indigenous school, I had to be prepared for the justifiable skepticism that I might encounter. I had to check my ego at the door and be sure that I was practicing not from a place of authority, but from the heart. I had to present my skill as an art therapist as an offering to the community. I had to be willing to prove myself over and over again, without taking it personally; understanding why things were this way. I did my best to let the community know that I was trying to educate myself, that I practice art therapy from an Indigenous lens as outlined in my proposed model; that I am Inuk (a different group of Indigenous people than they) but that I didn't think that, because I am Inuk, I understand what their people have experienced. Slowly, I began to build relationships and friendships.

Full Circle in Practice: An Aboriginal Model of Art Therapy

Full Circle: Toward An Aboriginal Model of Art Therapy (Vivian, 2013) has four central tenets:

1. *The natural world:* Developing a relationship with nature through the use of natural materials and being out-of-doors, in order to enhance a sense of groundedness that may lead to spiritual curiosity.
2. *Interconnectedness:* Increasing one's understanding of the connectedness of every living thing might facilitate insight into the client's role in relationships and the affects of his or her actions; exploring the concept of *that which serves to damage* and *that which serves to heal.*
3. *Art making:* Extending art making beyond the therapeutic space by integrating it into everyday life, thus allowing it to serve as a visual and symbolic representation of the endless journey of healing, with periods of reflection and recognition of imbalances and new growth. Art making may be done individually, with family, friends, or within a community.
4. *Balance:* Endeavoring to achieve balance among the following four realms, through the art activities noted:
   - *Emotional*—Providing for creative expression and intuitive art making; allowing the client to express, regulate, process, and understand emotions.
   - *Physical*—Exploring materials and techniques, kinesthetic art making, using natural materials.
   - *Spiritual*—Enabling the client to undertake a journey to seek his or her spirit; allowing for regeneration of spirit; regarding art as a spiritual practice; strengthening connections with ancestors and with nature.
   - *Mental*—Encouraging symbolic representation; allowing for an expulsion of energy or catharsis; providing a space for non-linear communication and opportunities to increase mindfulness, self-esteem, and self-discovery.

In my work I try to honor the seven sacred teachings: love, respect, honesty, courage, wisdom, humility, and truth; qualities that help to guide my ethical decision-making process. My role is that of accompanying the client on his or her healing journey. I do not represent myself as a traditional healer, Medicine person, or shaman. I do not attempt to provide my clients with traditional Indigenous healing techniques, but refer them to culturally appropriate resources.

Ethical Dilemmas in Practice

Although, like most people, I am trying to make a living doing what I love, I have to ask myself on a regular basis why I am doing something and who is benefitting. Being mindful of the exploitation and continued colonization practices that exist in Canada and elsewhere, I aim not to profit from the use of case material concerning people with whom I work, but, rather, to try to contribute to the overall dialogue about healing and reconciliation among the people of Turtle Island (North America).

MY ETHICAL DILEMMA

Teachable moments: How and when should I speak up?

My first post-graduate year, I took a job working at a shelter for Indigenous people in a large urban area. I was not employed as an art therapist, although I sought to use art therapy whenever I could and was able to do some art therapy in groups and with individuals (mostly children). One day I accompanied a family to a hospital so that one of the children could be seen by a doctor. My role was to help look after the other children while the child was receiving health care services. After waiting a long while, the children and I stood in the hallway while the parent asked questions at the nursing station. When the nurse saw me behind the parent, she came over and started to give me the answers, instead of responding to the parent.

How would you respond?

For the writer's response, see Appendix B, page 439.

MY ETHICAL DILEMMA

The many meanings of love: Is our response to the term "love" culturally considerate?

I was working with a young Indigenous child who had been through a recent trauma. It had been difficult for the child to finish the session and I had been working to develop a closing routine that would enable him to complete his artistic expression and leave the room feeling satisfied. In his final piece, the child clearly expressed the word "love" towards me. How should I handle this?

How would you respond?

For the writer's response, see Appendix B, page 439.

MY ETHICAL DILEMMA

The role of honesty in building the therapeutic alliance: How much would you share with your client?

A teenager with whom I was working asked me many questions about my own personal experience of art making for mental health. Having been trained psychodynamically, each time one of these questions arose, I would feel caught off guard. What would be the most appropriate way of handling this within my Indigenous framework, in keeping with the sacred teaching of honesty? The same teenager would frequently ask me to make art in session. What would it mean to make art alongside this person?

How would you respond?

For the writer's response, see Appendix B, page 440.

Moving Forward on the Path

As a first step, I suggest getting to know the history of the Indigenous peoples in your area. Using art, you can explore your own biases, curiosity, and questions about the Indigenous peoples near you, as well as what your own qualities of love, respect, honesty, courage, wisdom, humility, and truth mean to you. You can begin to build relationships with local Indigenous people and ask them about what you can do to help. Members of national and international art therapy organizations could create Indigenous working groups, to move the art therapy profession along the path to truth and reconciliation—not just in Canada, but across the globe. Educators and legislators could lobby for the inclusion of Indigenous history, values, and teachings in the curriculum of educational institutions, so that Indigenous students who live on and off reserve can see themselves reflected in what is being taught and, thereby, feel that their life experiences and those of their ancestors are valued. When this happens, we might see an increase in Indigenous practitioners working within their communities. I hope that this chapter has given you a starting point from which to consider the importance of Indigenizing art therapy. I write it not from a position of authority, but as an offering from one who is sharing what she is learning on her own path.

REFLECTIVE ART EXPERIENCES & DISCUSSION QUESTIONS

1. Create artwork that examines how your culture and sense of identity affect your practice as an art therapist.

2. Create artwork that examines privilege that you have experienced, or privilege that you have observed, in your art therapy practice.
3. Describe a moment when you could have acted as an advocate for a client but did not. Explore what stopped you.
4. Have you developed relationships with your nearest Indigenous community? Explore why you have/have not and how/why you might go about creating these relationships.

References

Vivian, J. (2013). *Full circle: Toward an Aboriginal model of art therapy*. Unpublished master's thesis. Concordia University, Montreal, Quebec, Canada. Retrieved from www.spectrum.library. concordia.ca/977982/

Confidentiality

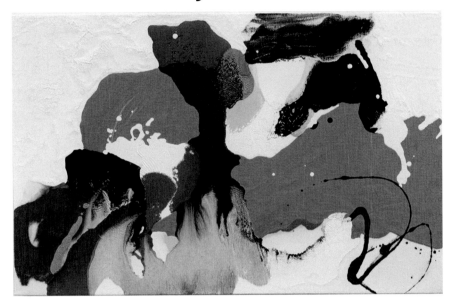

Sarah Vollman *(see color insert)*

12

A PART OF, YET SEPARATE

Ethical Issues Arising in Art Therapy with Combat Service Members and Their Families

Paula Howie

In his 1925 poem entitled "The Hollow Men," T.S. Eliot declares that there is "a shadow" that falls "Between the idea and the reality … Between the conception and the creation," as though this shadow might interfere with the implementation of ideas or with innovation (Eliot, 2014). As we consider ethical issues, however, perhaps it is helpful to linger on *the thought* before implementing an *action*; inaction may be the best course of action until we can decide upon a strategy and make a judgment as to how to proceed. Hesitation can give rise to thoughtfulness, rather than inertia, and provide those of us who work in health care with time to imagine creative alternatives to the course of action that initially came to mind. Interestingly, in Jungian theory, the shadow is described both as a dark, unknown side of the personality and as the place of projection and creativity (Jung, 1968).

Having worked in a military setting for nearly three decades, I have chosen to present in this chapter some of the ethical issues that may arise in treating combat veterans who have been diagnosed with major psychiatric disorders, including post-traumatic stress disorder (PTSD), and to highlight the importance of dealing with one's countertransference regarding the expectations of the setting, be it inpatient or outpatient.

When Ethical Principles Are Violated

In 2014, the Executive Director and the Ethics Chair of the American Psychological Association (APA), among other professional staff, resigned after being implicated for assisting in the use of torture on military detainees as part of the wars in Iraq and Afghanistan and with detainees at Guantanamo Bay (Ackerman, 2015). A report stated that APA leaders "colluded" with the US Department of Defense (DoD) and aided the Central Intelligence Agency (CIA) in loosening professional ethics and other guidelines to permit the participation of psychologists in torture, such as waterboarding and other atrocities perpetrated upon prisoners of war (POW's). How did this happen? How could anyone who was a member of such a highly regarded profession be caught in such a conflict of interest? How could so many people in the executive suite have known about this and condoned it?

Few people probably set out to violate ethical principles. As a matter of fact, some psychologists involved in the torture had asked their supervisors and the APA for guidance, because they thought that their treatment of detainees might be both unethical and inhumane. Even though some of these psychologists were civilians (we will see that military members are even more hamstrung in their choices), the report cites that these civilian psychologists did not want to jeopardize their employment or their pay. Of the 600 psychologists in the military, about two thirds are civilians. The DoD is a major employer of psychologists, who number about 7% of the APA. According to reports, these psychologists felt that they had few alternatives in defying this system; some believed that their presence might deter even rougher handling of prisoners by the interrogators. Whatever their rationales, it is apparent that the influence of the DoD, along with pressure from superiors and a lack of guidance from the APA, presented a perfect storm for abuses to occur (Ackerman, 2015)

Our ethics standards first derived from situations such as this. From 1932 to the 1970s, in what has come to be known as the Tuskegee experiment, black men, without their knowledge, were first infected with syphilis and then denied treatment for it, in order for clinicians to observe the course of the disease. During the Holocaust, German physicians experimented upon members of specific ethnic groups, Jews, gypsies, and others who were not part of the Aryan race. Although it would be easy to label as evil all who are involved in acts such as these, some of them—like some of the psychologists described above—might have gotten caught up in listening to those around them, rather than listening to and trusting in their own knowledge of what is right and wrong and what is good and bad practice.

Military-Specific Ethical Issues

In the landmark case *US v Levy* (1967), Dr. Levy, a dermatologist who was drafted during the Vietnam war, refused to obey a direct order to teach Special Forces Aidmen (medics), because they were being trained for combat roles and he asserted that "this eroded the distinction between combatants and noncombatants" (Pelegrino, Hartle, & Howe, 2004, p. 304). This situation placed Dr. Levy in an ethical bind because, as a physician, not only must he act ethically, but also he must anticipate that those whom he teaches will act ethically. He argued that the political use of medicine by Special Forces "jeopardized the entire noncombatant status of medicine" (Pelegrino et al., 2004, p. 304). Levy was court-martialed and sentenced to three years in military prison. This case set the precedent that a physician was a soldier first and the military organization would define for the military physician what was ethical and what was not (Pelegrino et al., 2004). The inequity between personal or discipline-specific ethical standards and military ethical standards is even more pronounced during wartime, when the line between soldier and physician becomes even more amorphous.

Although the uniform code of military justice and international law make it clear that the soldier must obey a "lawful command of his superior officer" (Pelegrino et al., 2004, p. 304), what one person considers lawful may be what someone else thinks is illegal.

Art Therapy in Military Settings

All art therapists currently working in military settings are civilians, because a military specialty for art therapy does not yet exist; this may change in the future. We need to keep in mind that being civilians in a military setting did little to insulate the psychologists caught up in the torture of prisoners. We must be ever vigilant and aware that we are working in a system with its own mores, rules, and culture (Howie, Prasad, & Kristel, 2013), some of which may conflict with our personal values and professional ethics. According to military ethicists (Pelegrino et al., 2004), the only reasons for denying soldiers the same ethical rights that they would have as civilians are the needs of the military mission as related to combat and to national security. Decisions concerning national security and combat readiness can be complex, though, and subject to interpretation.

Ethical Issues Confronted by Art Therapists in Military Settings

Providing a Safe Place

One of the basic tenets of therapy is the importance of providing clients with a sense of security, not only in the treatment setting and within the therapeutic relationship, but also in the belief that, except in certain carefully prescribed circumstances, confidentiality will be maintained. One of the most pervasive and detrimental ethical issues I have confronted in military settings is the difficulty in providing soldiers with such a space. Because we were part of the military system, we could not assure the soldier of complete confidentiality regarding what was said or what was conveyed by the artwork produced in therapy. As members of a treatment team, we were advised to tell clients that all members of the team had input into their problems, as all had the potential to help. In the art room, clients tended to become more relaxed and off guard while working with materials and would say things to us (civilian women) that might not be disclosed elsewhere, such as fear of injury or death, guilt over war crimes, and sexual preferences. It was incumbent upon the art therapist not only to remind soldiers of the limits of confidentiality, but also to maintain boundaries regarding some of the information disclosed (the Army's policy of "don't ask, don't tell" was in place during part of my tenure). Too much complacency on our part could work to the patient's detriment. We were a part of the military structure and, given that knowledge, the client could share what he or she chose to share.

We also sought to provide safety by setting up a culture of listening, of hearing one another's issues, of making space for each other, so that each person could feel protected and emotionally supported. This was necessary in order to enable patients not only to feel vulnerable during session, but also to feel powerful and self-directed, an especially important task for military personnel. Each soldier was encouraged to grow through acknowledging both strengths and limitations; the healthy aspects of the individual were focused upon and nurtured. Soldiers were encouraged to turn their focus inward for a short time, upon the subjective inner processes that served as emotional indicators for them, an experience that was especially difficult for trauma survivors (such as those with PTSD) who had learned to use avoidance and negation of the self as survival strategies. At the end of each session, clients were encouraged to evaluate their own experience. Providing a therapeutic space in which to process trauma within a context that was healing rather than re-traumatizing was a constant struggle, but I think we usually were able to keep the system away from the therapeutic work enough to allow soldiers to feel as though they could truly express themselves. In the final analysis, though, we—like all the other health care workers in military settings—were part of that system.

The Unintended Consequences of Doing our Job

As an art therapist, I may perceive something in a soldier's artwork that he or she does not want to impart verbally or might not be aware of because it is still contained within the realm of the preconscious. If, for example, I go on to discuss with the treatment team the latent suicidal ideation I've perceived in a client's artwork, this may impact the team's opinion as to that individual's combat readiness. If I then write these findings in the soldier's chart and the physician is ordered to release records to the soldier's commander, this could constitute a breach of confidentiality. A soldier's hospital stay may lower his or her security clearance, which might be a prerequisite for their job.

Howe (Pelegrino et al., 2004, pp. 348, 350) recommends being somewhat vague in writing chart notes; he even advocates leaving out some of the specifics of discussion with a patient if including them would be detrimental to the patient and not detrimental to the Army. We must realize that the notes we write about our patients and what we say about them at team meetings can have an impact upon whether those individuals remain in the military or are discharged from it. The art therapist must endeavor, to the best of his or her ability, to follow the principle of placing the patient's interest first, as would civilian medical professionals.

Conflicting Needs and Wishes

In the military, mental health diagnoses are some of the most highly compensated illnesses a soldier can have, compensated at a rate comparable to the loss of a limb. This can lead to a variety of scenarios: a soldier may want to be given a mental health diagnosis, in the hope of being medically retired from the military; a soldier might not want to return to a duty station but be deemed fit for duty; a soldier might want to return to active duty but might not be able, psychologically, to do so; a soldier who is determined to be unfit for duty might be so devastated by the loss of his military career that he becomes a high risk for suicidal behavior. These are issues we dealt with daily and discussed in treatment team meetings, although the physician had the final say about the disposition of the soldier.

Personal Responses to Working with Military Personnel and Their Families

Witnessing the physical, psychological, and cognitive injuries sustained by patients during combat can be traumatizing for health care workers, as can the stories of atrocities committed in battle. Ethical issues can arise from a conflict between the mission of the military and one's own feelings about war, military discipline, and the military culture. Supervision, a strong identity with a professional team, and a commitment to self-care may help ameliorate these disconnects.

Treating family members of soldiers can be challenging. Often, the people we saw were married to soldiers whose behavior was of interest to their command structure. The command would want to know if there was child or spousal abuse, which had to be reported anyway. However, there were times when unusual behavior was not reported. Howe (Pelegrino et al., 2004) encourages us to consider whether this behavior interferes with combat readiness or national security; if so, it should be reported. He gives an example of a therapist who saw the spouse of a general who was, by his wife's report, a serious alcoholic. The therapist decided not to report this as it was told in confidence and would have hurt the patient. On the other hand, one could assert that this was something that the mission needed to know, since someone of so high a rank might, at some point, be in charge of many troops. I'm not sure if I would have opted to report this had I heard something like it in my art therapy group.

MY ETHICAL DILEMMA

Should I break confidentiality?

A service member diagnosed with dysthymia, borderline personality disorder, and chronic pain for a service-related injury, had attended a long-term outpatient art therapy group for several years. She medicated her pain with legal and illegal substances and, consequently, had been hospitalized for drug and alcohol dependence and, on several occasions, for overdosing. She often appeared lethargic and unfocused in group; on occasion, she talked about her husband not being supportive. One day she called to let me know that she would not "bother the group any longer," which sounded like a veiled threat of suicide. When I asked if she would come in to meet with me or if she would go to the emergency room on her own, she said that it was difficult to ask for help and that she intended to deal with her feelings alone, at home. After she hung up, I was concerned that she might harm herself because of her past behavior and the fact that she had guns in her home. I was also aware that any decision I made could impact both our therapeutic relationship and her career.

How would you respond?

For the writer's response, see Appendix B, page 413.

Conclusion

In the process of trying to make decisions that are ethical, our judgment may be influenced by pressure from peers, supervisors, or superiors who have the power to rate one's performance, who have input into one's pay increases, and who can affect one's continued employment. Saying "no" can be difficult, even when we feel we are right in doing so and even though everything points to this being the correct choice. During times of great stress or pressure from those around us, even the most learned among us may make faulty decisions. Paying attention to our ethical compass, knowing when to say no and when to deliberate choices, and endeavoring to understand our ethical shadow are paramount to navigating the ethical dilemmas that we, as art therapists, are likely to encounter in any workplace, including those that are peculiar to the military setting. We are unlikely to find pat answers to all our complex questions in the law or in our profession's ethics codes. We might all do well to remember Howe's observation that "Ethics is often ahead of the law" (Pelegrino, 2004, p. 345)—and ahead of the codes.

REFLECTIVE ART EXPERIENCES & DISCUSSION QUESTIONS

1. You have a referral to work with someone who is in the military. Before the individual arrives—and, then, after the session ends—make a *mandala* (i.e. a circle) on 4" × 6" paper, using pastels. Compare these *mandalas*. How has hearing about your client's experiences impacted your ability to listen empathetically, your mood, your sense of safety? Make two *mandalas* each time you meet with this person and compare them over time.
2. Describe an instance when your client's goals seemed to collide with the goals of the setting in which therapy was taking place. Given this situation, explore your role.
3. Describe a work-related action that might be legal, but unethical.

References

Ackerman, S. (2015, July 14). Three senior officials lose their jobs at APA after US torture scandal. *The Guardian*. Retrieved from www.theguardian.com/us-news/2015/jul/14/apa-senior-officials-torture-report-cia

Eliot, T.S. (2014). *Poems: 1909–1925—Primary source edition*. Charleston, SC: Nabu Press.

Howie, P., Prasad, S., & Kristel, J. (Eds.). (2013). *Using art therapy with diverse populations: Crossing cultures and abilities*. London: Jessica Kingsley.

Jung, C. (1968). *Man and his symbols*. New York: Dell.

Pelegrino, E.D., Hartle, A.E., & Howe, E.G. (Eds.). (2004). *Military medical ethics, volume 1–2*. Walter Reed Army Medical Center Borden Institute, Producer. Washington, DC: Department of the Army.

13

'BUT I AM UNDERSTANDING THAT YOU MEAN TO SAY . . .'

The Use of Language Interpreters in Art Therapy

Elaine S. Goldberg

While art therapists are trained to be aware of and sensitive to diversity of race, religion, and gender, the need to address language differences in therapy is not mentioned in the American Art Therapy Association's *Ethical Principles for Art Therapists* (2013). Given the huge influx of immigrants from other countries in recent years, the clinical importance of using language interpreters is clear, albeit challenging. Just about every aspect of treatment is affected by the introduction of a language interpreter. Done well, the use of interpreters does not just enhance the art therapy process, it makes it possible!

Background

When individuals from Spanish-speaking countries were admitted to the large public psychiatric hospital where I worked in the 1970s, they were randomly assigned to inpatient units that had few or no Spanish-speaking staff or patients. Having taken a number of conversational Spanish courses in college, I invited them to participate in art therapy sessions. The kinds of conversations that were routine in the art therapy group that I conducted in Spanish with a bi-lingual, bi-cultural co-therapist were not typical of the interactions that other staff members were having with these patients. The artwork was rich and colorful, replete with beautiful images of South and Central America: tile roofs, animals, tropical flowers, rainbows, palm trees, and people dressed in the fashion of the countryside. Usually presenting as affectively flat and depressed, the patients came to life while talking about their artwork. Using art as an approach to self-expression seemed natural for them and, through their art and their words, they were able to address the profound losses they had incurred and begin a grieving process that could support a better adjustment to their new lives in the United States. The program was so successful that it was expanded to other language groups in the patient population. There were enough like-minded therapists and other staff to lobby for the formation of a Spanish-language day treatment program; henceforth, Spanish-speaking patients were admitted to a single inpatient unit where—besides receiving therapeutic services conducted in Spanish—they could gain support from, and socialize with, each other.

Individuals who have been subjected to the trauma of war, famines, and natural disasters in their native countries often suffer enduring scars from their experiences (including long-term separations from family members), putting them at higher risk for depression, anxiety, and post-traumatic stress. While many argue that immigrants have to learn English to participate fully in life in the US, as art therapists we have a duty to provide care and support, while respecting and honoring differences in our patients' therapeutic needs and goals. An integral part of this process is the provision of language interpreters, including sign language interpreters for patients who are hearing impaired. I am now working in hospital settings that provide live interpreters, video, and telephone interpreter services with language interpreters who are skilled in dealing with medical terminology (although they are not usually familiar with issues related to mental illness or the psychotherapeutic process). To use the phone or video service, the therapist calls to request interpreter services in the particular language needed and then the patient and the clinician communicate through dual telephones or, in my case, through talking via a phone interpreter on a speaker phone.

Ethical Issues in Conducting Art Therapy Using Language Interpreters

There are uniquely client-centered, therapist-centered, and interpreter-centered problems that can make it quite challenging to provide art therapy when using interpreters. The most glaring ethical issue is that the interpreter represents a third party who is present to all that occurs in the sessions. Interpreters in the hospital setting are bound by their own code of ethics, which includes maintaining the confidentiality of all that is said in the sessions (Hernandez-Iverson, 2010; National Council on Interpreting in Health Care, 2005). I believe that it is also the art therapist's responsibility to address directly with clients boundary issues, roles, and confidentiality with respect to the use of an interpreter. Situations in which interpretations are unclear or do not reflect the sentiment of the speaker (i.e., the client or the therapist) occur all the time. By talking, at the start of treatment, about the nature of interpreter services in therapy, the art therapist is establishing a climate of openness with the client and the interpreter that allows for spontaneous clarifications and corrections, promoting a best practice model.

Client-Centered Ethical Issues

Alem

An obviously exhausted, anxious mother accompanied her five-year-old boy, Alem, to my inpatient art therapy group. Alem was nonverbal due to the ongoing effects of a severe seizure disorder, but had been fluent and bi-lingual in English and Amharic prior to his illness. Although his mother spoke Amharic, she maintained that she understood English. The treatment team spoke to her in English and she answered in single word or brief phrases. In our sessions, her limited understanding of and ability to express herself in English became apparent. Since she clearly wanted me and others to perceive her as educated and competent, suggesting the use of an interpreter risked making her feel embarrassed and humiliated. When she understood that it would allow us to speak in more depth, without compromising her privacy, she was willing to try. This enabled us to work together more closely and she began to feel comfortable enough to acknowledge aspects of her child's care that she did not fully understand. It was only after the introduction of the interpreter that I was able to grasp the extent to which Alem had lost functional skills such as speech and fine motor skills. Eventually she gave me permission to let the rest of the staff know that they also needed to request interpreter services when working with her and her child.

Patients and/or their parents are often ashamed of their limited facility in English, so they do not acknowledge their limitations. Many speak some English—"survival English"—and may understand more of what is said to them than they can articulate. However, they often miss important details of what is said to them, even with the help of interpreters. Being observant and motivated to please, patients or their family members may grasp, nonverbally, what is expected of them. In a medical setting, for example, parents may demonstrate newly acquired skills in caring for their sick children, but their questions and their emotional reactions to the situations that they are facing might not get addressed. In working with an immigrant Latino population, I have observed that parents often cannot speak English, while their children, born in the United States, might not speak Spanish. Art therapy provides an avenue of nonverbal communication that can allow access to feelings and perceptions that otherwise might go unnoticed by family members. The art therapist has the task of finding a way, through the use of interpreter services, to bridge these gaps in communication, not only between the art therapist and the clients, but within the family group.

Patients are frequently reluctant to include a language interpreter in sessions. The very presence of someone (in person or via video or phone) who is hearing and repeating all that is being said complicates the dynamics of the session. The interpreter's gender, tone of voice, style, accent, or dialect may have particular meaning for the client or the therapist, and give rise to additional transference and counter-transference issues that the therapist must be mindful of, even if the treatment approach does not focus upon transference issues. In the hospital, language interpreters always begin sessions by directly addressing the client regarding their commitment to confidentiality and to the accurate interpretation of everything that is said. The art therapist must still consider the patient's comfort. Sensitivity to the nature of the client's problems and developmental and psycho-social needs can guide the therapist in setting up sessions with an appropriate interpreter, thereby creating a therapeutic space that the client is able to experience as a reasonably safe holding environment in which to share personal information. For example, in working with adolescents who have concerns about their bodies, sexual experiences, or trauma histories, the therapist has to be sensitive to the gender of the interpreter. I was working with a 15-year-old girl who suddenly began talking about feeling embarrassed about the surgical scars on her abdomen. The telephone interpreter was male and the client, while wanting to speak, looked extremely uncomfortable. I stopped the session at that point and asked to switch to a female interpreter; the client was much more at ease in that session and those that followed.

Therapist-Centered Ethical Issues

Early in a therapy session that I was having with a Spanish-speaking family with the assistance of a telephone interpreter, I realized that I was unable to follow what the interpreter was saying as she translated into Spanish what I had just said in English. When I noticed that the patient's mother looked as puzzled as I felt, I stopped the process and offered the interpreter a simpler version of my statement to convey to the family, which worked. Since I have enough familiarity with Spanish to recognize when what I have said is not being represented in the spirit and tone that I intended, at times I have asked an interpreter to restate what I said because the translation did not convey the emotional meaning that I intended. It is really important for the art therapist to pay close attention to the client's non-verbal behavior throughout the session, especially when the therapist does not know the client's language. If the client's facial expressions, posture, breathing, or the emotional expression in the art-work, itself, do not appear to reflect what the art therapist has said, the therapist may ask what the client understood was said and then correct any misunderstandings or misinterpretations.

The art therapist also has to establish the interpreter/therapist/client boundary in the session. When skilled interpreters desire to come out of role, they typically preface what they want to say by announcing that they have a question or a comment for me or that they would like to offer the client a suggestion regarding, for example, a community resource that might be useful. I find this level of involvement enlivening and helpful.

Interpreter-Centered Ethical Issues

Language interpreters who are of the same culture or country as the client can facilitate a connection between the client and me that feels quite natural. Regional differences in language, however, can leave interpreters perplexed; in these cases, I usually ask clients if what they are saying can be conveyed in different words. Occasionally, interpreters, who typically are college educated, have reacted to apparent differences between their own cultural and/or economic level and that of the client in a manner that was inappropriate. When, following a very long statement by one client, the interpreter provided me with only a brief, general phrase, I questioned him, whereupon he acknowledged that he had edited out what he felt was extraneous or inappropriate content. I find this selective interpreting to be especially frustrating, as it defeats an important aspect of therapy—that patients are encouraged to express themselves freely—and because word choice and inflection can be extremely significant. Interpreters are just as prone to being affected by transference and counter-transference as the art therapist and the client are. When, for example, interpreters have told me that what the client just said does not makes sense, I have insisted that they interpret what was said anyway. I have found it extremely helpful to have post-session process time with interpreters and, if possible, to work with the same interpreter over time. While the relationship is not co-therapy, it requires close collaboration and mutual understanding of boundaries and roles.

Conducting therapy through language interpreters can also feel cumbersome and inefficient. Many interpreters consider it a duty to repeat every word that is said, even when the client or therapist has understood what was said and would like to further the conversation. After a teen-aged patient started to roll her eyes because the interpreter insisted upon interpreting everything, I decided to let interpreters know when something does not need interpreting. Some are fine with this, while others maintain that they must interpret every word.

Miguel

Miguel, a bright, American-born eight-year-old boy, partially paralyzed by a rare viral illness but cognitively intact, was struggling with intense anger and aggression, drawing shark-infested waters and being behaviorally aggressive (e.g., cursing hospital staff). Close by, his parents were arguing loudly, ignoring their child. Mother, who came from a rural area of Central America and had a lot of folk/superstitious beliefs, was depressed and had developed some paranoid thinking, believing that she was responsible for Miguel's illness. Despite this, she was a competent caretaker, staying at his bedside 24-hours-a-day. Father, who was from a more urban environment and had more formal education, was rarely present. Alert and impatient, he expected his son to make a full recovery, which was not only unrealistic, but fostered a great sense of frustration and failure in Miguel, who was working to become more functional in his rehabilitation therapies. Father's lack of empathy was painfully evident; ignoring the artwork that Miguel was creating, he demanded, "So, when is Miguel going to walk?"

Father had actually requested a parent session, telling me in Spanish that his wife "was crazy and needed to be committed somewhere." I explained that she was not giving any indication of being a danger to herself or others, the standard for involuntary hospitalization, and that she was appropriately supporting their son. The language interpreter in this session, who happened to be from a different Latin American country, viewed both parents as irrational and did little to hide the contempt on his face. I frequently had to insist that he tell me what was just said and demand that he interpret my response, even when he protested. Since Miguel's response to his illness was complicated by years of hearing his parents bitterly arguing, it was especially important for me to keep in check the anger that I felt towards the interpreter and to focus upon my goal for the session, which was to engage both parents in supporting their son. Subsequently, I was able to focus more on working individually with Miguel, having collateral parent sessions with mother, as needed. He left the hospital, able to drive a power wheelchair and breathe with the help of portable oxygen. We continued to meet on an outpatient basis for several years. Miguel returned to a regular classroom and has performed at a high academic level.

MY ETHICAL DILEMMA

What should I do when the interpreter is bypassed?

Using an interpreter, I was conducting a family art therapy session with Mr. and Mrs. Diaz and their lovely 10-year-old daughter Rosa, who was born with a chronic deteriorating neuro-muscular disease that causes gradual loss of muscle control and mass, eventual paralysis, and death before adulthood. Rosa has normal cognitive abilities, so is well aware of the loss of her physical functioning and independence. Though now unable to walk, she has good eye-hand coordination and enjoys art, so is well-suited to art therapy. I was working with the family to support Rosa in maintaining the best possible quality of life while dealing with feelings associated with grieving and anticipated loss.

Rosa and her father are bi-lingual in Spanish and English, but their English can be difficult to understand. Mrs. Diaz speaks only Spanish. As the session began, Rosa started drawing, while Mrs. Diaz described (through the interpreter) the problems that Rosa was having at home and at school. Mr. and Mrs. Diaz started arguing about the cause of these problems, speaking so rapidly that the interpreter was unable to interpret. When the interpreter tried to speak, Mr. Diaz and Rosa pled their cases to me in English, leaving mother out of the conversation. The interpreter worked hard to stay in role, but turned to me in frustration, not knowing what to do because the family was ignoring his requests that they speak through him.

How would you respond?

For the writer's response, see Appendix B, page 408.

Conclusion

Arranging for an interpreter when needed, advising the interpreter of what is required, and talking with clients about issues related to confidentiality, roles, and boundaries when using the services of an interpreter are ethical responsibilities of the art therapist, whether they are directly addressed by the ethics codes of our professional organizations. While, as art therapists, we have an ability to view the patient's experience as expressed through art, we must be able to communicate with clients about what we are doing and why and they must be able to question and interact with us, in order to derive the most benefit from the process. While challenges may arise in working through language interpreters in therapy, these services are still the best way in which to bridge the language barrier. Of key importance is the therapist's ability to maintain open and clear communication among all those present and, whenever possible, to process with interpreters, following the session, any language–related difficulties that arose.

Editor's note: Shortly after this chapter was written, the Art Therapy Credentials Board released its *Code of Ethics, Conduct, and Disciplinary Procedures* (2016). Both the 2016 and the 2018 revisions include the following statement:

> Art therapists shall communicate in ways that are both developmentally and culturally sensitive and appropriate. When clients and/or therapists have difficulty understanding each other's language, art therapists shall attempt to locate necessary translation/interpretation services.
>
> *Standard 1.2.5*

REFLECTIVE ART EXPERIENCES & DISCUSSION QUESTIONS

1. Create art that expresses how you feel when you believe that others do not understand or are not responding appropriately to something you have said or needed.
2. Plan an art therapy activity for a client who speaks another language. Break down the instructions into simple, step-by-step sentences that could easily be translated.
3. What would you do if, after you said something brief in English, the language interpreter went on to engage in a substantial conversation with your client?
4. A client who is depressed and verbally withdrawn asks, through an interpreter, questions about her medical care or prescribed medications that she has not shared with her physician. What would you do?

References

American Art Therapy Association (2013). *Ethical principles for art therapists*. Alexandria, VA: Author.

Art Therapy Credentials Board (2016). *Code of ethics, conduct, and disciplinary procedures*. Greensboro, NC: Author.

Hernandez-Iverson, E. (2010). *IMIA guide on medical interpreter ethical conduct*. International Medical Interpreters Association. Retrieved from: www.imiaweb.org/uploads/pages/376_2.pdf

National Council on Interpreting in Health Care (2005). National standards of practice for interpreters in health care. Retrieved from: www.ncihc.org

14

ETHICS AND MORALITY ON THE STAND

Art Therapist as Expert Witness

David E. Gussak

A man stood accused of kidnapping his two children, murdering one, and attempting to kill the other. The prosecution sought the death penalty. The defense team worked to avoid this sentence by exhausting all appropriate resources and strategies available. This included using the artwork that the defendant had created over his lifetime; they believed it held answers that would assist in his defense. To obtain these answers, they contracted me, an art therapist, to provide expert witness testimony about the defendant's artwork and the results of art-based assessments, to determine if he had a mental illness at the time of the crimes.

This chapter presents a brief overview of Forensic Art Therapy, a description of the role I played as an expert witness in a death row murder trial, and an examination of the legal, ethical, and moral challenges that I faced. It concludes with a clarification of the contextual issues that may affect an art therapist's ethical and moral responses.

Forensic Art Therapy

Forensic art therapy juxtaposes art therapy principles, practices, and theory with legal tenets, procedures, and protocol. It is used in fact-finding endeavors and to assist in resolving legal matters that are in dispute (Gussak and Cohen-Liebman, 2001). It is investigative in nature rather than interventive (Cohen-Liebman, 1997, 2002; Gussak & Cohen-Liebman, 2001). Clients may be remanded by the court or referred by an investigative body to participate in an interview or evaluation (Safran, Levick, & Levine, 1990).

Marcia Sue Cohen-Liebman, considered the leading forensic art therapist, is responsible for coining the term *forensic art therapy*. She cites three advantages for using drawings in a forensic milieu. They can serve as *interviewing tools*, providing support to an investigation; as *charge enhancements*, providing context that can help to determine charges as well as to identify additional investigative areas; and as *evidentiary material* that is admissible in judicial proceedings (Cohen-Liebman, 2003; Gussak, 2013).

Cohen-Liebman developed specific investigative interviewing guidelines that evolved from the need for a common language/interview process for members of multidisciplinary teams investigating cases of child sexual abuse and would help bridge barriers intrinsic to multidisciplinary team investigations, such as differing burdens of proof. Her inclusion of free drawing made the procedure child friendly, as often children lack the ability to express verbally what they have experienced (Cohen-Liebman, 1999). Drawing often contributed to verbal associations and helped minimize the secondary traumatization which may occur in re-telling and, thus, re-experiencing the event (Gussak, 2013).

My Shifting Identity

Several years ago, I was contacted by a defense attorney and asked to serve as a consultant for a capital murder case, with the possibility of testifying in court. I was given limited information: that the prosecution was seeking the death penalty; that the defense team wondered whether their client might have a mental illness; and that the defendant had a long history of creating art. Although she had never worked with an art therapist before, the defense attorney believed that they needed someone to determine if the art they had collected from their client—over 100 images—would reveal a psychiatric disorder that had not been previously diagnosed.

I stressed that I was not a forensic art therapist and that, if they were looking for one, they could not do better than to contact Cohen-Liebman. The defense attorney said she had, but that Cohen-Liebman explained that, since she works primarily with child victims, providing support and testimony for someone who had killed a child would be a conflict. "However," she went on to tell the defense attorney, "if you want to work with somebody who is comfortable with someone who has murdered, contact Gussak." I recognized this as a dubious honor.

Although I had spent many years working as an art therapist with aggressive and violent clients in prisons and juvenile detention centers, had conducted research that investigated the effectiveness of art therapy in these settings, and had taught assessment in a number of universities, I had never testified in court as an expert witness. Although I was intrigued, I was cautious, as I was unsure how I felt about providing testimony for a murder defendant, let alone someone accused of killing his child. Upon reflection, I came to realize, and made it clear to the defense team, that I would not be testifying for or against the defendant; I would be testifying solely about his art.

I met with the defendant on two occasions to review his artwork and administer art-based assessments before being deposed by the deputy district attorney. These experiences culminated in a hearing before the judge and the public, which included testimony, cross-examination, and redirection, a process that lasted a few hours. My conclusion was that the formal elements of the defendant's art indicated that he suffered from a Schizoaffective Disorder at the time of his crime. Significantly, two other expert witnesses contracted by the defense—a psychiatrist and a psychologist (neither of whom I had spoken to prior to testifying)—independently reached the same conclusion. In his closing remarks, the judge acknowledged that it was likely that the defendant had a serious mental illness. The defendant received a sentence of 95 years.

I felt my identity as an art therapist shifting during this case. In order to provide the services for which I was contracted while maintaining my professional integrity as an art therapist, I had to ferret out and attend to the differences among legal, ethical, and moral issues.

Legality, Ethics, Morality, Oh My …

Legality

Initially, a *legal* hurdle needed to be overcome for me to testify; I had to secure expert witness status. In 1975, the United States Supreme Court, building upon earlier statutes, developed the Federal Rules of Evidence to clarify who could be an expert witness. *Rule 702: Testimony by Experts* (Bennett & Hess, 2006), or simply the *Daubert* rule [named after the first case in which it was applied, *Daubert v. Merrell Dow*], states that the presiding judge decides if someone's testimony is reliable (Lubet, 1998, p. 4). The ruling specifies that "…an opinion from an expert who is not a scientist should receive the same degree of scrutiny for reliability as an opinion from an expert who purports to be a scientist" (Bucklin, 2010, para. 4).

While this process might be relatively easy for a practitioner of an established profession, art therapists may find the scrutiny particularly challenging, due to the lack of familiarity with their profession. Hence, the court needed to consider several criteria prior to accepting me as an expert witness. Concluding that, as a clinician, I had experience with assessments and working with those with acute mental illness; as a researcher, I understood the reliability and validity of various procedures and was a meticulous reporter; and, as an educator, I provided information in a clear, succinct manner that could be easily understood by all parties, the judge accepted my qualifications as an expert witness.

Ethics

While issues in the legal realm tend to be black or white, ethical and moral considerations seem to come in shades of gray. Although I met the legal criteria, I had to make sure that I remained faithful to the ethical standards of my profession and my credentials as a registered, Board certified art therapist (ATR-BC). Several components of the *Code of Professional Practice* (2005)[1] of the Art Therapy Credentials Board (ATCB) directly addressed the ethical concerns I faced and, thus, affected my decision-making throughout the process. These standards were:

- Art therapists do not engage in therapy practices or procedures that are beyond their scope of practice, experience, training, and education.
- Art therapists should assist persons in obtaining other therapeutic services if the therapist is unable or unwilling to provide professional help, or where the problem or treatment indicated is beyond the scope of practice of the art therapist.
- Art therapists assess, treat, or advise on problems only in those cases in which they are competent as determined by their education, training, and experience.

- Art therapists, because of their potential to influence and alter the lives of others, exercise special care when making public their professional recommendations and opinions through testimony or other public statements.
- Art therapists do not distort or misuse their clinical and research findings.

Despite what the court deemed as my professional qualifications, I was ethically bound to understand my own expectations and limitations. I needed to be honest with myself regarding what I felt professionally competent to do. While the ATCB Code does not state that art therapists cannot render a diagnosis, since I was not licensed to do so in my home state or in the state in which I was testifying, I felt that it would be beyond my scope of practice. However, I felt competent to provide an educated assessment. I sought to resolve this ethical issue at the beginning of my testimony by making a statement, on the record, that I would assess but not diagnose.

MY ETHICAL DILEMMA

What happens to confidentiality in a courtroom?

The following ATCB standards provided me with a particular challenge in this case:

- Art therapists shall respect and protect confidential information obtained from clients including, but not limited to, all verbal and/or artistic expression occurring within a client-therapist relationship.
- Art therapists shall obtain written informed consent from a client, or where applicable, a parent or legal guardian before photographing the client's art expressions, videotaping, audio recording, or otherwise duplicating, or permitting third party observation of art therapy sessions.

Art therapists Agell, Goodman, and Williams observed that, "If we do our work well, artwork is as unique and individual as a fingerprint. We can leave names off work ... but if we're not encouraging stereotyped artwork, the patient is recognizable" (1995, p. 100). Thus, art therapists are diligent about obtaining release forms that describe how specific art pieces may be used, while ensuring that clients are aware of the risks to their confidentiality, despite art therapists' best efforts to protect their clients' identity.

This case was different. Once contracted to testify, I could not protect the anonymity of the client, nor was I expected to. The trial was public and the art became part of the unrestricted record. Legally, I did not need consent from the defendant to present my conclusions in court or to write about them following the trial. All that was needed was the authorization granted by the court, which was decided upon prior to my signing any agreement. Despite this, I felt uneasy.

How would you respond?

For the writer's response, see Appendix B, page 411.

In his proposed code of ethics for expert witnesses, Ambrogi (2009) stated that "an expert witness should assume that all communications with the client or with retaining counsel may be subject to disclosure through discovery and testimony, unless instructed otherwise by retaining counsel" (para. 7).

Because of the dissonance between the ethical responsibilities of the health care professional and those of the expert witness, several professional organizations (such as the American Academy of Otolaryngology-Head and Neck Surgery Foundation, Inc.) include standards for expert testimony within their codes of ethics. Unfortunately, most do not. Thus, it behooves an expert witness to be aware of the ethics of his or her given field, while also understanding the expectations of the court and the contracting attorneys. First and foremost, members of all professions should "accept only engagements that are within the expert's area of competence and training" (Abrogi, 2009, para. 11). Tanay (2010) points out that "unethical professionals would be ill-advised to go into forensic work, as it is much easier to be unethical outside the scrutiny of adversary proceedings" (p. 37).

During the deposition phase of the trial, the prosecuting attorney questioned my knowledge of the profession's ethical standards; he was right to do so. My knowledge of professional ethics and the extent to which that knowledge has been reflected in my behavior historically should be questioned. In turn, this underscoring of one's ethical competence can strengthen his or her position with the court.

Morality

Moral considerations required different deliberations. Throughout this process, I grappled with my own stand on the death penalty and my feelings about assisting a man charged with killing his child. Although I never indicated my stance on the death penalty during the trial, in order to address any moral conundrums, it was important for me to make clear—first to myself and then to the defense team—that I would testify neither for nor against the defendant; I would testify strictly about the art he had made. Some would see this as a question of semantics or a rationalization and perhaps it was a combination of the two, but it did allow me to present the best case possible while maintaining a sense of personal integrity.

This is not to say that I maintained objectivity; that would have been impossible. As Tanay (2010) observed, "The notion of a single impartial expert witness is an illusion" (p. 36). I obviously wanted my testimony to mean something—to contribute to the success of the defense. As Tanay stressed, "Neither ethics nor a sense of fairness demand that the expert witness walk down the middle in a legal dispute. On the contrary, it is the expert's contractual agreement that upon taking the witness stand, he or she will effectively testify in support of one side" (p. 37). When I agreed to work for the defense, I was expected to demonstrate how the art revealed that the defendant had a mental illness. It was up to me to decide if I would accept the contract. Once accepted, it was my responsibility to fulfill my contractual obligation.

Another issue I struggled with is my tendency to refrain from labeling a person with a diagnosis or illness. I feel that doing so is reductionistic and that it is likely that, once given a label, a person becomes forever identified with it (Becker, 1963/1991).

My own work as an art therapist has focused upon using art to allow participants to strengthen their identity and rise above the limitations placed upon them (Gussak, 2007). In contrast, the goal in this case was to grant the defendant a label. The hypocrisy was apparent—while usually I use art to humanize a client (in this case, to reduce the prosecutor's attempts to present him as a monster), I was now being asked to demonstrate that he deserved a particular label. The fact that I had to focus upon his art only as a reflection of his mental illness, not as reflective of any talent he may have had, caused an internal conflict with my identity as an art therapist. However, it would have been unethical and perhaps immoral *not* to do what was asked of me. If I were successful, I would help save the life of a man who, if mentally ill, was not fully responsible for his actions.

While the defendant knew that my testimony would focus upon his art—indeed, that I was hired to provide such testimony—being told what to expect and hearing the testimony are two different things. The art had been created by a person, a person who found my use of his art to indicate the existence of mental illness very painful. Although I was continually aware of this while testifying, the testimony could not be softened. I was not hired to provide therapy for the defendant, but to determine how his art could be used to support his defense.

To conclude, when art therapists find themselves having to serve a court of law, they are likely to find the realms of legality, ethics, and morality unexpectedly colliding. Hence, it is the challenge of the art therapist to disentangle and reconcile the various, and sometimes conflicting, expectations of their professional identity with the demands of the forensic system.

REFLECTIVE ART EXPERIENCES & DISCUSSION QUESTIONS

1. Although the terms *ethics* and *morals* are often used interchangeably, the author makes clear distinctions between the two. Create art that reflects your understanding of ethics and morals, including any areas where you believe they might overlap.
2. Diagram how you might go about determining whether a proposed action would fall within your scope of practice.
3. Describe a situation in which your professional ethics compelled you to make a decision that ran counter to your own moral code—and vice versa.
4. How would you respond to a situation in which you had to treat, assist, or provide testimony that might support someone whose actions you were morally opposed to? Explain and defend your rationale.

Acknowledgement

The bulk of this chapter is developed and borrowed directly and liberally from previous sources: the book *Art on Trial: Art Therapy in Capital Murder Cases* (2013) [used with permission from Columbia University Press] and the *Psychology Today* blog, Art on Trial: Confessions of a Serial Art Therapist (available at www.psychologytoday. com/blog/art-trial).

The author would like to thank his graduate assistant Ashley Beck for her assistance with this chapter.

Note

1 The ATCB Code of Professional Practice document that was current at the time of the trial and, thus, was used as my guide for ethical behavior, has since been replaced by the ATCB Code of Ethics, Conduct, and Disciplinary Procedures (20018).

References

Agell, G., Goodman, R., & Williams, K. (1995). The professional relationship: Ethics. *American Journal of Art Therapy,* 33(4), 99–109.

Ambrogi, R. (2009). Proposed: Expert witness code of ethics. Retrieved from www.ims-expertservices.com/newsletters/feb/expert-witness-code-of-ethics.asp#8

Art Therapy Credentials Board (2005). *Code of professional practice.* Greensboro, NC: Author.

Becker, H.S. (1963/1991). *Outsiders: Studies in the sociology of deviance.* New York: The Free Press.

Bennett, W.W., & Hess K.M. (2006). *Criminal investigation* (8th ed.). Florence, KY: Wadsworth.

Bucklin, L. (2010). Rule 702 of the Federal Rules of Evidence now incorporates the Daubert / Kumho / Joiner requirements. Retrieved from www.bucklin.org/ fed_rule_702.htm

Cohen-Liebman, M.S. (1997). Forensic art therapy. Preconference course presented at the annual conference of the American Art Therapy Association, Milwaukee, WI.

Cohen-Liebman, M.S. (1999). Draw and tell: Drawings within the context of child sexual abuse investigations. *The Arts in Psychotherapy*, 26(3), 185–194.

Cohen-Liebman, M.S. (2002). Intro to art therapy. In A. P. Giardino & E.R. Giardino (Eds.), *Recognition of child abuse for the mandated reporter* (3rd ed.). St. Louis, MO: G.W. Medical Publishing.

Cohen-Liebman, M.S. (2003). Using drawings in forensic investigations of child sexual abuse. In C. Malchiodi (Ed.), *Handbook of clinical art therapy.* New York: Guilford.

Gussak, D. (1997). The ultimate hidden weapon: Art therapy and the compromise option. In D. Gussak & E. Virshup (Eds.), *Drawing time: Art therapy in prisons and other correctional settings* (pp. 59–74). Chicago, IL: Magnolia Street.

Gussak, D. (2007). The deviant adolescent: Creating healthy interactions and re-labeling through art therapy. In D. Arrington (Ed.), *Art, Angst and Trauma: Right Brain Interventions with Developmental Issues* (pp. 132–149). Springfield, IL: Charles C. Thomas Publishers.

Gussak, D. (2013). *Art on trial: Art therapy in capital murder cases.* New York: Columbia University Press.

Gussak, D., & Cohen-Liebman, M.S. (2001). Investigation vs. intervention: Forensic art therapy and art therapy in forensic settings. *The American Journal of Art Therapy*, 40(2), 123–135.

Lubet, S. (1998). *Expert testimony: A guide for expert witnesses and the lawyers who examine them.* Chicago, IL: National Institute for Trial Advocacy.

Safran, D.C., Levick, M.F., & Levine, A.J. (1990). Art therapists as expert witnesses: A judge delivers a precedent-setting decision. *The Arts in Psychotherapy*, 17, 49–53.

Tanay, E. (2010). *American legal injustice: Behind the scenes with an expert witness.* Lanham, MD: Jason Aranson.

15

NO MAN, OR WOMAN, IS AN ISLAND— ESPECIALLY ON AN ISLAND

Practicing Art Therapy in the West Indies

Karina Donald

Come on, give me a hug! You get big job now, but I know you since you were a small little tiny child.

The prospect of returning to my native homeland in the Caribbean to practice art therapy after receiving my Master's degree in Art Therapy in the States raised many concerns. I was worried that my age would be a disadvantage, because in the West Indies the family has a matrifocal pattern in which the grandmother is the seat of wisdom (Seeman, 2011; Miner, 2003; Brunod & Cook-Darzens, 2002). Since I would be the first art therapist on my island, one of the Windward Islands within the Lesser Antilles, I assumed that my efforts to establish a practice would meet much resistance as the new ideas of a young professional would not be readily embraced. My greatest ethical concern, however, stemmed from the fact that the island has such a small population. Potential clients, colleagues, and other adults would remember me from previous encounters, know my address, family background, and typical social settings. How would I be able to implement what I had learned about the importance of therapeutic boundaries regarding self-disclosure, touch, confidentiality, dual relationships, and so much more? I did not want the Art Therapy Credentials Board (ATCB) to come knocking on my family's mahogany door—literally or figuratively— about unethical practice.

My first day on the job, working with families and young victims of abuse and neglect, I was surprised to find some of my concerns mitigated by my boss' recognition of the need to create policies for providing therapy. I was not just the first art therapist to work at the agency, but the only therapist of any kind to work there. On the island, spiritual interventions remained the first point of assistance for any kind of mental health issue. During the first two months, I interacted with staff and community leaders, learning much about mental health practice and other cultural issues of which I was unaware prior to my return. I also participated in drafting policies and procedures for the provision of therapeutic services.

Scope of Practice

You have a Master's, you can do everything

At the time that this chapter is being written, no local or regional credentials for mental professionals existed in my homeland. People such as I rely upon credentials obtained from countries such as the States, Canada, or England to prove the legitimacy of our disciplines. The first ethical issue I encountered arose from the assumption that my education and credentials granted me insurmountable knowledge about all topics related to mental health. As the only mental health professional at my workplace and the only art therapist in the nation, I unwittingly became the go-to person for complex cases for which I was mostly unprepared. Clients presenting with a wide variety of issues were referred to me. I also received many requests from coworkers and clients' parents to conduct assessments such as intelligence tests. Although as a young professional, seeking acceptance of her field and her place in it, it was flattering to be held in such esteem, I carefully explained what my training and my credentials qualified me to do and not do and referred those requests to the one available psychologist on the island.

When Cultural Expectations Meet Therapeutic Boundaries

In a paper for the Ethics class that was part of my art therapy training, I wrote, "Hopefully, I can negotiate the multi-dimensionality of roles when I return home, because I know my own culture." Although I now work in the land of my birth, I have found that the cultural assumptions that I held while I was growing up—such as the expectation that everyone on the island had a similar ethnic background and sexual orientation—are no longer valid (and undoubtedly never were). Cultures can and do evolve with time (Aronowitz, Deener, Keene, Schnittker, & Tach, 2015) and so must our cultural competency. For example, up until a decade or so ago, West Indian people sought mental health interventions only as a last resort (Lefley & Bestman, 1977). While I was away studying, mental health service was changing. School counsellors and counselling clinics were being introduced and West Indians were realizing that they needed a different type of assistance than a relative or a religious leader could provide.

As part of my discussion of confidentiality during my initial session with a client, I informed the client that I will not greet him or her in public. The same puzzled look appears on the faces of adult and child clients, alike, because in the West Indies it is culturally expected to greet a person after some form of interaction. To accommodate this expectation, I acknowledge the cultural value of the practice and clarify that, if the client initiates the interaction, I will respond, but I will not prolong conversation or respond to anything pertaining to therapy. To date, no one has refrained from initiating contact in public. In fact, most clients smile and greet me; young clients mostly giggle and shout my name from across the street.

It has been important for me to seek continuous feedback from other mental health professionals in order to learn how I can adjust my practice to meet cultural expectations and ethical standards. During the first two years, I met regularly, via

Skype, with a credentialed art therapist to assist in my professional growth. Over time, relationships with art therapists on three other West Indian islands blossomed into an informal online peer support group. Locally, I sought out formal and informal gatherings with other mental health professionals, such as social workers and a psychologist. I cannot thank those persons enough for their mutual encouragement, chats over lunch, and laughter.

Don't tell people "my business"

According to the Art Therapy Credentials Board *Code of Ethics, Conduct, and Disciplinary Procedures* (2018), I am expected to respect and protect the information that a client discloses in order to process his or her feelings. With limited resources available for mental health services and limited space available in which to facilitate the art therapy process—but great needs—this expectation often posed an ethical dilemma. Since my job entailed traveling to the northern part of the island one day of the week, to the western part on another day, and to the eastern part on yet another day, therapeutic spaces varied widely—so I had to innovate.

A small office in a rural area had no curtains on its windows to prevent others from observing art therapy sessions or satisfying their curiosity about who was attending, but turning the chairs so that my clients' backs would face the windows helped them feel more relaxed in the space and provided a degree of confidentiality. Isolated beach locations were used if an office was unexpectedly closed or when rooms at churches

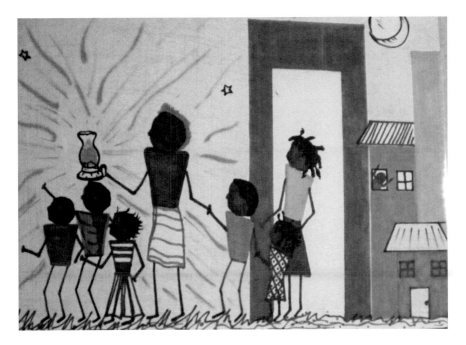

FIGURE 15.1 Searching for "a safe space."

or community-based organizations were unavailable. Whenever I used common spaces (such as a recreation room) in residential settings, I asked if staff would reschedule other activities, in order to create a safe space in which clients could express their feelings. If the common room needed to be shared, I developed art therapy directives that limited verbal art processing. Afterwards, brief post-group sessions were held in my car or at an empty bus stop to allow clients to make art or to talk about things that they were unable to share in the common room. Ensuring my clients' right to privacy raised ethical challenges—but sparked creative problem solving.

MY ETHICAL DILEMMA

Should I re-draw the boundaries of confidentiality?

At the end of a work day, two hours after completing a session with adolescent siblings in their home, I had returned to the guest house where I was staying when I received a call saying that the adolescents' caregivers no longer wanted them there and that I needed to find them another place to live. I was the only employee of our agency on this small island dependency of our country. The agency did have an emergency group home for children on another island, but the only way to get there was to take a public ferry that carried at least 80 persons to and from that island. Anyone who noticed me with the adolescents would assume that I was their therapist.

How would you respond?

For the writer's response, see Appendix B, page 406.

Miss, which person are you?

I have come to be known as the lady with the big bag, for I carry a large canvas bag full of art materials as I travel from one place to another. My bag piques curiosity and people find very creative ways in which to peep inside. The children prefer responding to art directives to using an open studio approach and love to create things that they can use, such as fans made from painted leaves larger than their hands. Because many of my clients have no storage space at home, they choose to leave their artwork with me, so my bag also contains completed artwork and work in progress. Art directives which involve paints, clay, glue, or other fluid media have to be completed at least 15 minutes before the session ends, to allow for drying in the Caribbean heat.

Although most people know me as the lady with the big bag, dual relationships are unavoidable on a small island. During an intake session, it was difficult to contain my shock when I discovered that my new client's caregiver—whom I have known since childhood—is related to a relative of mine. I tried to keep the focus upon my client's needs and not discuss our mutual relative. On informal occasions, however, my relative tried to get me to share details about therapy sessions with my client, but I persisted in redirecting the inquiry and spoke about my responsibility to maintain confidentiality.

Dual relationships also existed within my place of employment. Being easily accessible to colleagues, I was sought by staff who struggled with personal issues or were concerned about family members. I also became an in-house trainer regarding general mental issues, a member of the management team, and a clinical supervisor. My eagerness to help fostered my desire to take on multiple roles. Knowing that mental health services were limited or absent, I thought that I needed to be the cog in the wheel. Through online art therapy supervision, however, I was able to acknowledge my struggle to say no. Eventually, it became easier to politely decline requests or to ask other professionals to help.

I'm a good farmer—I'll pay you with some good food!

Bartering occurs primarily in rural settings in the West Indies. Historically, locals feel a sense of pride when they can give fruits and vegetables grown from their gardens in exchange for services rendered. In West Indian culture, gifts of fruits, vegetables, and flowers are symbols of appreciation. It is an insult not to accept gifts. Both adult and young clients offered me flowers as a symbol of gratitude for their art therapy sessions. One client brought in mangoes, clients' caregivers brought art supplies, others brought clothes and shoes for clients in need. I found these situations very awkward and struggled to decide how to handle them. During my first year of work, I accepted the gifts, shared them with co-workers, and added the clothing and shoes to my workplace's supplies for clients. After a client became disappointed when she did not see the flowers that she had given me (they had been discarded when they had dried up), I made a pragmatic decision to adopt a "no gifts" policy with future clients.

Miss, I need to know!

Some clients want me to share personal information because they are curious about the fact that I travel all over the island to conduct art therapy sessions; others want me to ease their uncertainty about my youthfulness. Still others insist that they need to know more about me because of religious affiliations or a desire to make a personal connection. Gentle but firm redirection usually is accepted, even by clients who are older than I.

MY ETHICAL DILEMMA

Should I alter my usual approach to self-disclosure?

A new client greeted me by observing, "Your last name is rare in this country ... are you related to [my father's name]?" She then answered her own question, "Yes! You are! You look like him!" I smiled and reminded the client about the purpose of sessions and the question was dropped. (Ironically, the truth of the client's speculation was confirmed when I was seen with my parents in a public place, but by that time her therapy sessions had ended.)

If her sessions had continued and she had persisted in asking if I were related to [my father], should I alter my usual approach to self-disclosure?

How would you respond?

For the writer's response, see Appendix B, page 406.

Small ting, gimme a touch nah?

In the West Indies, one's sense of personal space is much more limited than it is in the States. After having been introduced, whenever people meet, they hug. If two persons are talking and one steps back, the other one usually steps forward. Although initially I acted in a way that was culturally appropriate, I later explained to my clients that I have a different understanding of how to exchange greetings when people are in a helping relationship of this kind. Handshakes are accepted at the beginning or at the end of sessions. Hugs are accepted when part of a social activity outside of my professional work as a therapist, such as at a retreat, a community-based program, or a religious setting.

Let us pray

It was more challenging to redirect spiritual requests. Culturally, Christianity is interwoven into both formal and informal gatherings in the West Indies. Religious leaders are asked to give prayers at public gatherings and my clients expected me to initiate prayers at the beginning of their therapy sessions. When I declined to do so, they were insulted. One client was particularly insistent that we not only open, but also close our sessions with a prayer. My supervisor helped me to see the power struggle inherent in this dynamic, which proved useful to our work and allowed me to clarify my role as a therapist rather than a spiritual advisor.

Concluding Thoughts

Despite all the ethical concerns I anticipated when I returned to the West Indies to practice art therapy, I have found it surprisingly easy to redirect clients' personal questions and the issue of touch has not come up as often as I had expected. I no longer see my age as being a deterrent to West Indians embracing art therapy; I receive more requests for art therapy than I have time to fill. Ethical issues related to dual relationships, confidentiality, clients' rights, and scope of practice reveal themselves quite regularly and keep me on my toes. There are times when my knowledge of clients' needs, such as a place to live, and my desire to advocate for them poses an ethical issue for me, as the extent of the needs are daunting and resolving them is beyond my control. I also continue to feel the weight of being the only art therapist in my country. However, I make art as a way to process these experiences. I am, after all, an art therapist!

REFLECTIVE ART EXPERIENCES & DISCUSSION QUESTIONS

1. Imagine returning to your hometown to practice. What ethical challenges would you anticipate encountering there?
2. Your client is unable to pay but wants to give you items of a similar monetary value. Knowing your client's financial constraints, how might you address the issue of bartering?
3. Create art regarding your feelings about practicing art therapy with clients who have a cultural background that is (a) similar to yours, then, (b) different than yours. Discuss.

References

Aronowitz, R., Deener, A., Keene, D., Schnittker, J., & Tach, L. (2015). Cultural reflexivity in health research and practice. *American Journal of Public Health,* 105(S3), S403–S408. doi:10.2105/ajph.2015.302551

Art Therapy Credentials Board (2018). *Code of ethics, conduct, and disciplinary procedures.* Greensboro, NC: Author.

Brunod, R., & Cook-Darzens, S. (2002). Men's role and fatherhood in French Caribbean families: A multi-systemic 'resource' approach. *Clinical Child Psychology & Psychiatry,* 7(4), 559–569. doi: 10.1177/1359104502007004008

Lefley, H. P., & Bestman, E. W. (1977, August). Psychotherapy in Caribbean cultures. Paper presented at the Annual Convention of the American Psychological Association, San Francisco, CA.

Miner, D.C. (2003). Jamaican families. Extended matrifocal families can resourcefully respond to the child's needs for socialization. *Holistic Nursing Practice,* 17, 27–35. doi:10.1097/00004650-200301000-00007

Seeman, M.V. (2011). Canada: Psychosis in the immigrant Caribbean population. *International Journal of Social Psychiatry,* 57(5), 462–470. doi:10.1177/0020764010365979

16

WHEN "CLIENT" IS PLURAL

Confidentiality in Art Therapy with Groups, Families, and Couples

Mary Ellen Ruff

Ethical dilemmas arise in clinical practice with some frequency, but they are usually worked through with consultation, supervision, and a good working understanding of the ethical guidelines provided by our credentialing bodies—which, for me, are those of the Art Therapy Credentials Board and the National Board of Certified Counselors. When facing an ethical dilemma, I often hear a little voice inside asking, "Whose needs are being met?" and "What is in the best interest of the client?" The answer is not always straight-forward when, as in the cases described herein, the "client" is the group, the family, or the couple and the ethical dilemma involves confidentiality.

As an art therapist, I have had the opportunity to conduct group, family, and couples therapy in various clinical settings, such as inpatient psychiatric hospitals, day treatment programs, outpatient programs, and private practice. Confidentiality is an incredibly important component of any therapeutic environment. Although group members are not legally bound to keep each other's confidences, it is necessary to impress upon them its importance as an expectation and norm of the counseling experience. As group leader, I ensure members of the group that I will hold in confidence anything shared within the context of the group, except when there is a risk of harm to self and/or others; when there are indications of child abuse and/or neglect or elder abuse, neglect, or exploitation; or when I am compelled to disclose information by a court order.

MY ETHICAL DILEMMA

... while working with a group

Many years ago, as the program administrator of an intensive outpatient substance abuse program for adolescents, I found myself in multiple roles that could cause friction due to their competing needs. As administrator, I conducted the

orientation of new families, managed utilization review with insurance companies, supervised staff, and took care of any programmatic issues that arose.
As case manager, I advocated with school personnel for services, collaborated
with other involved professionals (e.g., psychiatrists, individual therapists, school
counselors), and maintained open lines of communication with parents regarding
their teenagers' care. As a therapist, I facilitated peer groups and multi-family
groups each week.

The program required teenagers to attend three groups each week, two
of which were peer groups, while the third was a multi-family group. If they
experienced a chemical or behavioral relapse during the week, the adolescents
would attend a fourth (relapse prevention) group. Teenagers worked through
phases of treatment as they progressed through educational and individualized
treatment plans.

My dilemma involved my work with a 15-year-old boy, "Scott," and his family.
Scott initially came into treatment after he incurred legal charges related to substance use and was ordered to complete a substance abuse treatment program.
Scott's father and stepmother routinely attended the weekly multi-family group
that was required as part of the program. In his peer groups, Scott often shared
the frustration he felt with his stepmother, describing the difficulties that both
he and his father were having in their relationships with her, and saying that
he didn't want her involved in his treatment. Anything Scott shared during
peer groups was not disclosed in family groups. In fact, peers were continually
reminded that groups were separate entities and that information did not transfer
from one group to another.

My multiple roles with Scott and his family created tension for me as I became
more involved over the months that Scott was in treatment. Not only was I seeing
Scott several times a week, but I was seeing both his dad and his step-mom in
the weekly family group. I was also in regular contact with his father regarding
insurance issues and Scott's stepmother frequently called with concerns about
Scott's behavior, suspicions of ongoing substance use, and questions about
Scott's participation in the program. Scott's father often appeared to be caught
in the crosshairs of the conflict between Scott and his stepmother, and I heard
much about that, as well.

At one point, Scott disclosed in peer group that he had suspected for a while
that his stepmother was abusing prescription medications. Initially, it seemed
as though Scott were deflecting some of the attention he'd been receiving for
being in treatment and was trying to implicate his stepmother in behavior that
would clearly create problems in the family. However, Scott continued to raise his
suspicions about his stepmother, describing the erratic moods, unpredictability,
and frequent angry outbursts that interfered with his desire to have any type of
relationship with her. Interestingly, the more he distanced himself from her, the
more frequent her calls to me became, voicing her concerns about his behavior
and her insistence that he was telling lies about her—despite the fact that no
information shared by Scott in group was ever disclosed to her. It was as if she
needed to make sure that I understood that she was a caring, concerned, and

responsible parent. Was this a classic case of parent/child "he said, she said?" or was there truth in each person's perspective? Was it my responsibility to figure that out? And was the rift between the two of them in danger of causing a split within the family that might impact Scott's treatment?

I was holding a significant amount of family information from Scott, his father, and his stepmother, conveyed through a variety of vehicles. Because each therapy group was considered its own entity, I needed to be very conscious of where specific information had been disclosed. For example, since Scott's peers were hearing about his stepmom's alleged substance abuse, I needed to hold that information during family groups, in order to protect the integrity of the peer group, as well as of the family group. When stepmom's behavior in the family group became increasingly histrionic (e.g., disrupting the process by abruptly lashing out at Scott and his father or erupting in fits of crying that were disproportionate to the discussion at hand), I had to consider what to do in order to protect that group without alienating any of its members.

How would you respond?

For the writer's response, see Appendix B, page 432.

MY ETHICAL DILEMMA

... while working with a family

I have worked with families in many different settings, but the ethical dilemma I am sharing here occurred with a family I saw in a family drug treatment court program. When Child Protective Services becomes involved with a parent due to complaints of abuse or neglect, the parent receives treatment through the Department of Social Services. When substance abuse is found to be a component of the behavior that contributed to that family's difficulties, the Department of Social Services refers the parent to the family drug treatment court. Once again, my position involved wearing multiple hats. As program coordinator, I testified in court hearings every two weeks about the progress and compliance of the participants. This included providing information about treatment attendance, drug screen results, visitation with children, employment or community service, and stability of housing. I also did case management, conducted weekly group therapy for all participants, and saw five people in individual therapy.

"Evelyn" and "Randy" came into the family drug treatment court program after the couple, who had two young children, was found to be in possession of marijuana. The children were removed from Evelyn's care and placed in foster care. Randy never engaged in the program and moved out of the area, voluntarily relinquishing his parental rights to the children and leaving Evelyn to work towards reunification on her own. Evelyn had to complete several requirements as part of the family drug treatment court program, not the least of which was substance abuse treatment and negative drug screens. She had to maintain stable housing, secure employment, and maintain weekly visits with her children. She also had to appear in drug court hearings every two weeks, at which time her progress in each of these areas was reviewed. I was Evelyn's individual and group therapist, as well as her case manager.

Evelyn was in full compliance with treatment, never gave a positive drug screen, and was able to find a job. She struggled with housing but got into a shelter that led to a transitional housing program. Evelyn was doing well and appeared to be on track to reunify with her children. Unfortunately, she began to struggle to maintain her newfound stability. She held a series of jobs, moving on after a few months, usually as a result of some conflict at work. There were issues with her housing program, also, and allegations that Randy was back in town visiting her there, which was against program guidelines. One thing that was consistent was Evelyn's strong devotion to her children and her commitment to regaining custody of them. As time passed, Evelyn seemed to have alienated herself from her children's foster care social worker, and it was becoming more and more clear that the foster care agency perceived her as a difficult and unfit parent. Evelyn's ongoing relationship with Randy, albeit sporadic, also created problems for her since his parental rights were no longer intact.

My ethical dilemma occurred when the foster care agency decided to petition for the termination of Evelyn's parental rights. I was very well aware of Evelyn's commitment to her children and her fulfillment of all of the family drug treatment court requirements. As her therapist, I felt as though I knew her more deeply than anyone else involved in the case, but my own agency was pursuing the termination of her parental rights, a decision I couldn't support. I was approached by Evelyn's attorney to testify at the termination hearing on Evelyn's behalf. I had to make a decision as to whether I supported my agency or my client. I needed to sort through my ethical obligations to my employer and my ethical obligations to my client. I also had to stand by my personal ethics and figure out whether these three areas overlapped.

How would you respond?

For the writer's response, see Appendix B, page 432.

MY ETHICAL DILEMMA

... while working with a couple

Couples present a unique challenge in that, when a couple seeks counseling, one or both members may be questioning the viability of the relationship and, therefore, may have different goals. When I begin working with a couple, I provide each person with an individual session in order to gather history and to clarify that person's perspective on the relationship and its future. This helps to create a framework within which therapy can be structured. Sometimes, couples agree to enter counseling in order to seek sanctioning for the dissolution of the relationship. Rather than focusing upon what their different goals might be, I try to encourage them to think about how they can create a healthful relationship, whether that includes staying together or not.

  "Ellen" and "Keith" initiated couple's therapy six months after they experienced the loss of their 17-year-old son to addiction. Initially, the work appeared to be focused upon their grief and how they could move forward together as a family. During Ellen's individual session, she disclosed that she had been unfaithful to Keith and that she was unsure whether she wanted to stay in the marriage. Keith disclosed in his individual session that he sensed Ellen's distance and that he was very committed to working through their grief in order to strengthen their relationship. They were clearly starting from different places, and initially it appeared as though the only thing they shared was their grief and their two other children, both of whom were in college. Ellen's disclosure left me holding information that could impact Keith's attitude towards the relationship. This information, however, didn't necessarily relate to the presenting issue, the grief that they were experiencing from the loss of their son. I needed to figure out how to create a therapeutic frame in which Ellen and Keith could work, while holding Ellen's infidelity until she felt as if she wanted to share it with Keith. I found that I needed to remain acutely aware of my counter-transference and how I worked with this couple, so that I could provide the space they needed to grieve and work through their relationship path, no matter what direction it led. My ethical dilemma arose when Keith confronted Ellen about her commitment to the marriage, asking her directly if she had remained faithful. Ellen denied Keith's concerns in our sessions, which left me conflicted about how to proceed. If the couple was my client, how was I to focus upon the needs of the couple, given the disparate needs of the individuals that comprised it? What was my obligation to Ellen and Keith individually, within the context of their relationship?

How would you respond?

For the writer's response, see Appendix B, page 433.

Concluding Thoughts

When "the client" is composed of multiple people, whether in a group, a family, or a couple, I often find myself privy to information that might be important for me, as a clinician, to know, but would be damaging to disclose to the group, family, or couple. Sometimes I think of the work, itself, as the coming together of a large number of seemingly disparate jig-saw puzzle pieces. When I look at some pieces, I seem to know where they're supposed to fit. I can almost see where they're going to connect, but it's just not quite time to pick them up. Holding bits and pieces of information for a group, family, or couple can feel much the same way. I like to try to guide clients to see those pieces for themselves, to disclose something when it's time, to make connections, to find meaning. There are few things more powerful than to see a group, a family, or a couple begin to perceive each other in a new light, to communicate more openly and honestly, and to work together to find solutions to the problems that brought them to therapy.

REFLECTIVE ART EXPERIENCES & DISCUSSION QUESTIONS

1. Create two pieces of art: one reflecting yourself and one reflecting an ethical dilemma you face with your group, family, or couple. After tearing or cutting the pieces of art into strips—but keeping the integrity of each image intact— weave them together to create a single image. Your finished product will show the interplay between you and the dilemma presented by your clients. Notice where strengths and weaknesses emerge and where you see the need for support or space for growth.

2. Think of yourself as the holding space for information, emotions, and other clinical material that your clients share with you. Using clay or Model Magic, create a representation of yourself as a vessel. What does the vessel need in order to contain all that it has to? How does the vessel allow therapeutic material to flow through it when it needs to? When working with a couple, how would you balance the needs of each member as well as the couple as a whole? How would you create the space for each member of the couple to remain an individual while working toward a common goal?

3. Personal ethics typically stem from our experiences within our family, culture, religion, or other defining components of our lives. Professional ethics develop through our experience in work settings or are guided by ethical codes related to credentialing and licensure. When your personal and professional ethics create friction, what resources do you use to work through the conflict and move forward in one direction or another? How do you prioritize one over the other?

17

YOUTH BEHIND BARS

Ethical Issues That Confront Art Therapists Who Work in Juvenile Detention Centers

Jane Scott

Juvenile detention, a separate placement for criminal offenders under 18 years old, was created by law in 1824. Since then, the number of juveniles in detention has fluctuated, with a peak of more than 115,000 in the late 1990's, decreasing dramatically thereafter (Office of Juvenile Justice and Delinquency Prevention, 2013). Detention centers are locked facilities that temporarily house youth who have been arrested and are being, or have been, charged with a crime. Detainment prevents youth from reoffending before trial or evading trial. They can be held from a few days to more than a year; they can be released directly to the community from detention; sentenced to time in a rehabilitative program; sentenced to "juvenile life" (until they are 21 years old) at a juvenile correctional facility; or, if their crime is serious enough, they can be sentenced for long prison terms after being tried as adults.

Mental Health Needs

Studies indicate that nearly two-thirds of the youth in detention have an undiagnosed mental health disorder (Grisso, 2008). Due to traumatic life experiences prior to being incarcerated, the rate of post-traumatic stress disorder (PTSD) among youth in detention is so high that it is comparable to that of soldiers returning from war (Buffington, Dierkhising & Marsh, 2010). A Justice Policy Institute paper states that "unmet mental and behavioral health needs" are at the top of the needs that administrators see in detained youth (Holman & Zeidenberg, 2006, p. 8).

Research shows that art therapy can help detainees reduce stress, increase self-esteem, express anger, and offer an empathic therapeutic relationship (Persons, 2009). Art programs restore choice and increase relaxation and engagement while detainees are incarcerated (Williams, 2002).

Ethical Issues That Arise in a Detention Center

Safety Trumps Privacy (Not to Mention Autonomy)

Safety was the top priority where I worked. Cameras installed throughout the building tracked the detainees' every move, other than when they were inside their cells. Corrections officers were with the detainees at all times—even during therapy. When seated, detainees could not stand up without asking; when sitting at a table, their hands had to be on the table's surface at all times; when walking in the hallway, they could not talk or look anywhere but forward, to prevent surreptitious communication such as by flashing gang signs. Before detainees arrived for art therapy sessions and, again, before they left the sessions, every pencil, eraser, oil pastel, and the like had to be counted meticulously. If even a pencil stub went missing, the entire building went on lockdown and every room and student was searched thoroughly until it was found.

Role Ambiguity: Art Teacher or Art Therapist?

While the corrections officers were the ones who were primarily responsible for safety and security, all staff in a detention center are part of a large, court-involved system dealing with high-risk individuals. I had the dual role of Art Therapist/Art Educator, which required a teaching license and a master's degree in art therapy. The ambiguous nature of my position presented its own ethical issues. My position description stated that my goal was "to help students develop skills to manage emotions and behavior" by using "art as therapy and psycho-educational experiences rather than projective psychotherapy." At the same time, I was required to mete out consequences for inappropriate behavior.

When Consequences Include Isolation: To Give or Not To Give?

As a member of the staff of a detention center, I was required to assign, and enforce, consequences for inappropriate behavior, which ranged from a simple redirection for minor behavioral issues to assigning isolation for larger infractions. For example, cursing in group was an infraction and, after a reminder, it warranted a sanction. This dynamic occurs in other court-mandated programs, as well; for example, substance abuse counselors must report clients who were mandated into treatment by the court if those clients continue to use substances. Being responsible for behavioral management within detention centers can raise a host of ethical dilemmas, however, particularly when one is required to assign a client to room isolation as a punitive act. In isolation, residents are confined to their cells for up to 72 hours at a time, without their mats and with only a small sliver of window to see outside their cells. They receive meals in their cells, and come out for recreation for only one hour a day. Numerous studies have cited adverse consequences of isolation for youth. Psychological damage, increased risk of suicide and self-harm, loss of education and rehabilitative activities, and impaired development can result from isolation (American Civil Liberties Union, 2012).

I observed the physical and emotional consequences of isolation on many occasions—when I walked by cells and heard teens in isolation screaming; when I was told about detainees who defecated, spit up blood, or self-harmed in their cells during isolation; and when I heard from youth about how they coped with isolation by singing their favorite songs out loud for hours or pounded the wall with the hope that a peer in isolation would answer with a sound.

To be part of the corrections system is to be linked to the controversial use of solitary confinement and all art therapists working in detention will have to grapple with this ethical issue. We may feel powerless to change the system, but we can advocate for change. I chose to give isolation only when I was required to do so by supervisors—mostly in the event of aggressive or sexual behavior toward a peer or me. There were times when detention staff would have preferred that I give a stricter consequence, but I tried to keep detainees out of isolation whenever possible.

When Crimes Are Disclosed During Sessions: To Report or Not to Report?

Upon intake, detainees were told that they had to refrain from speaking to peers, teachers, or staff about any aspects of their court cases or their "war stories" (crimes they had committed on the outside). When residents are involved in cases receiving media attention or in unusual or extremely disturbing cases, staff may be tempted to find out more about them. I have found that residents often disclose highly confidential information to peers or staff—without warning—during art therapy groups or via their artwork. Their incarceration (and what led to it) is the focal point of their lives and it can be difficult to engage in rapport building without at least the topic of their charges coming up. Youth want to talk to adults they trust about their cases. They feel guilt, anger, sadness, remorse, and a sense of injustice, and they want to voice these emotions. Developing a therapeutic relationship with a client while respecting the boundary imposed by the detention center can result in an ethical dilemma for the therapist.

Every detention center has different policies regarding confidentiality and disclosures of case-related material. Corrections officers—who were with the detainees throughout art therapy sessions—were lawfully responsible to report to the court. Therefore, if a detainee were to say, for example, that he/she was guilty of the crime he/she was being charged with, corrections staff would have to report it. Mental health counselors at our facility asked their clients sign a consent form which stated that confidentiality was protected to a high degree during therapy, but also gave clinical discretion to the therapist to disclose to the team information that was considered to be important in helping the client. What this meant for clients was that all matters regarding mandated reporting were not confidential, but other matters, such as past or current crimes (including homicide, gang involvement, drug dealing, and more) were not required to be reported. If the client had signed this consent form regarding the limits of confidentiality, mental health counselors could decide whether they wanted to share the client's disclosure with the team; however, in deciding to share the disclosure, their intention had to be to help the course of treatment, not for legal ramifications.

Although art therapists were designated as mandated reporters where I worked, policies regarding other aspects of confidentiality were not clearly defined. For example, we were not told whether we were required to report disclosures regarding crimes. As an employee within the court system, I was well aware that anyone could be subpoenaed by the judge at any time, so I would frequently say to my groups, "Don't tell me too much!" Even so, disclosures occurred.

Adam

An adolescent whom I will call Adam was in an art therapy group for several months. During a project that focused upon family, Adam turned to me and casually remarked, "When I stole the jewelry I got locked up for, my mom hid the money, so even if I do time it was worth it to help my family out. That's like $30,000 I gave them; I'll take 20 years for that."

I was completely caught off guard by Adam's disclosure and ill-prepared for it. I wasn't sure what to do, but, because the disclosure did not involve child abuse or danger to self or others, I chose not report it. Instead, I told Adam that he needed to be careful about disclosures because many staff would be obligated to report the statements to the police. He had no idea that his comments could be used in court and thanked me for making him aware of it. I also spoke in confidence to a mental health staff member about the situation and received guidance from that individual. As a result, I believe that the way I handled the situation was appropriate. I felt that it would not be fair to Adam to report his remarks, since the issue of reporting comments made by clients regarding their crimes had not been addressed in the facility's written material regarding the responsibilities of art therapists. Corrections officers were present when Adam made the disclosure, so I felt that it was an obligation of theirs if they deemed it important. However, I used the opportunity to set a new boundary with Adam that let him know I could not talk about or process crimes with him, despite my desire to support him. Finally, I made him aware of the limits to confidentiality while someone was in detention—information that he said he didn't know about. Had Adam's disclosure dealt with sexual abuse, or threat to self or others, I would have handled it differently.

MY ETHICAL DILEMMA

What should I do when I discover that information about a crime has been disclosed on a sheet of drawing paper?

Very early in my job at the detention center, a detainee whom I shall call John spent the art therapy group time doodling quietly on his paper. At the end of group, John looked up at me tearfully and asked if he could throw his paper in the trashcan. I replied "Yes," and asked if he were okay, to which he answered, "I'm good." When the group left a few minutes later, I noticed as I walked by the trashcan and peeked in (yet another ethical issue), that John had not drawn any artwork on his sheet of paper at all, but had written words all over it. I had assumed that he had thrown the sheet of paper away because he hadn't liked his drawing, but—deciding to read what he had written—I discovered that the reality for this 15-year-old boy was much worse. It turned out that John had been involved in sex trafficking and had written down information about his case. Aside from being extremely sad and heartbreaking to read, John had disclosed highly sensitive information on the paper, scrawling references to money and what appeared to be names.

I had to make a gut-wrenching decision: Should I turn John's letter in to the police and possibly become involved in providing evidence in a case of child prostitution or should I ignore what I had seen on artwork that, after all, a client had chosen to throw away?

How would you respond?

For the writer's response, see Appendix B, page 433.

A Final Note about Working in Detention Facilities

Attachment, trauma, and emotional regulation are the core issues that juveniles in detention face and an enormous part of our work in detention has to do with addressing them in therapeutic, ethical ways. Although the picture painted of juvenile detention by the media is peopled with cold, violent teenagers, the majority of the youth I came to know were usually quite respectful, very fun-loving, highly creative, and a joy to work with. I received many pieces of art with small notes attached, thanking me for providing an avenue for expression, and for being accepting and kind. While one should never forget the reason youth are detained—for lack of self-control and for breaking rules chronically or violently—it is a deeply fulfilling experience to work with this population. My hope is that art therapists who choose jobs in detention will offer youth a warm heart and a place for their voices to be heard.

Editor's note: A few months after this chapter was written, I opened a copy of *The Washington Post* (January 26, 2016) to discover that President Obama had taken measures to ban the solitary confinement of juveniles in federal prisons (Eilperin, 2016).

REFLECTIVE ART EXPERIENCES & DISCUSSION QUESTIONS

1. Create art that reflects how you feel about working for an institution which has policies and/or procedures that you do not think are ethical. Next, create art that depicts how you think your clients might feel about receiving treatment at an institution that has policies and/or procedures that they do not believe are ethical.

2. Have you ever felt conflicted about following an agency policy that you believed was not in the best interest of your clients? How did you deal with this ethical dilemma?
3. Most of us complain about behavior that we feel is unjust. Have these feelings ever led you to engage in advocacy work? If not, what kinds of issues might motivate you to do so?

References

American Civil Liberties Union. (2012). *Growing up locked down: Youth in solitary confinement in jails and prisons across the United States*. New York: Human Rights Watch. Retrieved from www.aclu.org/files/assets/us1012webwcover.pdf

Buffington, K., Dierkhising, C., & Marsh, S. (2010). Ten things every juvenile court judge should know about trauma and delinquency. *Juvenile Family Court Journal, 3*, 13–23.

Eilperin, J. (2016, January 26). Obama bans solitary confinement for juveniles in federal prisons. *The Washington Post*, p. A1. Retrieved from https://washingtonpost.com/politics/obama-bans-solitary-confinement-for-juveniles-8

Grisso, T. (2008). Adolescent offenders with mental disorders. *Future Child, 18*(2), 143–164.

Holman, B., & Zeidenberg, J. (2006). *The dangers of detention: The impact of incarcerating youth in detention and other secure facilities*. Washington, DC: Justice Policy Institute. Retrieved from www.justicepolicy.org/images/upload/06-11_rep_dangersofdetention_jj.pdf

Office of Juvenile Justice and Delinquency Prevention. (2013). *Juveniles in residential placement, 2010*. Washington, DC: Author. Retrieved from www.ojjdp.gov/pubs/241060.pdf

Persons, R. (2009). Art therapy with serious juvenile offenders. *International Journal of Offender Therapy and Comparative Criminology, 53*(4), 433–453.

Williams, R. (2002). Entering the circle: The praxis of arts in corrections. *Journal of Arts Management, Law, and Society, 31*(4), 293–303.

Conflicting Interests

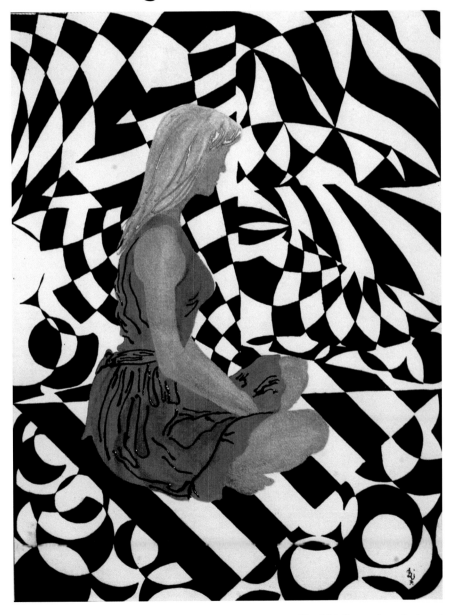

Bani Malhotra *(see color insert)*

18

AN AMERICAN ART THERAPIST IN FRANCE

30 Years of Teaching and Supervising European Art Therapists and Practicing Art Therapy

Elizabeth Stone

When I was young, I imagined living in a Paris garret, spending my days painting. Never did I expect to find myself living in southeastern France, long after that unrealized dream of my idealistic youth had been forgotten. A serendipitous vacation to Provence led to my leaving New York City, where I had been practicing and teaching art therapy, and supervising art therapists and student interns. Though I fiercely cherished my profession as an art therapist and, then, as a psychoanalyst, I didn't know how, or even if, I would be able to continue my career in my new surroundings. Eventually, I did build a new practice, but my new professional life began by teaching and supervising in Italy, Switzerland, and France.

Providing Training in Countries Where Art Therapy is Just Developing

A summer program in which I had been invited to teach generated enough interest to establish one of the first art therapy training programs for Italians, a collaborative effort of an Italian organization and the university where I had taught in the US. Upon meeting the eight students whom I was to supervise, I was surprised to find that their academic levels were markedly uneven; one or two had barely more than a high school education, although they were bright, creative, and motivated. Ethically, how could I train them to become art therapists when admission to the American program where I had been teaching required a minimum of a bachelor's degree? To complicate matters, there was a lack of educational equivalency among the professions from which art therapy candidates were drawn. Until 1990, an undergraduate degree was not required to teach elementary and middle school. In many European countries, the fine arts diploma awarded by *beaux arts* academies was not considered to be on a par with a college degree.

Was I to jettison prerequisite coursework altogether? Was working in a culture constructed differently from my own ample justification to alter standards? Was I was transgressing a code of professionalism to which I had tacitly agreed in the US? What did it mean, ethically, to impose, upon those of a different culture, my own standards regarding the content and quality of training, as well as the quantity of hours needed for coursework and internship? Although I was clearly not in my own culture, I was still in my own profession. I often felt as if I were in a kind of time warp that had propelled me back to the early days of art therapy in the States, when the field's pioneers—my mentors and elders—were just sorting out what the field was about. The newly trained art therapists and students in these European countries couldn't know the steps that would lie ahead, but I could often foresee that path, as a result of having witnessed the development of the profession in the US. Referring too much to what had been done there would be ethnocentric, as though I weren't encouraging the natural growth of art therapy in its own endemic way, while choosing not to address the many issues that would have ethical and clinical implications would be less than forthright of me.

A tangential but not unrelated dilemma was whether it was ethical to train art therapists to practice a profession that, according to their government, didn't exist. Art therapy remained unrecognized as a legitimate form of therapy because, under the law, only those with a degree in medicine or psychology could practice. Eventually, a measure of cross-cultural understanding enabled me to accept the situation as it was. I had to hope that, once the profession gained traction, grandfathering would eventually resolve the problem faced by those with lesser prerequisite qualifications. I often suggested that these students continue their academic education to be as prepared as possible for inclusion in eventual governmental recognition of the profession, if and when it should arrive.

Not all ethical dilemmas were based upon cultural differences, but to navigate the culture(s) in which I lived and worked, I had to understand them. The American Art Therapy Association's (AATA's) *Ethical Principles for Art Therapists* (2013) provides guideposts for working to achieve *Multicultural and Diversity Competency* (Standard 7), such as "Art therapists are aware of their own values and beliefs and how these may affect cross-cultural therapy interventions" (7.3). Also:

> Art therapists acquire knowledge and information about the specific cultural group(s) with which they are working and the strengths inherent in those cultural groups. They are sensitive to individual differences that exist within cultural groups and understand that individuals may have varying responses to group norms.
>
> *American Art Therapy Association, 2013, standard 7.5*

At the same time, I had to balance the above with my responsibility to the profession, as outlined in the Art Therapy Credentials Board's (ATCB's) *Code of Ethics, Conduct, and Disciplinary Procedures* (2018), namely, "Art therapists must adhere to the ATCB standards of the profession when acting as members or employees of third-party organizations" (1.5.2). This gave rise to an array of ethical issues.

A Sampler of Ethical Issues

Two Kisses on the Cheek ... with a Patient?

While a handshake is considered the appropriate greeting in any clinical situation in France, members of my cancer patient group kissed each other and me on both cheeks upon entering and leaving sessions. Although kissing patients is regarded as a boundary violation by US standards, may we view this parameter from a cultural and therapeutic, as well as an ethical, vantage point?

Despite my awareness of the precept prohibiting physical contact as a way in which to maintain therapeutic boundaries, once on the tarmac I realized that my evolving cross-cultural ease with French mores had changed my attitude as to what constitutes an appropriate response. In France, kissing on both cheeks signifies a friendly greeting between people who feel positively toward one other. Adolescents greet each other this way at high school, as do colleagues at work. My own physician greets me this way, though my dentist does not. I've also found the therapeutic bond with cancer patients to be a little different than that with other patients, since so much of the therapeutic focus involves the body and its vicissitudes. When a life-threatening physical illness is part of the therapeutic equation, its relationship to *life* is placed on a different plateau. Accepting the two kisses communicates a warm welcome. Though I do not exchange kisses with any client in my private practice, including those who are French, I've never worried that a therapeutic boundary was endangered by this practice.

Regulating the Fee Abroad ... What is Appropriate?

A dilemma regarding fee-setting arose when I created my private practice. Why would that dilemma be an *ethical* one? I knew that the going rate in France was substantially lower than in the US, especially for a seasoned therapist. On the one hand, I wanted my practice to work and the cost of sessions to be within reach. Insurance reimbursement was not an option for most of my clientele; only medical visits were reimbursed in France. Some of the expats in my practice were used to US fees. On the other hand, American fees would have shocked my French clientele. Some Americans working in France had already adapted to the French fee scale and would have regarded a US fee as being highly unfair. What part does my own financial need play in this equation? (And why does this question come last?)

I opted to charge fees that were consonant with what would be acceptable in France and included a sliding scale for students and others who could not afford the higher rate. On occasion, I realized that certain individuals could easily have afforded a substantially higher fee, closer to US rates, but I did not feel comfortable adopting the mindset of "sussing out" those for whom I could significantly hike fees. I could function only by making peace with myself and putting this issue behind me.

Providing Supervision through an Interpreter

To provide supervision in Italy, I needed to communicate via an interpreter. Although she and I developed a very close working relationship over nearly 20 years, since my words were always filtered through hers, the chance of error remained. If communication resulted in misunderstanding, confusion would usually show on my students' faces and I would backtrack to find out what had been unclear. I made it a point, not only when working with an interpreter, but also when working in French with students or patients, always to begin our work with this disclaimer:

> If I say anything that you don't understand or you say something that I don't understand, we must stop each other and ask to clarify what we didn't understand. We can work well together only if we scrupulously attend to this one rule.

The most difficult moments took place when, forced to respond to a delicate situation, I wondered whether doing so through an interpreter was fair and ethical, especially when a student was crying or, worse, had made a glaring error. Communicating "one person removed" might seem to lack an essential relational connection, yet, somehow, we did adapt. Because we were fortunate to have so skilled an interpreter, able to convey the necessary affective tone, we experienced the illusion that our communication was more direct than indirect, and an increasing depth of exchange ensued.

An Internship Placement with No Door?

Student field placements were difficult to obtain in another European country where art therapists were few and far between. As a supervisor, I worked with administrators to ensure that conditions such as the physical space were adapted to the special needs of art therapy. Although school, student, and placement contracts were signed before students could begin work, glitches did occur. Only by discussing in supervision what one student's room looked like did I learn that it had no door and that staff could walk through at any time. Eager to begin clinical work, the student figured that the issue could be addressed after he began his work, without serious impact.

Our own image of an art therapy space is not necessarily the same as that of an administrator, who is usually only minimally familiar with art therapy. Although we have to be realistic, adjusting our expectations regarding less than ideal spaces, we can insist upon certain "musts" below which the space becomes untenable therapeutically. Among the attributes of a "safe, functional environment" (Standard 1.8) listed in AATA's ethics code (2013) is the "allowance for privacy and confidentiality" (1.8.f). We cannot assume that the space is adequate unless we ask the student to describe it. For that reason, I always ask students to draw detailed maps of their spaces and their access to them, an idea Vera Zilzer taught us during the very first art therapy course I took. Without privacy, neither a sense of confidentiality nor a therapeutic alliance can be constructed. Only when this student obtained a closed space was I comfortable that he begin clinical work.

Wearing a Smock … an Ethical Dilemma?

A student I supervised was working with Martin, age four, who didn't want to wear a smock. He told her that he didn't get dirty. The student permitted him to paint without a smock and soon Martin became so absorbed that, instead of using a brush, he used his fingers, then a rag; before long, he was covered with paint.

As we endeavor to create a therapeutic atmosphere offering choices, insistence upon protocol can seem like a contradiction. I've learned that to construct a climate of safety, the clothing of clients (regardless of their age) needs to be protected from becoming soiled in art therapy. We tacitly communicate the symbolic *freedom* to create without fear of getting dirty when the smock/apron is donned upon entering the room. By not protecting this child's clothing, we invariably expose him to parental criticism or punishment and possibly sabotage his future desire to be involved with *messy* art materials. Wearing a smock is, thus, a therapeutic and an ethical issue.

An Intern's Concern about a Patient Goes Unheeded by Staff

A student interning at a psychiatric hospital came to her third supervision session distraught about the suicide of a patient. The student had observed this man to be closed and without affect during the week or two preceding his death. She had brought his artwork to the staff meeting and communicated her concern, but the staff had detected nothing noteworthy or alarming.

When we examined the artwork in supervision, her fellow students felt that the drawings looked like explosions. The intern explained that, on the contrary, when the patient was creating them, to her they felt more like implosions. She had sensed a great gap between his silence and the violence in his work.

On the one hand, it was important for me to address her guilt and sadness that she had not prevented his death; on the other, it was important to point out that, by being attuned to the relational process, her counter-transference enabled her to comprehend more about the meaning of the artwork by being so present for him in the session than simply identifying characteristics of the art product afterward. The contrast between his drawings and his affect informed and alerted her to a danger she could not avert.

Although the ethical dilemma here appears somewhat concealed by the clinical, a suicide always has an ethical dimension. Two aspects of it emerged for me. The first was that, as in many European programs, supervision took place only once a month in this program, due not only to the lack of funding for more frequent supervision, but also to the distance many students had to travel to get to classes. To bridge the gap, I gave students my contact information to use if needed between our supervisory sessions. However, the fact that a student would comply with the conclusion of the staff at her internship site, rather than seek out a second opinion, is understandable. Had she called me, what would I have said? How accurately could I have determined the degree of danger to be over the phone? In those days, instant Internet reception of imagery did not yet exist. This is why direct contact in supervision is so important.

The second ethical concern I derived from this vignette is that our profession has not yet elucidated an ethical principle regarding the way in which artwork is to be understood. Nevertheless, establishing an ethical mode of comprehension continues to be centrally relevant to our being able to do our work.

MY ETHICAL DILEMMA

When a religious patient creates transgressive imagery in art therapy, how should I respond?

Nadima, aged 36, was a recent immigrant to Europe from a strict Muslim country. A well-educated professional in her own country, both she and her husband had grown up in somewhat Westernized families. Her husband had lived abroad for many years before their marriage.

In her first art therapy session with my intern, she copied an unabashedly sexy woman from a magazine ad. Proud to have drawn the human figure for the first time, Nadima was eager to show it to her husband, although such a depiction was forbidden by her religion. Next, she made a collage using mixed-gender body parts, a tiger's head, buttocks, and phallic-like artifacts. The intern noted a lack of restraint in her art expression, the result of which was an assemblage of fragmentation and dismemberment. The content was atypical for someone of her culture, given the taboos she still practiced at home. Nadima appeared more fragile than the student had realized at first. Was she trying to prove that she could easily adapt to a Western view of culture and sexuality? Imagine that you were this intern's supervisor.

How would you respond?

For the writer's response, see Appendix B, page 434.

MY ETHICAL DILEMMA

When the presence of a painting on an art therapist's wall poses an ethical dilemma, how should I proceed?

When setting up my private practice, I was pleased to acquire a painting by an artist friend, Margaret Mortifée, which I hung on my wall. As a cancer survivor, she had painted a somewhat abstract nude bathed in blue light and then realized that her struggle over the way the right breast was painted corresponded to coming to terms with her feelings about the tumor in her own breast. I appreciated the painting for both its symbolic and aesthetic messages.

At first, my adult practice consisted primarily of women. Over the years, my clientele came to include more men, as well as people from a wider range of countries, including Islamic countries. Though no one questioned or commented negatively upon this painting, I began to wonder whether it was still appropriate to display it on my wall.

How would you respond?

For the writer's response, see Appendix B, page 435.

Concluding Thoughts

Reflecting upon these 30 years, the challenges have been many and humbling, but my experience abroad has offered me a wide lens through which to view and even to reevaluate my life and my work. Getting to know the many individuals with whom I have collaborated, in several languages, including students, clients, and colleagues, has changed the sense I make of my world. Having entered this cultural terrain essentially without ready-made guideposts, except those very substantive ones provided to me as an AATA member and an ATCB credential holder, I have been privileged to witness these worlds grow closer over the years.

REFLECTIVE ART EXPERIENCES & DISCUSSION QUESTIONS

1. Recall a time when, as an art therapy practitioner, educator, or supervisor, you felt out of synch with the prevailing way of doing things or the clinical approach to art therapy, due to cultural differences that went against the grain of your own ethical convictions. Draw the extent to which you felt that you could express those convictions honestly and how that made you feel.
2. Think of an occasion when you that felt you had a crucial clinical contribution to make to a treatment team regarding a client but found that staff weren't listening or disagreed with you and closed the discussion. Draw how you felt about not being able to convey the importance of your views. Does this stir up other such moments in your life when you felt not listened to? Make a second drawing, illustrating your counter-transference.
3. As an art therapist, educator, or supervisor, what are your expectations of yourself in handling ethical differences that arise as you realize that your art therapy standards of practice differ markedly from those in the prevailing culture?
4. Discuss the ethical dimensions of working within a hierarchical structure with respect to your position as art therapist, describing an instance from your own professional experience when you felt that your views were not taken seriously enough.

References

American Art Therapy Association (2013). *Ethical principles for art therapists*. Alexandria, VA: Author.

Art Therapy Credentials Board (2018). *Code of ethics, conduct, and disciplinary procedures*. Greensboro, NC: Author.

19

ART FOR SALE?

Using Client Art for Promotional Purposes

Lisa Raye Garlock

I am in the midst of an unexpected ethical dilemma. It started when an alumna of our program asked if we would show, in our art therapy gallery, artwork that a city-sponsored community organization had collected from groups that work with at-risk youth, adults in addiction recovery, and adults with disabilities or mental illness. On the face of it, it sounded like a good idea; it would allow us to support mental health anti-stigma awareness within the community.

I went to see the artwork at a local cafe and to choose 20 pieces to exhibit at our gallery. The pictures covered the wall, with no apparent thought to their placement. There were pieces that looked as though young children had made them (a watercolor of a crude house with a tree and fence); pieces that were disturbing because of subject matter (gang symbols, figures being choked); disorganized images that were hard to make sense of; and pieces that were heartfelt but poorly executed (images that were flat or copied from popular culture). The artwork had been made in a variety of settings, under the supervision of art therapists. Consent forms had been signed, which on the face of it should be enough, so why was I feeling so uncomfortable? Some of my first thoughts were:

- How is this serving the people who made the artwork?
- How is this addressing the stigma of mental illness?
- I don't want to show this in our gallery.

As the curator of a public art therapy gallery within a Graduate Art Therapy Program, it is my job to create a professional space that will not only showcase the artist identity of art therapists—something I feel very strongly about—but also be provocative, informative, and stimulating. We have two student shows a year (by incoming art therapy students and by those who are just about to graduate) as well as a themed, juried, or special guest exhibit each year. All must be related in some way to art therapy.

Thinking about exhibiting patient work raises many questions:

* Where does the work come from?
* Are there consent forms?
* Are they comprehensive and understood by the signer?
* What does the art look like?
* In what context was it created?
* What is the purpose of showing the work?
* How does it affect the patient who made it?
* Who benefits from showing it?
* What or whom does it promote?
* Is it for sale and, if so, who gets the money and how is it distributed?

As I looked at the pieces lining the walls of the café, I was concerned that it had been made because someone (art therapist, artist, counselor, or well-meaning volunteer) had encouraged the patients to create *something*. The patients might have had no interest in the directive or in making art, but complied because they felt pressured or coerced, because everyone else in the group was doing it, or because they were overmedicated. The creative process—making something from nothing—is important for many reasons, including engaging kinesthetically with materials, getting out pent-up emotions, communicating with self and others, reducing anxiety, improving mood, building self-esteem, making something meaningful. The creative act can be enough; exhibiting its results may be unnecessary. While Carl Jung (1954/1966; 1933) encouraged his patients to express themselves artistically and believed that spontaneous artwork was a key to healing, he gave the impression that it would be a disservice to his patients to let them think that they were artists. He seemed to think that the work was too important to exhibit as *Art*. Even though I'm a big proponent of everyone making art, of art exhibits, and of promoting art therapy, I found myself wondering if it would be ethical to show this client artwork. What do you think? How would you decide?

It is important to be attuned to right and wrong when it comes to protecting vulnerable clients and listening to our bodies can help inform our actions. When something feels wrong in relation to a client or that client's artwork, I feel it in my body. The feeling is similar to the stress response: an increased heart rate, sweating, a prickly sensation on my skin, rapid breathing, increased alertness, and an awareness that something isn't right. And, indeed, these were some of the feelings I had when I looked at the client artwork at the cafe. The stress response is designed to keep us safe, to help us react in dangerous situations. When I'm experiencing these sensations in the midst of an ethical dilemma, it can be confusing, as there is no actual immediate threat, but it is my responsibility to explore whatever is triggering this response and to determine the most ethical course of action. I often experience discomfort until I decide what to do. What I find confounding about ethical dilemmas is that sometimes this discomfort lingers even after a decision is made—and sometimes the ethical dilemma cannot be resolved.

MY ETHICAL DILEMMA

Shirley Mason's artwork: To exhibit or not to exhibit?

When we were offered the opportunity to exhibit the artwork of Shirley Mason several years ago, we jumped at the chance. Mason, an artist and an art teacher who had a diagnosis of multiple personality disorder, was the subject of the popular book entitled *Sybil* (1973) by Schreiber and Wilbur (the latter was Shirley's therapist). The book, which speculates that extreme abuse led Mason to develop 16 "alters," was later made into two TV movies. The artwork that was offered to us to exhibit was found after Mason's death and there was no way of knowing if any of the work was done in therapy. After we agreed to show the work, I read Nathan's book, *Sybil Exposed: The Extraordinary Story Behind the Famous Multiple Personality Case* (2011), which posits that the book entitled *Sybil* was largely fiction. Though it was her therapist, not Shirley Mason, who was responsible for the story, showing the artwork in our gallery suddenly raised a lot of questions for me:

- Did this artwork have anything to do with art therapy?
- Could it even be seen as related to trauma?
- What was this exhibit promoting?

Shirley Mason died in 1998, her therapist died in 1992, and Nathan's book was published in 2011. What was the truth? At this point in time, was it even possible to know? I wondered whether we should go ahead with the exhibit of Shirley Mason's work.

How would you respond?

For the writer's response, see Appendix B, page 407.

MY ETHICAL DILEMMA

Community-based artists' studios and art therapy: Is it a good fit?

Some of our art therapy interns were based at an artists' studio that was designed as a day program where adults with developmental and cognitive disabilities could focus upon art making. The organization maintained a website and arranged exhibits where the goal was to sell their clients' art. Many of the participants identified as artists; others had an interest in, or an affinity for, art. The process of working in a studio helped the artists to become better socialized, to express themselves more effectively, and to engage in meaningful work.

- Should art therapists work in this type of environment?
- Is making suggestions or giving directions about design, layout, colors, and technique contrary to the goals of art therapy?
- What about when the goal seems to be the sale of the artwork?

An open studio format within community-based organizations is another place where people create art and may have the opportunity to exhibit and sell their work. In one of these open studios, a homeless man, working with an art therapist, made art which then was exhibited. His work sold, which was exciting for him, especially since he needed the money. He created more work, but it didn't sell. Selling artwork is rarely easy, and it's usually difficult to make enough money from art to make a living. So is it giving false hope and setting unrealistic expectations to exhibit and sell client artwork? Will a client who may have delusions or isn't in touch with reality really understand it when his art sells and then doesn't and be able to handle it emotionally?

How would you respond?

For the writer's response, see Appendix B, page 408.

MY ETHICAL DILEMMA

Exhibiting art created in supervision: A good idea?

Several years ago, we organized an art project that involved on-site supervisors and their interns. Each person was given a silk mandala and could create imagery however they wanted—together or separately. The timing was such that it could be used as a termination art project about the supervisory experience. Everyone involved was asked to sign a consent-to-exhibit form; they were given the choice of having their mandala be part of a permanent installation or retrieving it after the initial exhibit. While most interns and supervisors readily participated, one supervisor was horrified by the idea of art therapists and art therapy interns making art to exhibit. As art therapists, is it our professional responsibility to make art, ourselves? Since exhibiting art helps to educate the public about what we do, is it our responsibility to exhibit our work as well?

How would you respond?

For the writer's response, see Appendix B, page 408.

Consent is Much More Than Just a Signed Piece of Paper

While our profession's ethics codes address the exhibition and use of client artwork (noting the importance of obtaining signed, informed consent to exhibit, photograph, reproduce, copy, or otherwise use client artwork, as well as ensuring the confidentiality of its creators), when endeavoring to treat clients and their artwork ethically, there is much more to consider. There are usually far more questions—such as the ones posed throughout this chapter—than answers and the answers will vary, depending upon the individual patients, the context, and the purpose.

I'm involved with an organization that does trauma work with survivors of gender-based violence. The founder is a psychologist with a keen interest in art therapy and she is very respectful of our field. One of the aspects of the treatment format is sewing story cloths. The story cloths are inspired by Chilean *arpilleras* that were originally made to tell the stories of oppression, torture, and the disappearance of people during the dictatorship of Augusto Pinochet. The making of the story cloths and the telling of the story in community is healing and empowering; the participants also have the option of exhibiting their *arpilleras* if they so choose. One outcome of the program is that participants may get to a point where they want to advocate for themselves and others, making their stories public through exhibitions. Historically, *arpilleras* were used for advocacy; today, that can be a next step toward putting trauma in the background and moving forward in life.

Alter-Muri (1994) gives an excellent example of the complicated process of working, over several years, with a client diagnosed with schizophrenia and the time, commitment, and perseverance it took to help the client move forward, through art making and exhibiting his work. Alter-Muri was clear about when exhibiting is important and should be part of the treatment plan, while cautioning that exhibiting artwork is not for all clients. Serving the client's best interests must be the priority. Shared decision-making and an understanding of the power differential is critical in choosing to exhibit client art (Leenstra, Goldstraw & Rumbold, 2014), as are in-depth discussions about what happens emotionally for the client before, during, and after artwork is exhibited.

Conclusion

Thinking back to the dilemma I described at the beginning of this chapter, after much thought I decided to select, for our gallery's exhibit, those pieces hanging on the café wall that included an explanation about the art and the creator's struggle with addiction, mental illness, or life challenges. These were pieces that indicated that their creators seemed to be engaged in the process; to be thinking about how the art related to their lives; and to have something that they wanted to say.

As I was hanging the work, the discomfort that I had originally felt did not subside. A colleague walked by and commented that the work was disturbing. Some artwork is meant to be unsettling, as was the case when I created—out of paint, ink, my own recycled artwork, and tape—a response to an ethical dilemma with which I was struggling (see Figure 19.1). Reflecting the tension between extremes—between white and solid black, between being torn apart and reconciled—it represents the

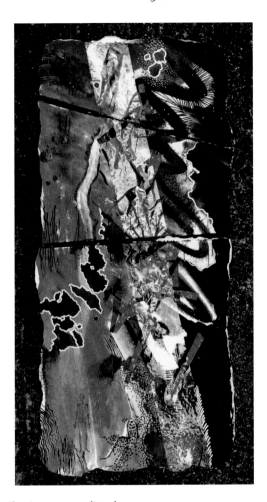

FIGURE 19.1 Art that is meant to disturb.

conflicting emotions and thoughts that occur during the struggle to decide what action to take.

If client artwork is unsettling, are the clients aware that it is? Are they trying to make a point or are they unwittingly exposing a confused psyche? There are unanswered questions about whether exhibiting the art that is made in art therapy can help address and reduce the stigma of mental illness or whether the confusion that is sometimes conveyed by the art can have the opposite effect, confirming stereotypical notions about people in need of help. In order to make real change, more work needs to be done collectively, over time, to increase both the clients' and the public's understanding of these artistic creations. It might be my ethical responsibility to contact the agencies involved in this annual project to discuss how best to educate and assist the public in understanding the effects of stigma, misunderstandings, and unconscious bias upon people with mental illness and other disabilities.

When I walked past the client work the following week, I thought that it fit well within the overall exhibit. It was hung in a balanced, appealing format, with a prominent sign explaining its purpose and where it came from. The exhibit provided an interesting juxtaposition of the art of art therapists-in-training and the art of people with whom they'll be working in their internships and future careers. People with mental illnesses have difficulty "fitting in" society. Here, their artwork, at least, does fit in. Are these thoughts rationalization to relieve my discomfort? Am I being patronizing? What will I do next time this type of dilemma presents itself? Sometimes the best we can do is to ask ourselves the right questions.

REFLECTIVE ART EXPERIENCES & DISCUSSION QUESTIONS

1. Have you ever had a client who insisted upon showing his or her artwork to the public, even though it was graphic or extremely personal and had the potential to harm the client or trigger a viewer? How did (or how would) you respond?
2. Meditate on an ethical dilemma you've faced relating to client artwork. Consider what made you uncomfortable and note where and what feelings you experience in your body. If an image comes to mind, draw it; if none comes to mind, create an abstract image related to your physical sensations.
3. Imagine that you (or your interns) are training at a school for children with special needs. Noted for the artwork that their students make, the school exhibits, sells, and gives it to visitors and funders. You discover that it is not the students but the aides who are creating the artwork. How would you respond?
4. Make a scribble drawing, recalling an ethical dilemma you've experienced; note any sensation in your body as you recall the dilemma. Look at the scribble from all directions. If any images reveal themselves, bring them out with colors and line, and consider what they may convey in relation to your dilemma.

References

Alter-Muri, S. (1994). Psychopathology of expression and the therapeutic value of exhibiting chronic clients' art: A case study. Art *Therapy: Journal of the American Art Therapy Association.* 11(3), 219–224.

Jung, C.G. (1933). *Modern man in search of a soul* (W.S. Dell & C. F Baynes, Trans.). New York: Harcourt, Brace.

Jung, C.G. (1966). *The practice of psychotherapy: Essays on the psychology of the transference and other subjects* (2nd ed.) (R. F. C. Hull, Trans.). Princeton, NJ: Princeton University Press. (Original work published 1954.)

Leenstra, S., Goldstraw, S., & Rumbold, B. (2014). Thinking about the arts as evidence. *Journal of Applied Arts & Health.* 5(2), 227–234.

Nathan, D. (2011). *Sybil exposed: The extraordinary story behind the famous multiple personality case.* New York: Free Press.

Schreiber, F., & Wilbur, C. (1973). *Sybil.* Washington, DC: Henry Regnery.

20

ART THERAPY IN CHILE

The Ethical Challenges and Dilemmas of an Emerging Professional Practice

Pamela Reyes H.

My work over the last 18 years has taken place mainly in the academic field, training and supervising art therapists doing research and psychotherapy through art, and within the community. Before that, I practiced art therapy in a wide variety of settings. To understand properly the ethical dilemmas that I will describe, it is necessary to provide some background regarding the particular context in which the experiences occurred, because art therapy, like any other professional field, is affected by the environment in which it takes place, in terms of its mission, its requirements, and its limitations.

Art Therapy in Chile: Contextual Challenges

Practicing art therapy in Chile requires a great deal of flexibility, creativity, and sensitivity towards the environment. First, art therapy is not a recognized profession in Chile. There are graduate training programs in art therapy, but, in Chile, training in psychotherapy—and art therapy is considered a form of psychotherapy—is geared toward professionals in psychiatry and psychology. The accreditation of training programs in psychotherapy is regulated by the Comisión Nacional de Acreditación de Psicología Clínica (the National Commission of Accreditation in Clinical Psychology).

Second, although the first graduate training in my country dates back to 2002, there are important differences among the three graduate training programs. For example, with regard to the number of hours of direct professional specialization practice required during training, 160 hours are required at one master's-level program, 650 hours are required at the other, and 60 hours are required at the postgraduate level course. Such differences have consequences for the development of a professional identity and, therefore, for the ethical formation of professionals trained in Chile. Furthermore, learning through practice constitutes an important forum within which to develop a reflexivity that promotes an appreciation of the priorities and needs of the particular context in which the work of art therapy is taking place.

The Asociación Chilena de Arteterapia (the Chilean Art Therapy Association) has 23 members, approximately 12% of the art therapists trained in art therapy programs within Chile or abroad (mainly in Spain and the United States). From the very beginning, the Association established a code of professional ethics based upon those of the American and Spanish art therapy associations, emphasizing its vision of art therapy as a form of psychotherapy. The Asociación Chilena de Arteterapia has no legal authority to exert ethical supervision of art therapists in Chile, a situation that is shared by other professional associations, such as the College of Psychologists of Chile (Pasmanik & Winkler, 2009).

Because of these conditions, art therapists have had to undergo important adaptations in terms of academic curricula, as well as professional practice, and have faced significant ethical challenges derived from uncertain, ambiguous, unstable, and demanding professional conditions. In spite of these ambiguities, the country is in need of professionals with integral and interdisciplinary approaches to take up various tasks in the health, education, and social fields. That is where Chilean art therapists are increasingly finding their niche and where we are constructing a specific professional practice.

Art Therapy in Mental Health Facilities

MY ETHICAL DILEMMA

How do I weigh the patients' right to privacy against the institution's desire to exhibit their art?

My initial activities in the field of art therapy were working in outpatient units, as well as in psychosocial rehabilitation, with people suffering from serious mental disorders (schizophrenia and other psychoses). In my first work experience, I faced pressure from mental health institutions to organize art expositions of the creative work made by patients in various art therapy workshops. Without making a distinction among the frameworks in which the different art therapy processes were carried out, I was asked, sometimes insistently, to show the work of my patients to their relatives, to the community, or to the institution, itself, at various social events in and out of the facility. Generally, these requests stemmed from a lack of knowledge of what the process of art therapy entails and the difficulty other professionals had in distinguishing art therapy from art education. On the one hand, the expositions could be a means by which to promote the social inclusion and destigmatization of people suffering from mental disorders, in that the visual work could serve as a bridge to connect viewers with the patients' visions of the world. Since they were also records of live, significant experiences within the context of a psychotherapeutic relationship and framework, I was faced with a breach of privacy and of the trust and security placed in the relationship and in the process of art therapy.

> **How would you respond?**
>
> *For the writer's response, see Appendix B, page 430.*

Furor Curandis vs. Collaboration

Since art therapy is a novel field in this country, it is sometimes seen as a curative alternative for patients who have not been treated successfully by verbal psychotherapeutic modalities. As a new treatment alternative, art therapy is fertile for the emergence of an ethical dilemma in the health field known as "furor curandis" (the false belief that therapists are able to cure or heal *any* kind of mental health problem under *any* circumstance).

A 20-year-old girl was brought by her mother to my private practice; she had quit the university and was staying at home, almost never going out. She had a mental health background in infancy and, when she was 13 years old, she was diagnosed with anorexia nervosa and depression. She self-harmed. She had a complex family history with an absent father, so lived alone with her mother. The only thing that affected her moderately was art. Her medical diagnosis was bipolar disorder, but, in spite of numerous referrals, she would not accept psychiatric support.

During twice-weekly art therapy over a period of ten months, the young woman recovered gradually, her everyday activity level an important indicator of her progress. She even considered going back to the university. Progress was also seen in her artwork, especially in its spontaneity and creativity. After one year of treatment, her mother reported that she had noticed food restriction, a symptom that had not appeared previously during our work. Her daughter was beginning to lose weight and there was a suspicion of anorexic behavior, which, in view of her background, turned her into a high risk patient. So far, I had dealt with the patient alone, conducting art therapy interventions with her and occasionally including her mother in family sessions. We had been able to identify complex situations and generate an adequate therapeutic alliance, which had constituted a successful art therapy process up to that point. After analyzing the patient's situation and the health risks that had appeared, my supervisor and I decided that it was now necessary to put a work team in place; a psychiatric evaluation would be essential in safely supporting the therapeutic process. In this young woman's case, art therapy had allowed her to make gains, but had not been sufficient to enable her to maintain and fully recover her health. I could not continue supporting her alone but needed to be able to draw upon the resources of other professionals. Unfortunately, neither she nor her mother would accept my recommendation. Ethically, could I continue to work with her under these conditions? What were my limits?

Following my supervisor's advice, I explained to my patient that I could continue working with her only under the condition that I be part of a multi-disciplinary team effort to help her. Her refusal led me to terminate our work together. I believe that recognizing our professional limitations and the conditions necessary to conduct our work in art therapy is a fundamental, and continual, exercise. I need to have a safe base upon which to develop the art therapy process, especially with patients whose problems are complex. In the analysis of this particular case, the figure of the clinical supervisor emerges as a cornerstone of an adequate therapeutic system and, therefore, as the safeguard of ethical behavior.

Art Therapy in Prisons

Perhaps one of the most extreme experiences I've had in relation to ethical dilemmas has been in the supervision of art therapy student interns in my country's prisons. The conditions in Chile's prisons are particularly deprived, with overcrowding and a culture of prisoner treatment that has been denounced by the country's human rights reports. Within this context, my students began their internships in a prison unit where women were imprisoned with their children who were under two years old. As soon as they reached the age of two, the children were separated from their mothers and the women were transferred to a regular prison where they would serve the remainder of their sentences. The children were returned to their families of origin; if there were no family members available, they would be delivered to institutions that care for minors. Thus, the art therapy students were inserted into a large social project aimed at promoting the resilience of, and the parental link between, young children and mothers who had been deprived of their freedom.

Although the art therapy activities were meant to offer individual and group support for the mental health of these women within an *art as therapy* framework, week after week, we were impacted by the precarious conditions in which we worked. The first difficulty arose from the need to find a safe place to store the artwork created during sessions. Although we had all the necessary authorizations and a place to store the art materials and the art, every week we would return to find the artwork damaged or broken. This would generate intense feelings of despair in my students, which we would need to work through. Often, at the last minute, the duties of the participants in the art therapy workshops would be changed, preventing their attendance at group. Although the group workshops were carried out in the shared spaces of the prison unit (the cafeteria or the yard), we would also offer open art workshops, which mothers could attend with their children, working individually, jointly, or collectively. During this activity, the women would talk about their everyday problems, share the care of their children, or learn some new art technique, which meant a great deal to some of them. Although we know that learning art is not a particular objective of art therapy, it constituted a significant experience for the women, as their life histories were marked by social and cultural abandonment and negligence, both materially and spiritually. The vigilance of the prison guards was constant, but when, on occasion, they seemed a bit more distant, the women related more freely, talking, at times, about the precarious conditions in the prison.

As the four-month art therapy workshop drew to a close, the women proposed making a collective mural in the dormitories, reflecting the growth of the group. The additional permits to carry out the activity were requested and the design and painting of the mural began. The images referred to the women and their histories.

The production of the mural took approximately one week. While the group was celebrating its accomplishment, without prior notice, a guard entered the group and removed from one of the mothers a boy who was about to turn two years old. The mother was immediately taken to the common prisoners unit, in a different prison, while her child was placed with a family who would take care of him. This generated a collective degree of anguish, grief, and uncertainty that is difficult to fathom. In the following days, a violent search of the unit took place by guards looking for weapons, cell-phones, and drugs. The group mural activity ended in this disruptive context.

This experience made my students and me, as their supervisor, question the sense of what we were doing, as there was such strong dissonance between the social and therapeutic support that we envisioned and the violence of the environment in which we were trying to help it take root. The greatest ethical dilemma was that our interventions had sensitized and opened up the women, within a place that provided no support for personal growth, but rather the opposite. We even asked ourselves whether our interventions could be manipulated by a system that wanted to show positive behavioral rehabilitation but could not (or would not) change its conditions. In setting up interventions in this field, the importance of appreciating the unique social, cultural, and psychological complexity of the prison environment cannot be overestimated.

Art Therapy in Response to Natural Disasters

On February 27, 2010, Chile suffered one of the most intense earthquakes and tsunamis of the last 30 years. As an art therapist, I worked first as a volunteer for the Ministerio de Salud (The Ministry of Health), helping to set up resources in the communities and to place health teams in localities affected by the emergency; later, I worked as a member of psychosocial projects that were assisting in the recovery of these communities.

These kinds of disasters attract a large number of helping volunteers and organizations at both the national and international levels. Especially during the first stages of a post-disaster emergency, everybody wants to help and collaborate. But, as we know, the risk of this immediate, short-term voluntary aid lies not only in the *over-intervention* bestowed upon some recipients while others go wanting, but also in the difficulty in articulating and organizing the different levels of territorial collaboration required not just in the emergency stage, but throughout the long-term recovery of the communities in question.

Because of this, I found it challenging to respond to calls from international and national organizations which were offering art or other mental health therapies to support our communities during the emergency. An ethical dilemma arose in me when I asked myself how I would respond to offers of what I call "express" (brief, externally designed) interventions that, nevertheless, (a) depend upon local field work to implement them and (b) do not consider the capacity of the locals (individuals, as well as social, religious, governmental groups) to face the crisis. Moreover, most of the mental health interventions proposed were derived from a counseling and/or individual and group psychotherapy model, not from a socio-community vision. On the one hand, my dilemma was technical, in that I asked myself what the value of such post-disaster psychosocial interventions would be; on the other hand, I questioned the type of social commitment that generated such a brief intervention with a population that had been so violently affected by the disaster.

That questioning made me look for alliances with different teams within the country, teams that would not simply provide relief, but would invest in the creation of recovery-oriented psychosocial support programs that would last at least two years. I believed that communities had the right to expect that the interventions, programs, or projects that they were offered were supported by sustainable evidence and that the psychosocial interventions would develop the local capacities necessary to maintain the achievements of those interventions. This is particularly relevant in post-disaster socio-natural interventions, where recovery implies reinforcement of the social web of the affected community.

Concluding Thoughts

In reflecting upon the various ethical dilemmas that I have faced in my professional practice as an art therapist in Chile, I have observed a guiding thread, an axis that crosses my ethical dilemmas and the way in which I have sought to resolve them. I recognize in my statements a given notion of *person*, a vision of the other who is suffering. That "other" is the one who is asking me for help in my clinical therapeutic practice or the ones who are calling for aid, as in the communities affected by disasters. In both cases, I am dealing with an "other" who is suffering, and confirming that suffering puts me in a situation of responsibility that I think is fundamental to guiding the ethical practice of the art therapist. I became *aware*; an echo of the ideas of Emmanuel Levinas: "For others, in spite of myself, from myself" (Orange, 2012, p. 92).

REFLECTIVE ART EXPERIENCES & DISCUSSION QUESTIONS

1. Create an image in response to the "Art Therapy in Prisons" case presentation and add three free association words. Think about how your own work is linked to the ethical dilemma described in this case.
2. Cut out words and images from magazines and create a collage in response to the settings described in "Art Therapy in Response to Natural Disasters." Ask yourself what you would do in this situation.
4. Do you think that the "furor curandis" dilemma is a risk only for young art therapy professionals or can it be a risk throughout your entire career?
5. What other ethical dilemmas can be seen when institutions ask us to expose (in institution-sponsored exhibits and the like) artwork that was created by clients in art therapy?

References

Orange, D. (2012). *Thinking for clinicians: Philosophical resources for contemporary psychoanalysis and the humanistic psychotherapies.* Santiago, Chile: Cuatro Vientos Edit.

Pasmanik, D., & Winkler, M.I. (2009). Searching for orientation: Guidelines for teaching professional ethics in psychology in a context with a postmodern emphasis. *Psykhe* (Santiago), 18(2), 37–49. https://dx.doi.org/10.4067/S0718-22282009000200003

21

'I AM NOT DISORDERED, I AM SPECIAL'

Ethical Issues Faced by Art Therapists in the Evolving World of Children with Special Needs

Laurie Mowry-Hesler

For 35 years, I have had the privilege of working as an art therapist and Marriage Family therapist in five different kinds of settings designed to treat children who struggle with psychological and/or developmental issues. This chapter focuses upon ethical issues that have arisen due to the context within which treatment has taken place, the goals and expectations of treatment, and even the definition of treatment. It describes ethical issues that I have confronted in my work with children in residential treatment, community-based services, special education schools, home-based settings, and private practice. It is my hope that these "snapshots" will present a picture of how the treatment of children with a variety of clinical issues has evolved over time.

The Evolution of Treatment of Children with Mental Health Issues

From the 1970s through the 1990s, beneficent treatment meant that children struggling with social/emotional, behavioral problems were treated within public schools, psychiatric hospitals, residential treatment centers, or group homes. Children were diagnosed and labeled; treatment teams collaborated upon drawing up "Master Problem Lists," spelling out areas of deficiency. Special education schools were just emerging for the treatment of children who were labeled "Emotionally Disturbed" or "E.D."

Children whose home lives subjected them to abuse or neglect were often removed from their homes and placed in foster care (sometimes for several years at a time) or provided with institutional care (usually far from home, making it difficult for family to visit; often lasting one or more years). The objective was to promote the child's well-being through removal from an "unhealthful" environment and placement in a "healthful" environment where corrective treatment would be most effective.

Over the years, the labels and conceptualizations used to identify a child's issues have shifted away from problem-centered to child-centered. Recognition that a child's identity is not rooted in the problems they face and cannot be summed up by a diagnostic label became central in viewing the child as a person who has strengths as well as weaknesses; this helped define treatment as a means by which to overcome adversity by attaining a state of well-being and resiliency. Today, the terminology and methodology of treatment have evolved to reflect a more comprehensive approach. Treatment for "special needs" children is believed to be most effective when they remain within their support systems—and when those systems receive the services required to promote health. Removal from the family and community of a child struggling with psychological and/or developmental issues is seen as a last resort, to be considered only after all other treatment services have been exhausted.

Residential Treatment

During the 1970s–1990s, art therapists became integral parts of many treatment programs, providing adjunctive therapy. From the mid- to late 1980s, I was an art therapist within an Expressive Therapy Department at a large residential treatment center that had been built as an orphanage in 1888 and been operational until the mid-1900s—representing another bygone era of caring for disenfranchised children.

The converted facility housed 150 children from 4–10 years of age, who lived in six cottages of 25 children each for 6–12 months. All residents were considered wards of the court and had been placed in residential care due to physical abuse, sexual abuse, or neglect. For most, reunification with their biological or foster family was the goal; for others, the goal was adoption or group home placement. Most of the children exhibited severe behavioral issues due to neglect, abuse and/or mental health.

Ethical challenges

The Expressive Therapy Department was housed in a separate building that had been the laundry/boiler room and infirmary for the orphanage. The renovated space was designed for art, music, movement, and recreational therapies. The art room occupied the former laundry/boiler room—a vast, open space with exposed pipes. How could such an echo chamber be turned into a therapeutic milieu that reflected warmth and safety for individual and groups of small children who would occupy only a fraction of the room? The answer came in the form of hanging plants, sectional furnishings, and a floor newly painted in colorful segments that divided the room into areas for clay work, painting, and drawing.

Multidisciplinary services were offered to maximize therapeutic impact, but ethical issues related to autonomy arose frequently, due to the children's status of "wards of the court." Consequently, few parents were involved in their children's treatment; for those who were, it was limited to an hour of therapy weekly or biweekly. Thus, decisions made on behalf of the children were made by a collection of professionals who were virtually strangers to those children. Family or ethnic culture was not well known or understood. It was difficult for children to make attachments in the absence of their parents and they often struggled to understand the reasons they were taken from their homes. Unintended consequences of attachment issues were created or reinforced. Some residents formed attachments to the expressive therapists due to the trust developed in therapy and to viewing the afterschool programs as an enjoyable component of their day.

In addition to the children's confusion regarding their placement (or displacement), families, also, were confused and disconnected from their children's experience in treatment. They struggled with shame and resentment when professionals, whom they distrusted, offered "health" to their children. The Expressive Therapy Department attempted to address these issues through family art therapy. The process offered a better understanding of family dynamics, but raised other ethical issues, such as how to maintain a clear understanding of who the client was and how to protect the child's confidentiality. The family often wondered about their own confidentiality, with regard to the rest of the treatment team. Thus, families struggled with guardedness and mistrust.

A struggle for autonomy and a family disenfranchised

Reggie was a four-year-old African American male who—along with his two-year-old brother and an infant brother who was born addicted to crack cocaine—had been removed from his mother and grandmother, due to neglect. The mother was an addict; the grandmother was a crack dealer. Bullet holes riddled the outside of their house, while, inside, there was little food, few furnishings, and no sheets or blankets on the beds. The children could not bathe, due to wet clothing being kept in the bathtub. Initially, all three boys were placed in foster care together. However, due to Reggie's severe behavioral reactions, he was removed and placed in residential care. I was assigned as his case manager and individual art therapist. Each week, for months, Reggie would ask during art sessions, "Why did the policeman take me away from my mommy and grandma?" For this four-year-old, the way he had been living with his family was "normal." Now he was faced with living far from home, away from his family, with a group of 25 children older than he (making him a potential target of predatory behavior), never seeing his grandmother or mother, and visiting with his brothers only once a month. He often appealed for help to return to his family.

Clarity regarding my role and boundaries as a helper versus a therapist was important. It was challenging to explain the goals of treatment to a four-year-old child and instill hope for his future when it appeared to be so unclear. It was difficult to explain that the intervention had been made for his benefit and that no malfeasance was intended, because he did not recognize the deficits or dangers of his home, only the severing of his relationships.

Fidelity was also a very important ethical value in my work as an art therapist in residential treatment. Vigilance in demonstrating the clinical importance of the art process and the power of the artwork itself was very important, particularly since the Expressive Therapy Department was also responsible for activities such as coordinating special events and holiday celebrations. Maintaining a strong presence on the treatment teams, establishing family art therapy assessments as part of the intake protocol, and providing family art therapy helped to underscore the clinical legitimacy of the field—and helped to prevent our department from being labeled as the "activities" department.

Community Art Therapy Services

Near the end of the 20th century, support of the family system and recognition of human resiliency resulted in the increase of community-based services, reducing the need for residential services. The goal was to keep children within their homes and communities. More day treatment, in-school, and afterschool programs were developed for "at-risk" children, a term which often replaced the "E.D." label. As a contracted art therapist working for a community-based agency in an urban setting, I offered individual and group art therapy in public preschool programs for "at risk" children; in therapeutic schools for adolescents who were transitioning from juvenile detention centers back to their communities; and in afterschool programs and summer camps for high-risk youth.

Ethical issues: Safety and treatment integrity

Many of the challenges I faced doing contract work seemed to be endemic to urban areas where resources are limited and must be stretched to meet the needs of many. For example, creating functional and safe environments for art therapy was challenging due to inadequate space. The few vacant classrooms had little to no heating or cooling. At one location, I converted a large equipment closet into a therapy room. Rooms far from the child's homeroom made transitions to and from the classroom a safety issue, due to the unpredictable behavior of some children. Often, I had to provide and transport the art supplies, which limited the variety of media I could offer in sessions. Assuring privacy was difficult due to groups having to meet in cordoned-off areas. Limited storage space for artwork resulted in therapists storing artwork, ourselves, to ensure its protection and privacy. I endeavored to resolve these issues by developing alliances at each site with professionals who, having recognized the important role that art therapy played in treatment, would advocate for better conditions to be provided. The biggest lesson I learned from doing contract work was the necessity for the art therapist to have a stake in the contractual process, in order to ensure safer conditions on site and to establish the integrity of the services offered.

Special Education Schools for Children with Developmental Issues

With the rise of Autism spectrum disorders in the 21st century, private specialized schools were established to focus upon the impact of developmental issues related to school performance and socialization. The objective was to offer an alternative to public school systems that struggled to offer adequate services, such as speech and language therapy, counseling, adaptive physical education, occupational therapy, and expressive therapies that targeted not only educational delays, but also social and emotional delays, in order to treat the whole child. The philosophy was that educational success should not come at the expense of other developmental issues. A child who can find success through better peer interactions, better articulation of thoughts and feelings, and better expression of his or her talents, tends to perform better academically.

As an art therapist and art teacher, I worked in a special education school in a suburban area, with preschool through high school students who presented primarily with speech and language delays. The objective was to offer art education from a therapeutic perspective to a population diagnosed with Pervasive Developmental Delays, as well as Asperger Syndrome or mild Autism. Sensory integration issues greatly impacted a large percentage of the students. Individual art therapy was offered to students who did not respond well to verbal therapy.

Ethical challenges: Privacy and well-being

Ethical issues arose in relation to the promotional use of students' artwork. I worked with a middle school student who drew only stick-figure battle scenes for almost a year, until one day, in a life-drawing unit, he was given a mirror and asked to draw a self-portrait. The result was a stunningly realistic likeness of the adolescent! His parent was thrilled to discover her child's artistic talent and the school wanted to highlight it. I tried to mitigate this issue by designating specific projects for the creation of promotional artwork. Even then, caution was needed to screen for personally sensitive reflections in the art. I also invited visiting artists to help the children do projects that would be displayed in the school and/or in the community. A side benefit of both remedies was that they proved to be esteem-building.

Due to the fact that many of the students struggled with verbal expression, art was a powerful tool for self-expression and self-advocacy. Nikki, a 12-year-old child who had immigrated from Africa, was almost non-verbal, offering only one-word responses to questions. When in trouble—and unfortunately he was often in trouble for explosive behavior—he completely shut down verbally. After one such episode, he was brought to the art therapy room to work through the incident. Nikki loved the comic character Spiderman and drew many comic strip recreations during his individual sessions with me. Utilizing this concept, he was asked to draw what had happened in segments, like a comic strip. He dramatically drew the beginning of the story (being picked on by another child in his class), the middle (the child hitting Nikki with a ball when the teacher was not looking), and the end (Nikki hitting the instigator back). Consequently, this form of self-expression was implemented in treatment to compensate for Nikki's inability to use words to advocate for himself, as well as to promote his sense of well-being and autonomy.

Home-Based Services

In an effort to continue addressing Special Needs issues within the context of the family and community, home-based services began emerging in the early 2000s. Since the "identified client" is often both the family and the child "at risk" of being removed from the family, the objective is to go into the home to gain a better understanding of family dynamics and how the special needs child is functioning within the system. Embracing the dual role of primary therapist and art therapist, I worked on a home-based Autism specialty team. Familial evidence-based therapy, with art as the modality, was often the approach utilized. The Family Art Therapy assessment was implemented to determine the strengths and weaknesses of the family system.

Ethical challenges: Dual roles and professional integrity

The special needs of children can place strain on the family unit, requiring interventions to help the family better support their child. Other times, family issues contribute to the child's inability to overcome challenges, as in the case of a family in which all three children were diagnosed with Autism, while the mother struggled with hoarding issues. Recognizing the children's artistic abilities, the creative process was utilized as a means by which to aid decision-making and problem solving through family art therapy, establishing the art as a clinical document instead of decoration for the kitchen refrigerator. Working with the mother helped bring order to the home, so that her children could experience a safe place where therapy could take place and healthier family interactions could develop. The art process also greatly helped in promoting the understanding and the autonomy of the children, who needed an alternative means of communication.

MY ETHICAL DILEMMA

What difference would a few decades make?

Remember Reggie, the four-year-old child with whom I worked in residential treatment during the 1980s? Imagine that you are working with him now. In light of current ethical values/codes and treatment objectives, present a conceptualization of the case, as well as treatment recommendations.

How would you respond?

For the writer's response, see Appendix B, page 423.

Lessons Learned

The past should inform the present and, ultimately, the future. Now, as a private practitioner, I not only feel as though I've walked along the continuum of treatment approaches for children who have special needs, but also have the luxury of incorporating lessons learned from these varied therapeutic venues. Being clear about just who my client is, while supporting the family system (thus enabling that child to thrive *in situ*), and protecting the child's right to privacy are ethical values born of challenges faced in the midst of therapeutic work with clients. These lessons aren't the final answer, however, for current ethics codes will be challenged by future dynamics, requiring fresh approaches to new ethical dilemmas. How will you be part of the process, as an agent of change?

REFLECTIVE ART EXPERIENCES & DISCUSSION QUESTIONS

1. On one sheet of paper, draw a picture of some of your clients and add some of the terms that you have heard used to describe or define those with whom you work. On another sheet of paper, convey how you would like to see your clients addressed. Discuss how to bring that about.
2. Draw a picture of a setting in which you had to conduct art therapy sessions even though it was particularly unconducive to therapeutic work. Draw a second picture depicting what you did (or what you could have done) to try to "rehabilitate" that setting.
3. Think about providing home-based art therapy services. What kinds of ethical concerns come to mind? How might they be addressed?

22

IF NOT FOR THE GRACE OF GOD, THERE GO I

The Ethical Challenges of Providing Art Therapy and Other Services to Those Who Are Homeless

Gwendolyn M. Short

During the 35 years that I worked for a county health department, I was detailed to six programs within the addictions/mental health division. Although I had worked intermittently with "the homeless" in each program, the four years that I worked at a community outreach and treatment services program gave me the opportunity to work directly with people who were homeless. I said "opportunity," because the privilege of getting to know so many individuals shattered any preconceived notions I might have had about people who, at some point in their lives, found themselves to be without a home.

As an art therapist whose role was that of outreach worker and case manager at the program, my job was to search for the mentally ill homeless, providing them with a road to treatment and wrap-around services. In the city, people who are homeless may be seen pushing shopping carts laden with all their belongings or sleeping on park benches or steam grates. In the suburbs, homelessness can look very different. My partner and I were charged with going out into the field—which encompassed the vast corners of the county and all parts in between—not only urban areas, but also rural areas and woodlands. Although my unwritten role was that of a problem solver, the very first problem I needed to solve was my own attitude about the homeless people whom I was about to encounter. I learned to get past their appearance—and the intense smell of urine or other body odors that could, at times, make my eyes water—because bathing is not a priority over basic survival. Body odors can also be a deterrent to abuse by others or an indication that the mind has gone far beyond being concerned with cleanliness. Whenever showers were requested, however, we made arrangements for them. Our role was not to judge these individuals, but to gain their trust and get them the resources they needed. Respect and courtesy were key in helping them to understand that were not there to hurt them, but to help if we could. I felt it was important always to address, and refer to, individuals by Mr. or Mrs. before their surnames. When someone refused an offer of help, we continued to try to keep the lines of communication open, hoping that one day they might avail themselves of these services that they were entitled to.

When working with people who were homeless, we made sure that we always had bus tokens, a few dollars for coffee or a burger, gift cards to shop for necessities, forms for applying for picture identification cards or Social Security Cards, birth certificate information, and enough gas in the car to transport someone if it were needed. Most importantly, we had the phone numbers of helping agencies and the Homeless Hotline for shelter. A large city nearby provided small laminated cards showing the location of soup kitchens and shelters in relation to well-known points of interest, for those who had difficulty reading written directions. The county car we drove could double as an office for privacy and provide a little comfort from the elements.

Where Do We Find the Homeless?

The task of locating mentally ill or addicted homeless people can be daunting. Though, at times, they would approach us on their own, assistance usually came via phone calls from family, friends, or concerned citizens. Thus, a regular "day at the office" saw us scouring the streets of the county, looking for individuals who would meet our criteria for services. Some of the obvious places to look were shelters, soup kitchens, 24-hour establishments, wooded areas, and somewhat secluded areas off the beaten path. We had to be prepared for the unusual on any given day. On one occasion, responding to an anxious call from a mother, we located her daughter in an abandoned car in the southern part of the county. It was winter, after a snowfall, and the car was parked about 100 feet away, on a parking lot that was covered by a thick sheet of ice. My partner and I clung to each other as we slowly crept across the ice to the car. Spotting a young woman inside, slumped over, we knocked on her window, hoping that she had not frozen to death. Suddenly a man appeared on the other side of the car, angrily questioning why we were there. Scared beyond belief, I started talking fast, explaining that her mother was concerned about her and that we had come to check on her and see if she needed anything. When told that she was OK, I said that we needed to talk to her. At that point, the young woman rolled down the window and said that she was all right. Upon our return, a few days later, they were nowhere to be found.

Another time we received a call concerning someone who was living behind a fire station. When we arrived, we saw a fence that formed a V-shape and, nestled within it, a carefully erected, tarp-covered abode, complete with a regular-sized red door at the front. The door was there for a reason, so I knocked on it and, out from the side of the structure, came its occupant. We learned that he was quite comfortable with his situation and didn't need anything, but he agreed to call us if that changed. On another occasion, we were alerted to the fact there was an encampment under a bridge in the northern part of the county. We arrived to find a well-worn path heading down the steep hill that ran beside and underneath the bridge. In this case, my fear of inclines prevented me from risking skidding down that hill and falling and, thus, having the homeless have to try to help me, so my partner scurried down there, returning a short time later to report his findings.

Establishments that are open 24/7, especially laundromats, are popular with the homeless as they enable them to keep off the street at night. One day, in response to a call, we went to a particular laundromat and, following the description we were given, attempted to locate a young lady. As soon as our eyes met, she took off walking, then running, away from us. We followed as best we could in our county car, but she was able to lose us by ducking into yards and alley ways. We finally gave up our pursuit and returned to our office. Later, we found out that we had been pursuing the wrong person! I never said the job was easy.

Shelters

Although many people who are homeless avoid shelters, fearing a lack of privacy, theft, or violence, there are various types of shelters in the county. A men's shelter houses those 18 and over; a women's shelter accommodates single women, mothers, and children, including boys up to age 11 (the day that a boy turns 12, however, his family is no longer eligible to stay there); a family shelter houses families in individual apartments; a domestic violence shelter houses women and their children in a clandestine location; some hotels are made available for shelter residents. The Warm Nights Shelter, which a faith-based community operates from November to March, provides cots and van transportation for people who are homeless. Like many shelters, participants have to vacate the premises at 7:00 am and may return at 7:00 pm. Each Sunday, participants pack up their belongings and take them with them, as the cots are then transported to another church in the county which will provide shelter, and sometimes showers, clothes, and warm meals. Shelters are a place where we may not only look for those whose family or friends have contacted us out of concern, but also meet prospective clients and assess their need for services.

Soup Kitchens

In partnership with other churches and some corporations, a Methodist church in the county served hot lunches Monday through Friday from 12:00 to 2:00 pm. Each day, one of the churches or businesses would provide the hot lunches for those who stood in line for the free meal. Some of the churches would also hand out bag lunches for participants to take with them. My partner and I would stand in line to get our lunches and then mix and mingle with everyone there, seeking out those who might be in need of our services. I felt that it was more beneficial to be among the people than to stand on the sidelines, as observers. It was our way of quickly building trust and familiarity, and participants would often bring friends to us to resolve a problem or simply ask for a little help. The Soup Kitchen also provided a place to arrange to meet with folks who were trying to get in contact with us; at times, we would bring hungry clients there for a meal. There were also food banks, which gave out free food, but not hot meals.

Art Therapy with Those Who Are Homeless

Shelter Ladies with Children

Although I was allowed to provide art therapy services to the ladies on a voluntary basis, most would agree to come only if they brought their children with them; then, they would not want to express themselves with their children present and, if a topic became too difficult for them to discuss, they would focus upon their children. The beauty of having an intern was that we could split the session, having my intern work with the children while I worked with the adults. Since we were all in the cafeteria, the moms could keep an eye on their children, while focusing upon themselves. Since a separate table was set up for each group, far enough away from each other that it afforded the moms a degree of privacy, some took the opportunity to release pent-up feelings that would not have been appropriate for their children to witness. One of their favorite techniques was to pick an item from a list of household items, such as *stove*, *tub*, *broom*, *bed*, *curtains*, *cup*, and *lamp*; write a few sentences about the item; and then create a drawing that included the item they had chosen. This simple technique allowed them to think positively about their lives beyond the shelter; many ladies stated that it enabled them to hope for something better than the shelter.

Group Home Boys

Some might not consider boys in group homes to be homeless, since they are being housed and cared for by an agency after having been removed from their families, but, because some families don't want them back, some boys have no home to return to.

Clarence was a boy small in stature but big on following the leader. Even the beginning of his journey into the judicial system came about as a result of Clarence taking the blame for someone else's misdeeds. He was in awe of his fellow group home mates and tried to gain acceptance by mimicking the others. Art therapy offered him a way to distinguish himself.

Clarence was the only group member who decided to create a life-sized portrait. Usually very active, he laid perfectly still while I traced his outline onto brown craft paper, seeming to enjoy the process. Once completed, he was asked to complete the portrait by filling in the outlined space any way he chose. Studying his figure, Clarence carefully selected magazine pictures that appealed to him and glued them onto the craft paper, clearly ecstatic about the results. Choosing to place in the area of his heart a picture of a canoe with people paddling down a river, he proudly told me that he liked camping and the outdoors. I wondered whether the picture might also represent the shared journey that he was making with his house mates. When, with great pride and confidence, he shared his portrait with his group home mates, they listened attentively; it appeared as though Clarence had risen to a new level of respect with them.

Later in the year, Clarence lost his mother and was allowed to attend her funeral. He entered the next art therapy session clutching the funeral program. The group helped him to grieve his mom's death and he was able to pay tribute to her in his artwork, writing her name and filling the entire page with flowers of her favorite color. Again, his peers were very respectful and supportive; all of them had lost their mothers temporarily and Clarence's permanent loss seemed to make them acutely mindful of the pain of separation.

James was about to leave the program and return home. He was very enthusiastic about his hometown football team and usually portrayed them in his artwork. Since he had shared with the group that he also loved to cook, I decided that, as a final project, each member of the group would make an apron (something that James would be able to take with him). The project included measuring, cutting fabric, and learning basic sewing skills—which, I explained, everyone needed to know, so that they would be able to hem their pants, sew on loose buttons, or stitch up a tear in their clothes. The boys measured each other, cut out the pattern, and carefully hand-sewed the pieces. James came to every session, carefully worked to complete his apron, and beamed with pride as he modeled it for the group. This was his own creation and the valuable skills he had learned in the process (including the importance of following directions) had allowed him to produce something he could treasure. He left his last session a more confident young man.

MY ETHICAL DILEMMA

How should I respond when staff members limit freedom of expression in art therapy?

In contrast to the art therapy sessions at the group home described above, at another group home staff would hover over the boys during groups, noting anything they drew that was drug related and threatening to write them up for it—a measure that would terminate any up-coming weekend passes to go home. The practice of having non-clinical staff sit in on group sessions—let alone monitor the boys for conduct that they deemed inappropriate—was unacceptable; allowing non-art therapists to set rules for the way in which art therapy groups would be conducted was unethical; and the house rule that forbade drugs or drug paraphernalia to be depicted in pictures (or any reference to be made to drugs) was untherapeutic, as many of the boys came from the drug life (using, selling, or just being present when it occurred). How would I be able to engage therapeutically with the boys, encouraging their efforts to explore, understand, and work to find ways in which to resolve their concerns, if what they expressed was so severely censored? How could the very practice of art therapy be redefined by staff, inhibiting the expression of clients' thoughts and feelings? Yet, I could not encourage the boys to pursue these themes when doing so would set them up for reprimand and or punishment. At the same time, I was new to the setting and was present only once a week to conduct groups, while staff were responsible for managing what went on in the group home day in, day out.

How would you respond?

For the writer's response, see Appendix B, page 434.

Conclusion

If not for the Grace of God, there go I. Homelessness can happen to anyone, at any time. No one knows what uncertainties life will bring. Each individual I encountered had his or her own story about the journey into homelessness, whether it stemmed from a natural disaster, an illness, the loss of a job or a loved one, or the inability to survive on what the person earned on the job. I worked with individuals who had degrees, former business owners, and those who had merely fallen on hard times. Homelessness can exacerbate any mental illness and not knowing what to do can lead to drug and alcohol use and abuse, to mask the pain of what led to homelessness. A good outcome was helping someone to become stable on medication or clean and sober, to get into an appropriate treatment program and/or obtain a job, and to find appropriate, stable housing. These are the goals we worked towards every day and the joy we felt when they were reached was priceless.

REFLECTIVE ART EXPERIENCES & DISCUSSION QUESTIONS

a. Draw a picture of a homeless person.
b. Draw a picture of that person before he or she became homeless.
c. Draw a picture of that individual as someone who, formerly, was homeless.

1. Jot down your observations about each rendering. Reorder the pictures as: b, a, c. Any further thoughts?
2. Some cities have passed ordinances that enable outreach workers to pick up people who are homeless and transport them to shelters when the weather drops below a specified temperature. What are your thoughts about this?
3. How do you feel when, on the sidewalk or in a car, you see individuals who appear to be homeless? How do you react if some of those individuals ask you for money? If you respond differently to different individuals, what plays a role in your decision-making process?

23

'IT'S NOT EVEN MY FAULT'

Ethical Issues Encountered in Providing Art Therapy for Those Who Have Been Injured on the Job

Donald J. Cutcher

A family bread-winner experiences a 7500-volt electrocution at her workplace, the electrical current traveling down her left arm, through her torso, and out her foot. This results in significant physical injury, the development of reflex sympathetic dystrophy syndrome (RSD), and diagnoses of traumatic brain injury and post-traumatic stress disorder.

A young man is electrocuted via a lightning strike to the building in which he was working, the current traveling through the telephone handset he was holding and into his head before exiting his lower body. This causes significant heart damage, as well as a decrease in the functioning of other organs, the development of syncope, and problems with memory recall and sequencing.

Treatment Delayed

For 10 years, I worked with clients who had experienced physical injury and/or psychological trauma in the execution of their job duties. Often, the trauma/injury resulted in clients not being able to return to their specific type of employment—or any type of employment. This affected not only the families' income and lifestyle, but also the workers' self-image and relationships. A need to rely upon permanent benefits from the workers compensation corporation comes with its own problems, including its effect upon the self-esteem of the former worker.

The extent of this population is unknown, due to several factors. After an initial period of hospitalization and surgery, and sometimes physical therapy, many individuals try to return to work in the same field, without benefit of therapy. Even when that is not the case, the system frequently fails to provide assessment and treatment that is timely, comprehensive, and of sufficient duration to address the long-term effects of the injury. It is not unusual for people to wait 2½–5 years following their injuries to receive notification that their claim for therapeutic services has been approved. One of my clients waited for 25 years, not giving up on his desire to have his injuries recognized and remediated. Some get tired of waiting; others don't even apply.

Long-Term Effects of Job-Related Injuries

Significant electrical injuries result not only in immediate effects, but also in long-term effects, including major organ deterioration. Primeau, Engelstatter, and Bares (1995) and Bryan, Andrews, Hurley, and Taber (2009) document the delayed or progressive decline of cognitive and emotional functioning after electrical injury. Clients require the provision of on-going treatment, not a short-term intervention, to develop coping mechanisms and accept limitations on life goals and activity.

The family bread-winner described in the first vignette continued to try to support the family by returning to work in the same field, after an initial period of hospitalization and surgery, as well as physical therapy to prevent contractures of her extremities. She did this despite a significant fear of any electrical episodes, including lightning or any contact with electricity. When her employer was absorbed by another company, it resulted in constant appeals of service approval by the new employer, including denial of psychological services. This would result in service disruption for months at a time, while the case was appealed. Marital discord ensued, due to a lack of communication and a decrease in intimacy, due to pain and emotional withdrawal. This resulted in feelings of rejection, anger towards self and injury, and a lack of understanding by others in the client's immediate environment.

How Art Therapy Can Help

In addition to the creation of drawings and scribbles, art therapy included the use of technologies to compensate for the decrease in the patient's immediate memory recall and the increase in her frustration over her inability to do simple recall or even to retrieve words to express personal needs. We made use of additional techniques such as visual journaling, visual scheduling programs, and written documentation to help keep the patient focused upon her abilities rather than her deficits. The client was also introduced to visual relaxation techniques that took little time to implement and—a feature that was important to her—would not be evident to others. These were especially useful to her during painful physical therapy sessions, when exposed muscles and tendons had to be stretched and manipulated to prevent further deterioration. Of significance in this case was the patient's constant fear of not being able to provide for her family, as it was ultimately determined that she could not meet the minimum job expectations, even with modifications, which resulted in the loss of her job and in reliance upon state benefits. Coinciding with this was the consistent reduction in, and denial of, services by the system, which impacted the consistency of the patient's improvement, as well as her acceptance of the results of the injury. Her therapy provided her with a healthful environment in which she could document her fears and her anger and develop what she titled her "game plan," which she would present to her legal representative as well as her family members.

The man who was electrocuted while he was speaking on the phone at his workplace began treatment in art therapy years after he had been injured. He had participated in verbal psychotherapy, but stated that he could not be open during the sessions. In all those years, he had never shared his feelings regarding the actual trauma and had blocked all verbal communication regarding its impact. A turning point occurred in art therapy when, despite much trepidation, the client was able and willing to draw the image of a large, bold, lightning bolt above a small, lightly drawn figure and to begin to have a conversation with it, emotionally relating what it had cost him: how it had robbed him of his future and instilled a fear that he felt would never totally go away. Later he said that, until that moment, he had never confronted the image that was locked in his head, but that now he was capable of looking directly at it.

Another Population Affected by "Hidden Trauma"

A police officer is transporting an inmate who is feigning paralysis; the inmate attacks the officer, causing multiple injuries that necessitate significant surgeries. This results in the loss of the profession, as she is retired from the force for medical reasons. The officer experiences nightmares, revivification of the trauma, and fear of the attacker targeting her in the future, which causes self-isolation and fear of being in public.

A corrections officer attempts to stop an inmate from harming himself; in the process, he is exposed to the inmate's bodily fluids, putting his health at risk. During the process of trying to execute his job, he is badly injured by the inmate, resulting in medical retirement, which, in his words, has robbed him of his purpose and replaced it with a constant revivification of the emotional trauma, as well as an exasperation of the pain resulting from the physical trauma.

Another population affected by "hidden trauma" are those in law enforcement and corrections, who, during the execution of their duty to protect or prevent injury, can be injured, themselves. These clients have what are titled "hidden injuries" in that they are not physically apparent. Because of this, they might be denied services by a bureaucratic system that provides them with a 15-minute hearing in which to convince a hearing officer of their need for services, a need that must be justified by written documentation. These clients are often seen as malingering, but when one researches their history, it is evident that they have experienced catastrophic injuries that cause constant, debilitating pain or that the visual memories that they hold are so overwhelming that just taking a forward step can cause significant anxiety.

The use of visual imagery and expression/resolution through fabric arts enabled the police officer to gain the self-control needed to depict and share her trauma within a safe environment. She was also able to illustrate and explore concerns about her safety within the community. After having been injured, the corrections officer became very confrontational and reactive in negative ways to those within his personal and community environments. He had tried "traditional therapy," which he said had increased his anxiety. His use of visual and written expression provided him with the ability to structure his responses in a way that would avoid further decompensation during his interactions with family and coworkers.

In the course of executing their jobs, law enforcement and corrections personnel can also witness horrific scenes that become imprinted upon their memories, creating trauma that, if unresolved, can lead to further trauma, based upon fears. For example, a client employed in law enforcement witnessed the death of his peers in vehicle accidents and, afterward, was asked to assist in clearing the sites. In therapy, the client talked about having nightmares of images of body parts, about an inability to develop healthful relationships, and about an increasing fear of engaging in any social activity. In therapy, we focused upon the client's changed perception of himself. While he had initially portrayed himself as a strong individual, he now had an image of himself as weak and worthless to others.

Confronting Ethical Failures of "the System": Patient Reactions, Therapist Reactions

Malchiodi (2013) points out that the creative arts therapies present a positive option that is often not permitted by funding agencies, which rely upon traditional forms of therapy—when therapy is provided at all. Even when limited therapeutic services are provided initially, an ethical dilemma that is continually presented during therapy is the consistent reduction and denial of services. Most clients require the provision of on-going therapy to develop coping mechanisms and to accept limitations upon activity and changes in life goals. Even if they were approved by the hearing officer during formal hearing processes, long-term services were usually denied by the funding source or were appealed for additional due process by the employer or the funding source—a process that can delay a decision for up to a year, due to timelines for the filing of appeals and the scheduling of additional higher level hearings. Patients often reacted to this with regression, withdrawal, apathy, or a sense of resignation. At times this led to the client deciding to settle the case for a lump sum, to avoid hearings and the feelings of disrespect and humiliation that so often seemed to accompany them.

When a client is receiving financial benefits from a funding agency but the therapist must act as his or her agent because the client isn't coming to therapy or exhibits a lack of commitment to therapy, it can affect the therapeutic relationship and the mutual trust that is developed between therapist and client. Art therapists rely upon their clients to act jointly with them to facilitate change and to improve client functioning, but what happens if those clients—who have already sustained substantial physical, psychological, and neurological injuries and whose conditions are continuing to deteriorate— feel unmotivated or depressed? What happens when this situation is compounded by inconsistent efforts on the part of third party payers to provide the resources that these patients require—or when years elapse before treatment can even begin?

MY ETHICAL DILEMMA

Why is it that I seem to be doing all the work?

It can be frustrating for a therapist when, in spite of continuing investment in the therapeutic work and continuing efforts to secure additional therapeutic sessions from third party payers, clients don't show up for sessions, don't call, or don't respond to our communications. This is only enhanced by our knowledge of how crucial therapy is to the continued improvement of the clients who are not showing up. It can feel as though we care more than the client does.

How would you respond?

For the writer's response, see Appendix B, page 402.

It's Not My Fault, Either! Counter-transference Kicks In

As patient advocate, I was required not only to support, through documentation, the need for requested services, but also to advocate for those services by consulting with the client's legal representative, the funding source, and the state workers compensation bureau representative. This would result in writing letters to the hearing officer to justify the need for the service, based upon the approved allowance for the claim. When those services were not forthcoming after months of seeing clients whom, ethically, I was bound to serve, without the ability to be reimbursed, I felt as helpless as the clients and as frustrated with the reviewers/the system, which seemingly looked only at dollars instead of client needs. I felt that they were needlessly withholding services that were essential to the well-being of my clients. At the same time, given the apathy with which many of my clients responded to the denial of services, based upon their experience of the hearing process and, at times, the futility of the process, I found myself feeling a lack of support from the clients towards the work that I was trying to help them accomplish.

How did I cope with these feelings? I would rely upon peer consultation/support and also look at the progress that was evident in the clients, themselves. I could see the success of the therapeutic process in clients who would leave sessions feeling empowered and having new strategies that they could employ; in clients who were able to seek additional training or education and return to competitive employment with a sense of self-worth and a more positive self-image; and in the clients who spoke, during their last session, about gains they'd made from therapy and told me that I'd fought as hard as they had to secure what they needed. I recall one client who knew she was unable to return to competitive employment, but said that it was okay because she knew that she had made every effort to do so. To this day, she still sends little cards about feeling positive and appreciating what she has gained.

Conclusion

When working with a population such as those who have sustained work-related injuries, art therapists are frequently required to serve in multiple roles, such as those of therapist, case-manager, gatekeeper, and client advocate for managed care funders. Regarding the latter, many funding agencies, for example, require initial assessments and on-going outcomes reporting to show the effectiveness of the therapeutic process and to measure change and improvement/regression. These tools not only provide for the monitoring of the consistency of the client's attendance, but also can be used as an interactive tool with the client to establish goals and objectives to reach measureable goals, thus strengthening the therapeutic relationship. However, this is a role that many art therapists have not had to participate in and have not had the training/education to understand, utilize, and evaluate its components.

The interaction and clarification of the multiple roles in which art therapists find themselves is an area that is either not covered or insufficiently covered in many graduate art therapy programs. Providing more guidance in the business aspect of art therapy and developing training models that can ensure that art therapists are able meet multiple job responsibilities/business expectations is essential. So, too, is the continuing need, post-graduation, for peer group and professional supervision on a formalized basis, as art therapists expand the populations they serve and the kinds of settings in which those services are provided, such as community-based practices. It would undergird the role of the art therapist as a multi-disciplinary team member who must not only respond to multiple ethical challenges, but also navigate the use of multiple ethical guidelines.

REFLECTIVE ART EXPERIENCES & DISCUSSION QUESTIONS

1. Diagram how you visualize the various roles you hold at your workplace (e.g., their similarities, differences, areas of overlap, boundaries).
2. Describe how you would explain to the clients with whom you work the various roles you hold.
3. Create art that reflects your response to administrative policies or procedures that seem to challenge, rather than facilitate, your ability to do your job.
4. How do you explain to clients the administrative policies/procedures that effect their treatment when you, personally, do not agree with those policies/procedures?

References

Bryan, B., Andrews, C., Hurley, R., & Taber, K. (2009). Electrical injury, Part II, Consequences. *The Journal of Neuropsychiatry and Clinical Neuroscience,* 21(4), iv–lv.

Malchiodi, C. (2013). Defining art therapy in the 21st century. Retrieved from www.psychology today.com/blog/the-healing-arts/201304/defining-art-therapy-in-the-21st-century

Primeau, M., Engelstatter, G., & Bares, K. (1995). Behavioral consequences of lightning and electrical injury. *Seminars in Neurology,* 15(3), 279–285.

24

MY TOP TEN ETHICAL PET PEEVES

An Art Therapist Reflects Upon a Career Working in Psychiatric Settings

Charlotte G. Boston

During a nearly 35-year career in art therapy that includes working as a clinician, a supervisor of interns, a faculty member, and a Board member of both the American Art Therapy Association (AATA) and the Art Therapy Credentials Board (ATCB), I have encountered a wide range of ethical issues. In this chapter, I share my "top ten ethical pet peeves" in working as an art therapist in psychiatric hospitals, along with the practical solutions I have developed over the years. I include a tool which might come in handy when a course of action has to be determined quickly. My peeves are listed in no particular order of importance (or aggravation)!

My Top Ten Ethical Pet Peeves

Peeve #1: BOUNDARIES, Pulleeeze!

The issues that concern me most are the poor boundaries of some staff and interns of various disciplines. Rather than attending to patients' needs, all too often I've observed them attending to their Smart phones, chatting about personal relationships or sharing weekend plans, or talking about patients in open spaces where others may hear—sometimes even laughing about something a patient did. They come to groups late, leave early, or dart in and out while group is in session. They are nowhere to be found when the room needs to be set up or materials put away. During group time, they leave their cell phones on; chart, read, or take notes; and treat patients' questions as intrusions. They give students and staff who are doing the right thing a bad name, by association.

Solution options. As the art therapist, you are in charge of your group. You set and enforce the group rules. If it is a patient's first time in art therapy group, you orient the patient. Likewise, you orient staff and interns before group begins, briefing them on group procedures before any infractions occur and outlining what they can do to assist you or the patients during group. Create an art therapy fact sheet that succinctly defines the discipline and lists "dos and don'ts" for students, fellows, doctors, and anyone else who might observe (or even co-lead) your group; carry copies with you to give to staff or interns who show up unexpectedly. Ask observers to sit separately from each other, to minimize side conversations. I don't hesitate to redirect anyone whose behavior is distracting. Nip it in the bud! If I have to redirect someone twice, they have to leave. Assert yourself politely and professionally, but assert yourself.

Peeve #2: "What's THAAAT?" Co-leading Woes

Closely related is the issue of co-leading art therapy groups with staff who don't know what art therapy is or what is appropriate behavior in art therapy groups. Just the thought of this makes me want to shake my head and make them magically disappear until I can pull them aside to have "the talk." Some co-leaders talk far too often (and far too much) while patients are trying to concentrate upon creating art. Instead of appreciating the art as an expression of the inner self, they make comments such as: "That's pretty!" or "Why don't you add some bright (or, worse, *happy*) colors to your drawing?" or the dreaded, "What's THAAAT?" Some even grab a pencil to show a client how to draw something! Others become so invested in creating art, themselves, that they become oblivious to patient needs. Incidents like these are most likely to occur in settings where art therapy is new or when a new wave of staff "did not get the memo" about the in-service on art therapy etiquette. Ignorance is still out there causing mischief.

Solution options. Besides creating a list of "dos and don'ts" for co-leading groups (see Peeve #1), give prospective co-leaders a copy of Judy Rubin's article entitled, "Art Therapy: What It Is and What It Is Not" (1982). Give an in-service to staff. If you will be co-leading groups with a non-art therapist, establish your boundaries; clarify each person's role and expectations; plan the group, identifying related assignments BEFORE sessions; and schedule time to process, after group. Provide a "go to" folder of self-directed art tasks and/or directives, in case you are absent.

Peeve #3: You call this a "THERAPY" group?

Yalom (1975) cites 6–8 members as a reasonable number for a therapeutic group. In some settings, however, art therapists are expected to run groups of up to 25 or 30 patients if there's a high census. How therapeutic can that be? In addition to the sheer number of participants, the acuteness of their mental illness and the varying levels of their cognitive abilities make it challenging to provide everyone with the attention they need.

Solution options. Advocate for your patients! Make sure administrators know that art therapy groups involve not only interacting verbally, but also providing patients with art directives or group projects geared toward their specific needs; assisting those who have difficulty getting started or implementing their ideas; fostering a supportive environment in which members show appreciation for one another's work as well as words; and ensuring that there is time for everyone to present and process his or her art. If each patient isn't given the support needed to participate fully—because he or she has to compete with 24 other patients for the art therapist's time and attention—is the institution adequately meeting its patients' therapeutic needs? Sounds like an ethical issue to me.

Consider using an open studio group format. Patients are free to come and go, usually based upon their attention span, but I provide music, circular (*mandala*) outlines, and other pages that provide the beginning lines of an image or a simple directive to help patients get started. Although many of these published or online sheets may be duplicated as needed, you can make your own. Also available are easily controlled materials such as markers, oil pastels, colored pencils, letter stencils, basic object/animal stencils, dot-a-dot paints, and paper. If insight-oriented art therapy groups are larger than they should be, I use concrete themes; those who prefer, and are able, to work more abstractly have that option. If there isn't enough time to allow everyone to discuss and process their artwork, I may have to select a few volunteers.

If all else fails, adjust your expectations regarding what can be accomplished. If everyone is engaged in an art-related task and completes it even partially, if everyone interacts even minimally and you observe their affect, that is noteworthy information regarding a patient's status.

Take note of the fire code; every room has a maximum capacity of occupants. Identify this number and monitor group numbers. If a worrisome pattern develops, inform your supervisor, the administrator in charge, and the safety officer.

Peeve #4: Am I an Art Therapist or WHAT??

"Other duties as assigned." We're all familiar with the clause that appears at the bottom of our job description. It's not unusual for non-art therapy staff to assume that your creative ability qualifies you to make "decorations on demand" for the facility or have your clients make "holiday" artwork. And why not throw in transporting clients, chaperoning field trips, serving meals? It's one thing to clear or clean the area you will use for your art therapy group; it's another thing to serve trays, get linen, or make copies, just because you are there (unless, of course, it's part of your job).

Solution options. When you are interviewing for an art therapy position, ask what duties other than art therapy you might be expected to fulfill. When you're offered a job, go over your job description and ask questions about your duties. If, then, you're asked by staff to make decorations, offer to provide them with the necessary materials or to order art supplies and *how-to* books. You might direct them to relevant YouTube videos or demonstrate how to make a template for the project, to get them started. You can also remind them of your role, reassuring them that they are well able to meet the task as a team; this way, no one person has to complete the entire task. They might even discover someone who has a knack for "decorating"!

Peeve #5: So You Do Art Therapy, Too?

Sometimes we come across non-art therapy colleagues who claim that they, too, "do art therapy." Some even interpret client artwork whenever it is presented at team meetings.

Solution options. First, get a sense of what they think art therapy is; maybe they just don't know. You might, then, mention your training. They might not be aware that the ATCB regards a Master's degree in Art Therapy (with a hefty number of supervised clinical internship hours) as entry level to the profession. Gauge the level of their interest. Enrolling in a "Survey of Art Therapy" course would not give them the credentials to practice art therapy, but it would allow them to discover whether they'd like to pursue study in the field. If they insist upon calling what they do art therapy, inform them that—if they are "doing art therapy" in one of the growing number of states that license art therapists and provide title protection—they are violating the law. They could also be reported to their own professional association, as most ethics codes don't allow members to function outside the scope of their competence. Tell colleagues who ask you to show them how to do art therapy that it would be unethical for you to do so, but you might be willing to consult with them on cases, at your discretion.

Peeve #6: Who are you?

What happens when decisions made by the hospital, based upon a patient's given name, do not reflect the patient's sense of identity? Upon admission, a tall, fully developed adolescent, whose history identified her as a transgender male and included the fact that she had had genital reassignment surgery, was assigned a male roommate. Hospital policy was that patients were assigned rooms according to gender—apparently their gender at birth. This decision made an already uncomfortable situation more uncomfortable, adding an additional obstacle to the patient's treatment.

MY ETHICAL DILEMMA

Hospital policy and the patient's needs

When hospital policy and the patient's needs conflict, how should I proceed?

How would you respond?

For the writer's response, see Appendix B, page 400.

Peeve #7: Is It STINKY?

Picture yourself facilitating an art therapy group with pre-kindergarten children. You smell something putrid, but the kids happily continue to create. You inconspicuously move around to identify which child is the source of the odor, but the child will neither acknowledge his predicament nor leave the group to change clothes. You can't ignore the smell because it's distracting and affecting others.

The child with the stinky pants is you, if you won't bring up certain issues with your supervisor. Even if you behave as if everything's fine, your supervisor is aware of their presence. Whether you feel that your supervisor has treated you unfairly or a fellow intern is getting on your nerves, the stink of the matter won't go away until you acknowledge that it's there.

Solution options. Supervisors have been through what you're going through and are invested in guiding your professional development. If you store up issues, rather than addressing and exploring them, the real world may not be as accommodating. Use your on-campus supervision, but first give your on-site supervisor the courtesy of addressing issues directly with him or her. A sulky demeanor and passive aggressive behavior speak volumes; more importantly, the work suffers. By facing your fears, a misunderstanding might be clarified or a problem might turn out to be smaller than imagined. At least, you will have availed yourself of a significant learning opportunity.

Peeve #8: Do Your Homework!

Have you ever failed to respond to a demeaning comment about race or ethnicity? The absence of a response is, itself, a response and it sends a loud message. As a group leader who is obligated to maintain a safe, respectful environment, the impact of failing to stand up for patients can be devastating. In this very diverse world in which we live, "I didn't know what to do" is unacceptable.

Solution options. Review your multicultural training. Concepts such as privilege and microaggressions should have been embedded in your art therapy coursework and continuing education. Did you do your homework? Assess your knowledge and skills in this area; if they are lacking, crack the books! Establish respect as Rule #1 in your group. If anything is said or done that's threatening or demeaning, you must proactively deescalate the situation. If group members aren't willing to come to a mutual agreement, give the aggressor some space, or time outside the group, to cool off. An issue might need to be clarified or apologies made. Consider addressing the issue metaphorically, through a team building or group task.

Peeve #9: Your Momma is so …!

As a child, hearing those words meant there was going to be a fight, because it was a "no-no" to talk about someone's momma. How do we react when staff or administrators make demeaning comments (often in humorous form) about art therapy?

Solution options. Calm your emotions so you can hear objectively and respond professionally. You might respond as you would in an art therapy group if a patient said the same thing. You might testify, giving an example of how art therapy made a difference in someone's life. You could employ humor: "You're joking now, but you'll be looking for me when the patient won't talk to you" or "If you can't name five benefits of art therapy, you can't talk about it." (If you use that last one, be sure you can rattle off 10 benefits in quick succession!) You could provide art therapy literature or, if appropriate, invite them to observe an art therapy group.

As Michelle Obama so eloquently put it, "When they go low, you go high."

Peeve #10: Warm Fuzzies for Art Therapy

Some patients have such a positive art therapy experience or develop such good rapport with you that they wish to give you something or to continue contact.

Solution options. Acknowledge the patient's feelings, but inform them that it's against hospital policy for therapists to have a relationship with patients outside of treatment. If you sense that they might be interested in art therapy resources in the area, have them contact their case manager (and ensure that the latter has up-to-date information). While clarifying that personal gifts cannot be accepted, let the patient know of the context within which gifts (such as art materials for patient use) might be received by the unit.

Ethics 101: Never Do Anything You Can't Tell Your Momma About

The Ethics Formula Evaluation Test (EFET)

Over the years, so many students have asked me if something were ethical or unethical that I developed a way to help them make that determination, particularly when a decision about a prospective course of action had to be made quickly. The EFET, which is still in development, is meant to be a practical support—not to take the place of intensive professional study, well supervised experience, and a keen awareness of ethics codes and applicable laws. Lest readers think that the section heading raises yet another ethical issue—that of breaching confidentiality—no, I'm not advocating that we tell our mothers about work-related decisions!

Using the EFET, then, when we are considering a specific course of action, as part of our deliberations, we might ask ourselves:

> *Would my decision harm or negatively affect the individual?* If yes, add 2 points.
> *Would my decision harm or negatively affect others?* If yes, add 5 points.
> *Would my decision harm or negatively affect the agency?* If yes, add 3 points.

After totaling the points: 0–5 points would indicate behavior within an ethical range, and 6–10 points would indicate behavior within an unethical range.

Let's consider an example. Fifteen patients sat around a table in a room with enough space for ten. The art therapist stood at the open door, distributing art supplies from an art cart in the hallway because it would not fit inside the room, asking patients to slide the materials down the table, as it is too crowded for her to walk around it. Patients were asked to represent, within the circle that patients traced on their paper, a loss that they had experienced and to surround the circle with lines/shapes/colors that might soothe the pain, hurt, or distress. The patients quietly began to create. Ten minutes into the process, a patient began to sob loudly. Group members gave him tissues and the person beside him offered words of support. When I asked if he wanted to stay or to speak individually with a therapist, he continued to draw. Then he began to wail. When staff came to the door to see what was wrong, I was informed that the patient had lost both his parents to a fire the week before. The patient was grieving. He had not cried since the loss.

Those nearest the patient patted his shoulder and provided encouragement. Others looked uncomfortable; some stopped drawing. Wiggling my way along the space between the chairs and the wall, I asked, again, if he wanted to leave; he shook his head no. I had a dilemma. The patient was not a danger to himself or others and wanted to stay. Would allowing him to remain be fair to the others, since, as someone in crisis, the focus of the group would be upon him? Would I have adequate time to process the impact of this upon the group? Would the needs of the other group members be met if only a few were able to share their work, due to the group's size and time constraints?

I decided that the patient should stay. Creating art seemed to be cathartic for him and might allow him to sublimate some of his grief. By accepting the gift of his peers' support, he'd given one to them: enabling them to recognize the value of what they had to offer. Gradually, his crying became softer. Everyone who had stopped drawing returned to work.

To apply the EFET formula to my quandary, I would ask myself:

> *Would my decision to allow the patient to remain in group negatively affect him*? Not likely; 0 points.
>
> *Would my decision affect others negatively?* Yes; 4 points. Some of the patients looked distressed; the patient's sobbing might have triggered a reaction in them and the focus upon the grieving patient might have kept their own needs from being addressed.
>
> *Would the hospital be negatively affected?* No; 0 points. The patient was not a threat, no one was harmed, the room was left intact. The total score of 4 was within the ethical range. I would be able to tell my momma about this decision and not be ashamed.

I asked the group to complete their artwork within five minutes. In the 15 minutes remaining, I asked three volunteers to share their art, briefly summarized the group, encouraged patients to check on each other (just as they'd supported their peer), and urged them to let me or program staff know if they wanted to discuss their issues or needed more closure.

Concluding Thoughts

I hope that this light-hearted attempt to categorize the myriad serious, complex ethical dilemmas that present themselves to art therapists will be of help in your professional development. Although we know that most ethical issues defy ready solutions, I hope that those I shared will get your own creative problem-solving juices flowing.

The work in which we are engaged is endlessly challenging—but endlessly rewarding. My best wishes to each of you as you pursue it!

REFLECTIVE ART EXPERIENCES & DISCUSSION QUESTIONS

1. Draw two circles, large enough to overlap by two or three inches. Using lines/shapes/colors, symbolize your facility in one circle, yourself in the other circle, and, in the overlapping space, yourself within your facility.
2. Symbolize your supervisor. Symbolize yourself. Symbolize the blending of your symbols/your relationship. Journal about each. Consider areas of harmony and areas of conflict.
3. How do you handle issues at work that you can't control? Which battles would you engage in? What resources can you call upon? Who is in your support network (e.g., colleagues, professors)? Whenever you are facing a challenging situation, consider what you can control and what you cannot control.
4. How do you respond to racially charged comments directed toward you in public? At work? At home?

References

Rubin, J.A. (1982). Art therapy: What it is and what it is not. *American Journal of Art Therapy*, 21, 57–58.
Yalom, I.D. (1975). *The theory and practice of group psychotherapy*. New York: Basic Books.

25

SEPARATION OF CHURCH AND STATE

Parochial Politics, Third-Party Payers,
and Art Therapy for an Individual with
Complex Trauma, Eating Disorder, and
Dissociative Identity Disorder

Michelle L. Dean

Eating Disorders: The Arduous Journey

Individuals who suffer from eating disorders are often confronted with the reality of a long and costly journey to recovery. The length of recommended treatment for sustained recovery is often as long as eight years for some and several decades for others, which may include multiple medical and inpatient psychiatric hospitalizations at specialized eating disorder treatment centers (Anorexia Nervosa and Related Disorders, 2015). Residential programs cost on average $30,000 a month and many patients require three or more months of treatment, often at a facility far from home. Even after leaving a specialized eating disorder program, patients will need years of follow-up care (Alderman, 2010; Parker-Pope, 2010), reaching as much as or more than $100,000. Outpatient therapy, which includes specialists such as a psychiatrist, physician, nutritionist, and psychotherapist, contributes to ongoing costs associated with recovery. For many, the costs of recovery are comparable to the costs associated with a college education from an esteemed private university in the United States, so any financial assistance can be welcome whether it be from family members, insurance companies, or other support networks such as charitable means like a religious organization or agency.

Costs of Third-Party Payers

Newer healthcare laws have attempted to address the disparity between coverage for treatment for mental health and medical care by creating a kind of reciprocity between what is commonly reimbursed for medical care and psychiatric care. While these efforts have helped, they often do not do enough to address the complex psychological issues underlying many of the behavioral symptoms and thus, funding for treatment is often focused on symptoms or behaviors rather than the complex underlying psychological problems that contributed to eating disordered behaviors in the first place, including complex trauma. Insurers typically will not cover long-term treatment and some routinely deny adequate coverage of eating disorders (Parker-Pope, 2010), leaving the individual and their family or support system with these costs.

Providers of mental health care are also in a conundrum, as they are expected to be professionals, run their business by upholding the highest level of expertise through on-going training and education, as well as a practice like other medical professionals with much of the same rising expenses, all while supporting themselves and their families. Additionally, many providers have seen an increase in their credentialing standards over the last decade, including more stringent requirements, additional education and supervision, and expertise to work with individuals who demonstrate complex and, at times, psychologically and medically volatile conditions. Those who take insurance reimbursement payments for outpatient sessions have experienced a decline in payment for services over the years. Reduced reimbursement rates, or limited session limits, have left many providers faced with the dilemma that, in order to make ends meet, they must see more clients in order to earn what they were once paid years ago. Many must live with the declining rates of reimbursement or leave insurance panels and work as a fee-for-service practice. Like many clinicians, I have chosen to work outside of the system of insurance panels, setting rates that are commensurate with my experience, expertise, specialized training, and practice location, offering sliding-scale fees when needed. This arrangement allows the treatment length, frequency, and duration to be a part of a clinical dialog that does not involve a third entity—a party who has an economic incentive to limit or deny services that will directly affect the course of treatment, but lacks intimate knowledge of the patient and often does not have experience, expertise, or specialized training with the population. While assistance with the costs associated with mental health treatment can be welcomed, they can also come at a cost. This chapter describes how the actions of one such third-party payer impacted the treatment of a young woman with trauma, an eating disorder, and dissociative identity disorder.

The Story of Rachel: The "Lord" Giveth and the "Lord" Taketh Away

One day, I received a call from a minister who had seen a flyer about my services.

"I understand you work with people with eating disorders, complex trauma, and abuse such as sexual and physical abuse, is that right?" he asked. When I affirmed his understanding of my expertise, he proceeded to tell me about a parishioner in his church who was struggling with self-harm and restricting. He said she had been seen initially by one of the church's Christian counselors but that her issues and symptoms were beyond her skill level due to their potential lethality. The minister, feeling he had exhausted his typical options for parishioners in need, sought care for Rachel outside of his flock.

During our first phone call, the minister said:

> Rachel is a woman in her mid-thirties who has had a long history of trauma; her trauma started in her early childhood at the hands of her father but extended to other family members in incestuous relationships. She has severe dissociative episodes, to the point where she would disappear for days, returning with what

appeared to be multiple self-inflicted injuries. Other times, she would call after "coming to" in another part of the state with no awareness as to how she had driven for more than five hours to get there.

He also expressed his concerns for her compromised physical health due to her restrictive eating disordered behaviors: "She is so thin, she sometimes nearly passes out (an indication of orthostatic hypotension)," he said. "Will you see her?"

It was clear that the degree of traumatic sequelae was severe and Rachel was in serious need of ongoing psychiatric care. I agreed to meet with Rachel and asked that she call to set up an appointment. The minister thanked me, adding that "Rachel has a hard time trusting others, so I hope she will trust you enough to open up to talk about what is going on." I agreed that trust is very important if a therapeutic alliance is to be established. I explained that trauma, especially when inflicted by family, often inhibits one's ability to trust others and to find meaningful relationships. I also explained that Rachel would need to feel comfortable working with me, in order for a therapeutic relationship to develop over time.

The minster then said, "Oh, there's something else. Rachel is on Medicaid for her psychiatric disorder and is considered disabled, unable to maintain reliable work outside of the church." He explained that, in return for the work that Rachel provided to the church, mostly clerical, the church was willing to contribute monetary aid to her housing and medical care. The church would be compensating me for my services. Since they supported several church members in this manner, he asked if I could provide a sliding scale fee for Rachel, intimating that there may be other members of the congregation who, too, could benefit from my services. I agreed to reduce my standard fee by a third.

The following week, I met with Rachel, a tall, thin woman whose gaunt face belied her youth and the weariness on her visage was shadowed by the long hair that fell over her eyes. Her slender frame was held tight as she gripped her journal across her chest and sat on the edge of the seat in my office, anxiously bouncing her leg. As she quietly told part of her medical and mental health history, I became aware of the chronic and severe nature of her illness, which spanned 20 years, and had required multiple hospitalizations for both mental health and physical illnesses. She explained that her child-like alters kept her locked in her home, at times in her closet, for extended periods of time, feeling anxiety stricken or depressed with little or no contact with others except when church members would make house calls to check on her. She refused to eat or drink for long stretches of time as a means of piety, purity, and control. Without the intervention and support of the church and some of its members, Rachel would have most likely been completely alone in a city far from where she grew up, purposely severing the ties to her perpetrating family.

Rachel was apprehensive about discussing prior abuse, falling silent and becoming avoidant when I inquired about the extent of her experiences or her intense reactions when, on occasion, family members attempted to find her through internet searches and other means. Weekly, our appointments continued, building rapport and trust. Slowly, she began to share about the loss of her mother as a child, the lack of protectors growing up, and her abuses at the hands of family members, most significantly, a family

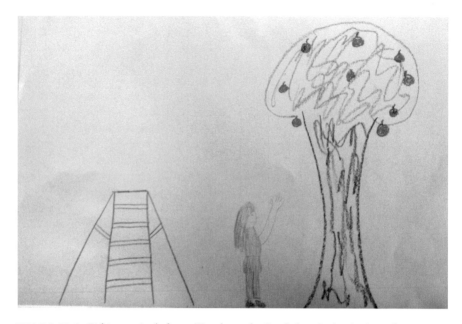

FIGURE 25.1 *Picking an Apple from a Tree*, drawn by Rachel at the beginning of treatment.

member who was a preacher and was inexorably intertwined with her childhood church. He twisted biblical passages to create a rationale for abuse.

Rachel's inability to care for herself or reach for nurturance was evident in her behaviors and her art. Rachel drew Figure 25.1 at the beginning of our work together, in response to my invitation to draw herself "picking an apple from a tree." Rachel's reluctance and inability to obtain nurturance is reflected in her inability to extend her arm fully, as well as in the tree's towering height, which keeps the apples out of reach. She spoke of her frustration about not being able to reach other goals in her life, just as the apples were out of the reach of her grasp in the picture. Her ambivalence about self-care was apparent, and the traumatic sequelae would often plague her with debilitating physical and emotional distress.

Our work consisted of building a relationship of trust, support, and caring. We worked to identify triggers to eating disordered and dissociative symptoms, as well as to creating safety in her life through her relationship and her self-care. On occasions, we addressed her understanding of church, religion, spirituality, and its corruption at the hands of her perpetrator. We discussed the difficulty in taking in nourishment when it seems poisoned and tainted, as it was often tied to sadistic abuse rituals. Contextually, her quest to understand the role of abuse within a church was triggered by the multiple child abuse allegations and their cover-up by high-ranking officials that were frequently on the national news. She shared her struggles and understandings of human suffering and attempted to find a belief system that allowed her to enjoy her life and not restrict or self-harm as a means of punishing herself or purging incompatible thoughts. Our work was complex and not always easy going. When her weight plummeted a year into our work together, it meant a re-hospitalization.

The minister was concerned and needed to be reassured that re-hospitalization did not mean that that Rachel was not making progress and that the therapy was not helpful. I spent some time educating the well-meaning minister about complex trauma, post-traumatic stress disorder, eating disorders, and dissociative identity disorder. We continued our work together along with the medical doctor and nutritionist checking in with the minster as needed. We worked together for four years, making great strides. During that time, Rachel became much less dissociative, and her anxiety lessened. She worked on articulating more of her needs and feelings by writing poetry and creating artwork in addition to the art we created in our therapy session. She joined discussion groups on the Internet that supported survivors of abuse and shared her experiences through an anonymous blog. She joined several groups within the church, partly because she was persuaded to do so if she wanted her funding to continue and because being more social would help with her tendency to isolate. Although her eating disorder would be classified as chronic, improvements were made there, too. Her low weight stabilized and the destructive behaviors lessened. We were approaching what may have been a midway point in therapy, where the relationship was solidified and the crises dissipated to a manageable degree. It was at this time that changes began to occur within the church. A new minister was appointed and she began to question how monies were being allocated to their parishioners in need.

The new minister wished to speak with me about Rachel's treatment. Rachel, untrusting of what might be said in her absence, was invited to be a part of our meeting. With Rachel's input, I explained to the new minister many of the same issues and concerns that I had shared with the previous minister. She listened politely, nodded her head during our meeting in seeming agreement, but when she left, I had an uneasy feeling that something was amiss.

MY ETHICAL DILEMMA

What should I do in this situation, considering the multiple factors that are at stake?

In our next session, Rachel informed me that we could continue our work together if I signed a Statement of Religious Conviction, meaning that I had to sign a form stating that I took Jesus Christ as my Lord. It was explained that the new minister insisted that all recipients of their charitable funds would need to sign such a statement. It was a part of their protocol, and I had not been asked to participate in it before. It was not my religious beliefs that were key to Rachel's treatment and recovery but my expertise—the same expertise that was more than adequate under the previous minister who had initially requested my services. I felt conflicted. While discussions ensued about the therapeutic relationship and the importance of specialized care and consistency, it was clear that the new minister intended to cut off funding for Rachel's treatment by offering to pay only for a Christian counselor within their parish. The minister made arrangements for the funding to gradually decrease over four months. This reduction left Rachel with the decision to continue her treatment with me by finding paid employment, which would jeopardize her disability benefits, or to go with the Christian counselor recommended by the new minister. I offered to reduce my rate further, but the conflict seemed too great. It seemed as though no matter what it was, she could not afford it. Ultimately, she felt that if she did not go with the recommendations of the minister, she would lose the support of the church, her other subsidies that the church was providing for her, help with rent and car repairs, and feared the church might shun her. We discussed how the dynamics of staying replicated many of the power dynamics that contributed to her staying in an abusive family system.

We both felt outraged and powerless to change the situation. I questioned the good it might do to discuss my own religious background, in all of its complexity, with the minister, in case doing so would somehow change her judgment of me. For myself, I questioned if the knowledge of being a descendant of missionaries who came to this country seeking religious freedom would make a difference in her opinion of me. I wondered if my upbringing as a Protestant, absorbing the teachings of my Methodist and Brethren parents would make her see me in a more favorable light—or, perhaps, the knowledge that in my early twenties I converted to Catholicism and was baptized and received communion by the very archbishop who was currently being brought up on charges of harboring child abusers in his church (BishopAccountablity.org, 2004). And I wondered if my quest to understand more about religion and spirituality through seeking knowledge about these religions and others would have convinced her that I was worthy and met the standard that would enable me to continue our work together—as my intention was to help one of her parishioners, by helping to heal the trauma had been perpetrated by the hands of a church official, a family member.

I reviewed the Code of Ethics of the American Counseling Association (2014, p. 5) and found that Standard A.4.b. states that:

> Counselors are aware of—and avoid imposing—their own values, attitudes, beliefs, and behaviors. Counselors respect the diversity of clients ... and seek training in areas in which they are at risk of imposing their values onto clients, especially when the counselor's values are inconsistent with the client's goals or are discriminatory in nature.

Additionally, in order to promote multiculturally competent and ethical practice, one must continually increase his or her understanding of the diversity among the clients with whom he or she works. Such diversity is defined by Webster's Dictionary as "a state or instance of difference; a diversity of opinion" (Merriam Webster, 1956, p. 243); it was about being different or having differences, including different religions.

How would you respond?

For the writer's response, see Appendix B, page 402.

Conclusion

This chapter is not about debunking the value of religion or spirituality in a person's life, which can be essential. It is about what happens when a third party, who is undertaking the financial obligations of treatment, whether it be a religious-based organization, a parent, or an insurance company, promotes a particular theoretical, philosophical orientation or economic agenda that takes priority over the treatment goals and therapeutic relationship. These priorities can create conflict and recreate dynamics that are reminiscent of power struggles, splitting, and in worst-case scenarios, like Rachel's, a recapitulation of traumatic experiences through the rupture of attachment and relationship, loss of expression, individualism, and agency. And while assistance with health care costs is often necessary from a third-party payer, understanding the costs—both overt and covert—is crucial, as they may impact not only the therapeutic dialog, but also one's personal integrity and beliefs.

REFLECTIVE ART EXPERIENCES & DISCUSSION QUESTIONS

1. Discuss a time you were asked to say or do something with which you were not comfortable because it either did not feel right or was a conflict to your personal, moral, or ethical beliefs. Create a response piece of art related to this experience.
2. Today, if placed in the same situation, how would you navigate this request? If you have found you did something that did not sit well with you, due to clarity around your personal, moral, or ethical beliefs, what would you do to right this situation?

References

Alderman, L. (2010, December 3). Treating eating disorders and paying for it. *The New York Times.* Retrieved from www.nytimes.com/2010/12/04/health/04patient.html?_r=1&ref=health

American Art Therapy Association (2013). *Ethical principles for art therapists.* Alexandria, VA: Author.

American Counseling Association (2014). 2014 ACA code of ethics: As approved by the ACA Governing Council. Retrieved from www.counseling.org/resources/aca-code-of-ethics.pdf

Anorexia Nervosa and Related Disorders (ANRED) (2015). Treatment and recovery. Retrieved from www.anred.com/tx.html

Bishop-accountability.org (2004). Cardinal Bevilacqua's management of abuse allegations assessments of the Philadelphia grand juries in 2003, 2005, and 2011. Retrieved from www.bishop-accountability.org/reports/2005_09_21_Philly_GrandJury/Bevilacqua.htm

Merriam Webster (1956). *Webster's new collegiate dictionary* (2nd ed.). Springfield, MA: G. & C. Merriam Co.

Parker-Pope, T. (2010, December 3). The cost of an eating disorder, well. *The New York Times.* Retrieved from http://well.blogs.nytimes.com/2010/12/03/the-cost-of-an-eating-disorder/?_r=0

Multiple Roles

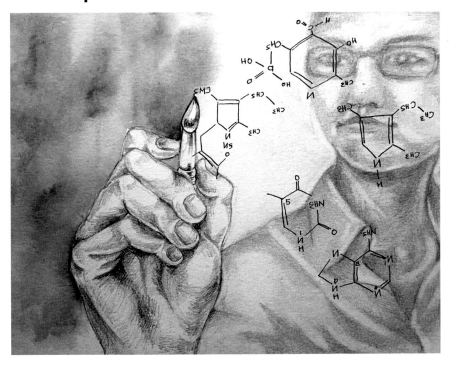

Min Kyung Shin *(see color insert)*

26

ACTUALLY, HONG KONG *IS* A SMALL TOWN

Art Therapy and Multiple Relationships within a Community

Jordan S. Potash

Early in my art therapy career, my professional and personal communities rarely coincided. I went to my agency or studio in one county in the morning and then retreated to my home in a different county in the evening. Perhaps I would see a client on the subway or in a store, but not often. All of this changed when I went to live in Hong Kong for eight years. Although 7.2 million people live in Hong Kong, the expatriate community is relatively small, with estimates around 300,000. This number decreases when one is participating in communities based on shared nationality (60,000 Americans), religion, or interests. For example, the Jewish community in which I was involved numbered about 4,500 people.

Although the largest city in which I had ever lived, Hong Kong felt more like a small town. The interconnectedness of social circles was illuminated when a friend casually commented upon how much more confident her friend's child had become since working with me. Suddenly, my professional and personal lives collided. Up until then, I had not realized that these two people knew each other, let alone knew each other well enough to confide about participating in art therapy. My neatly compartmentalized world dramatically changed.

Multiple Relationships

My experience falls under the ethical category of multiple (sometimes referred to as dual) relationships, which the American Art Therapy Association (AATA), in its *Ethical Principles for Art Therapists*, defines as follows:

> … when an art therapist is in a professional role with a client and (a) is simultaneously in another role with the same client, (b) is simultaneously in a personal relationship with a client in the professional relationship, and/or (c) promises to

enter into another relationship in the future with the client or a person closely associated with or related to the client.

American Art Therapy Association, 2013, Principle 1.4

In short, a multiple relationship exists any time an art therapist has a relationship with a client that is in addition to the therapeutic one, whether the former is concurrent with or sequential to the latter. The nature of the non-therapeutic relationship might be social (e.g., that of a relative or friend) or professional (e.g., that of a business partner, colleague, or contractor).

In addition to defining multiple relationships, Principle 1.4 offers advice for managing them:

> Art therapists refrain from entering into multiple relationships with clients if the multiple relationships could reasonably be expected to impair competence or effectiveness of the art therapist to perform his or her functions as an art therapist, or otherwise risks exploitation or harm to the person with whom the professional relationship exists.

It concludes:

> Multiple relationships that would not reasonably be expected to cause impairment or risk exploitation or harm are not unethical. Art therapists recognize their influential position with respect to clients, and they do not exploit the trust and dependency of clients.

The *Code of Ethics, Conduct, and Disciplinary Procedures* (2018) of the [American] Art Therapy Credentials Board states that exploitative relationships "include, but are not limited to, borrowing money from or loaning money to a client, hiring a client, engaging in a business venture with a client, engaging in a romantic relationship with a client, or engaging in sexual intimacy with a client" (Principle 2.3.4).

Being mindful of multiple relationships ensures the integrity of the therapeutic process, guarantees that clients are not taken advantage of, and protects therapists from malpractice allegations (Freud & Krug, 2002). For these reasons, Goldstein (1999) suggests replacing the term multiple relationships with "boundary violation," to refocus our awareness upon how various relationships may affect the professional one. The aspirational values contained in the Preamble to AATA's ethics code can help guide art therapists to make decisions based upon what is right for a client in a specific situation (Hinz, 2011). In particular, art therapists can respect client decision making (autonomy), emphasize harm reduction (nonmaleficence), bolster well-being (beneficence), foster integrity (fidelity), consider fairness (justice), and respect imaginative problem-solving (creativity). When determining if a multiple relationship is problematic, art therapists should be aware that "the burden of proof shall be on the art therapist to prove that a non-therapeutic or non-professional relationship with current or former clients, students, interns, trainees, supervisees, employees, or colleagues is not exploitative or harmful to any such individuals" (ATCB, 2018, 2.3.3). Thus, it is incumbent upon the art therapist to have open conversations with clients and supervisors when multiple relationships present (or are likely to present) themselves, in order to ensure that multiple relationships are warranted.

In certain situations, multiple relationships are unavoidable. Clinicians may participate in agency endorsed community-building activities, such as recreational or social gatherings, and professionals working in advocacy organizations may find that clients also hold organizational roles (Freud & Krug, 2002). Art therapists occasionally navigate among providing art therapy, facilitating recreational art activities, serving as an art educator, and relating as a fellow artist (Moon, 2015). The potential for extracurricular relationships often occurs for therapists working within their cultural, racial, religious, or social communities. Similarly, therapists who live in small communities find that "social overlap is difficult to avoid," particularly when the therapist may be the "only available option for treatment" (Burgard, 2013, p. 70).

Ethical Issues

Shared Expectations

I was excited to accept a friend's invitation to a new restaurant. She had booked a private room for a small group. When I was shown to my seat, I found myself sitting directly across from the parent of one of my clients. As she and I were part of the same cultural organization, we had run into each other on several occasions, during which we had talked briefly about non-therapy matters related to community events. Given the intimate nature of the dinner and the room, there was no opportunity to have only a short interaction.

One way of managing multiple relationships is to make sure that the client and the therapist have shared expectations of the relationship (Freud & Krug, 2002). This includes having similar values regarding the nature of the work and a shared understanding of the likelihood of multiple relationships. In such situations, it is imperative to reinforce confidentiality and the difference between *being friendly* and *being friends* outside of the therapeutic setting. From the start of our work together, the client's mother and I quickly became aware of the fact that we were in the same community. The parents even liked it, as it suggested a common worldview. More so, they thought it was helpful for their child to know that attending art therapy is not a shameful activity. The parents did not necessarily tell others that they were working with me, but the fact that their child would see me was not a problem for them. At the dinner, we initially had a quiet laugh about the situation and then talked about the dishes being served, as well as other topics that we would each discuss in any casual situation.

Role Differentiation

I received a call from a man who wished to refer his cousin. The caller was glad to have found me as he was looking specifically for an art therapist and had hoped for an American and a man. At the time, I was also working at a university as an instructor and, a few months after accepting the case, I was invited to participate in a curriculum planning meeting for my department. Part-way through the discussion, I looked up and saw the man who had made the referral. I was introduced to him as a respected artist who would begin to work with our program.

Although the man was not my client, he was intimately connected to my client. As the only American man who was an art therapist practicing in Hong Kong, I did not feel that I could end the relationship with the client given my new professional relationship with the client's relative. Likewise, I was not willing to give up my teaching responsibilities. Burgard (2013) suggested several strategies to determine if a multiple relationship is harmful, including: assuring that therapist and client have a mutual understanding of the relationship, identifying conflicts that may arise, and noticing shifts in power dynamics. To resolve the situation, I first had conversations with both the client and the referral source regarding my separate roles in the therapy and the education spheres. We then agreed that we would limit our conversations and interactions to those appropriate for the given role. For work matters, the referee agreed to direct most of his projects to another colleague, so that there would not be even the appearance of impropriety. I let my client know that, if the situation became uncomfortable, I was open to conversation and suggestions as to how to proceed.

Art Objectivity

While I was working with a particularly challenging adolescent, she was preparing to participate in an art show at her high school. As part of the exhibit, she had created an installation related to some of the themes that we discussed together in art therapy. Occasionally, she would tell me about her creations for the show and it was very clear how important they were to her. The more she told me, the more intrigued and excited I became that she was finding a way to apply our work in her life. The week before the show, she invited me to it as a fellow artist.

Thompson (2009) described ways in which art galleries offer opportunities for clients, art therapists, and members of the public to come together within a shared space in order to relate to each other and the art in a new way. Typical power dynamics are flattened as everyone engages each other as artists and appreciators of art. However, art therapists have to be careful that they are not seduced by meaningfully expressed or well rendered art, as they can lose sight of their professional objectivity (Klorer, 1993). To make sure that I was making a choice that would benefit the therapeutic relationship and not just my artistic curiosity, in supervision I discussed the potential for multiple relationships. In so doing, I was able to ensure my own impartiality, in order to participate in the exhibit in a way that would allow the client to feel supported. Prior to attending, I also discussed with my client and her parents their expectations of me at the event and how we would describe our relationship should either of us run into someone that we knew.

Non-clinical Engagement

When I advertise my services as an art therapist, I stress not only their psychotherapeutic value, but also the wellness applications of engaging in creativity. My work with one client over a few years focused upon assisting her in her efforts to attain a healthy lifestyle and to meet her career goals. Soon after our work together ended, I saw the client at an expressive arts workshop delivered by an international expert.

Multiple relationships can become problematic for professionals working in non-clinical settings, such as those focused upon advocacy, case management, educational assistance, and vocational training (Freud & Krug, 2002). The same may be true for art therapists who work in certain community art studios or arts and health settings. Halverson and Brownlee (2010) found that therapists in a small community frequently based their decision to be involved in a multiple relationship upon the type of service offered; they were more likely to engage in multiple relationships with clients who participated in services that were less psychotherapy-oriented.

As my role with the client mentioned above had centered upon facilitating a creative process that would help her to obtain her professional goals, I saw no harm in our attending the same workshop. During a break, I made sure that we talked about our changed roles and each other's comfort with the arrangement. I assured her that, even though our work had not been psychotherapeutic in nature, it still fell within the bounds of confidentiality, so I would not mention our past relationship with any of the other training participants.

MY ETHICAL DILEMMA

How can I best support a client's community arts initiatives?

It had been one year since an adult client and I first started to work together. Having come in due to reoccurring depression and uncertainty about the general direction of his life, he had made substantial progress. Although he was better able to manage his feelings and increase his support network, it was his commitment to art making that he credited as a major source of his improvement. At first limiting his art making to the sessions, gradually he began to use a sketchbook at home and then to dedicate a space there to work on larger pieces. As he devoted more time to his art, he began to be recognized as an artist. Given his experiences with me, he wanted to organize community arts programs that would engage people in making art for their own well-being. His projects started small, but eventually grew in scale and scope. With increased reach, he solicited the help of arts educators and professionals as volunteers. The director of my agency asked me and other colleagues to participate in one such event as facilitators. She thought that we, as art therapists, would have a lot to contribute.

How would you respond?

For the writer's response, see Appendix B, page 427.

Conclusion

Given the complexity and inevitability of multiple relationships, particularly in small communities, there is a great need for formal education and open discussion about this issue among mental health professionals (Halverson & Brownlee, 2010). When handled appropriately, multiple relationships do not need to disrupt the therapeutic encounter. In fact, when managed well, they can even strengthen it.

REFLECTIVE ART EXPERIENCES & DISCUSSION QUESTIONS

1. Using watercolor, select one color to represent yourself and another color to represent your client. Brush clean water over the entire surface of a sheet of paper. Apply to one side of the paper the color that represents you and, to the other side, the color that represents your client. While the paper and paint are still wet, pick up the paper and rotate it in different directions. Take notice of the areas where the colors intersect, cross, and mix. Where one color overpowers the other, what can be changed to rebalance the colors? Where the others blend, what can be changed to reassert some differentiation? How can these artistic strategies inform practices for navigating multiple relationships within a shared space?
2. Create an image to represent your social map. Indicate social, cultural, religious, and other organizations—as well as geographic, retail, recreational, transit, and other areas—you frequent. Indicate in which ones you are likely to encounter clients; in which ones it is possible for you to encounter clients; and in which ones it is unlikely that you will come in contact with clients.
3. The only plumber in your town comes to your studio for assistance in coping with a challenging life circumstance. You are the only art therapist in town and are likely to need the plumber's professional services at some point. What are some considerations to discuss in order to reduce the possibility of exploitation, as well as discomfort or confusion, regarding multiple roles?
4. As a recognized arts professional, you are invited to be a juror for an upcoming arts exhibition. After accepting the role, you realize that one of your fellow jurors is a current client who is also a practicing artist. Which aspirational values can help you to navigate and ensure role differentiation?

References

American Art Therapy Association (2013). *Ethical principles for art therapists*. Retrieved from http://arttherapy.org/aata-ethics/

Art Therapy Credentials Board (2018). *Code of ethics, conduct, and disciplinary procedures*. Retrieved from http://atcb.org/Ethics/ATCBCode

Burgard, E.L. (2013). Ethical concerns about dual relationships in small and rural communities: A review. *Journal of European Psychology Students*, 4(1), 69–77.

Freud, S., & Krug, S. (2002). Beyond the code of ethics, part II: Dual relationships revisited. *Families in Society*, 83(5), 483–492.

Goldstein, H. (1999). On boundaries. *Families in Society*, 80(5), 435–438.

Halverson, G., & Brownlee, K. (2010). Managing ethical considerations around dual relationships in small rural and remote Canadian communities. *International Social Work*, 53(2), 247–260.

Hinz, L.D. (2011). Embracing excellence: A positive approach to ethical decision making. *Art Therapy: Journal of the American Art Therapy Association*, 28(4), 185–188.

Klorer, G. (1993). Countertransference: A theoretical review and case study with a talented client. *Art Therapy: Journal of the American Art Therapy Association*, 10(4), 219–225.

Moon, B. L. (2015). *Ethical issues in art therapy* (3th ed.). Springfield, IL: Charles C. Thomas.

Thompson, G. (2009). Artistic sensibility in the studio and gallery model: Revisiting process and product. *Art Therapy: Journal of the American Art Therapy Association*, 26(4), 159–166.

27

AVENUES AND BARRIERS OF DUAL ROLES

Ethics and the ART Therapist as Researcher

Richard Carolan

As an art therapist who has practiced for more than 30 years, I appreciate our profession as one that is concerned with the suffering of the soul and is dedicated to ethical practice. Yet, as art therapists, have we looked carefully at the ethics of art as a way of knowing? The purpose of this chapter is to reflect upon ethics, art therapy, and research.

Ethics and research both address issues of epistemology and ontology, practices of knowing, and conceptions of truth. The ethical principles of a profession codify the collective wisdom of that profession in the form of best practices in serving the public. A key principle regards the role and responsibilities of the practitioner, as conflicts and exploitation can occur when the practitioner or researcher has more than one role in relationship with participants. Ethical issues for researchers in art therapy might also concern the methodology that the researchers choose and what they identify as evidence.

Relationship with Self

Perhaps the most fundamental dual role that, in some ways, is unique to the art therapist is that of the artist and scientist. The basis of ethics is care of the soul (Moore, 1994), which many associate with the role of the artist. Ethical issues, however, usually come to the foreground through legalistic procedures that call to the scientist. It could be argued that the ethical practitioner is one who limits him- or herself to evidence-based practices—that is, one who operates in accordance with guidelines that have been scientifically established as having valid and reliable results; thus, the practitioner would strive for predictability; the researcher would use scientific methods, the language that the natural sciences accept as the best measure of truth.

The Artist's Way of Knowing

Then, the artist arises with the notion that knowing in the scientific sense sometimes serves to shackle the process of discovery, and that care of the soul requires going beyond what can be described in scientific terms. In *Philosophy in a New Key* (1942) and *Feeling and Form* (1953), Langer wrote that she believed in positivism and all that it has contributed to understanding and development, but that, in her quest for knowing and understanding, she was not willing to stop at the limits of positivism. Indeed, it might be absurd to think that what we know is limited to what we can explain. A five-minute conversation with a child will put that notion to rest; it is obvious that the child knows so much more than he or she can explain.

When we are searching again (*re-searching*) an area that has to do with human suffering, an important question arises: *Is it our ethical responsibility to limit our evidence to just that material we can translate into the language of science, disallowing the artist's voice, or is it more ethical to report results from the artist's understanding along with that of the scientist?*

The Practicing Art Therapist

It might help to understand this dilemma more clearly if we look at it from the perspective of the practicing art therapist. I think that it is appropriate to assume that all ethical practicing art therapists are researchers. Not only are they not oblivious to, or uninterested in, the efficacy of their interventions, they look with intention at what they determine to be evidence of the effectiveness of their interventions, changing them if they do not have the intended impact. The question then becomes how does the ethical art therapist determine the efficacy of their interventions? Do they use the scientific method or a different way of knowing? I suggest that the ethical art therapist uses a combination of scientific approaches and other ways of knowing. Although most art therapists probably do not conduct pre- and post-tests, they do make note of behavior, as well as of the formal elements of the art. They formulate goals and a means of measuring progress towards them.

The ethical art therapist also, I believe, uses other ways of knowing as measures of progress: trusting the felt sense of the other person, the notions that arise within the art therapist in relation to the person with whom he or she is working; an empathetic knowing. The images that are created in the art therapy sessions also are likely a basis for the art therapist knowing about the internal experience of the participant. The art therapist may be aware of a non-linear integration of multiple contextual factors that are present in the process of creating the image, in the image itself, and in the ways in which the artist reacts with the created image that cumulatively facilitate a *knowing* that may serve as a primary basis for the next step in the therapeutic work. This, I suggest, is the *artist's knowing*. Is it ethical to use only reductionistic processes as a means of knowing and communicating knowing or should we also use more associative means of understanding and communicating? Does the ethical art therapist operate from the stance of the scientist, identifying truth as that which can be explained using the accepted language of science and evidence or does the ethical art therapist researcher require the organization and communication of the artist's ways of knowing?

Relationship with Other

There is a notion that, as researchers, we should have no previous relationship with research participants. The ethical premise of this concern is that the previous relationship with the research participant might skew the participant's or the researcher's behavior in a manner that might impair the accuracy of the results. We are very preoccupied with this issue of "contamination;" we are unable to accept that there is no absolute objectivity, that we all come with pre-established lenses through which we view the participants, the process, the purpose of the study. It might facilitate a more meaningful reflection if we considered not how much but, instead, *in what manner* the research impacts the results.

There are two critical ways of measuring the meaningfulness of results: their validity and their reliability. The emphasis on reliability has to do with the consistency of the research process as a basis of confidence in the meaningfulness of the results. Validity concerns itself with the accuracy of the results compared to what results the research was designed to gather. A clarifying example can be found in the protocols for administering assessments such as the WISC intelligence test. When a participant asks the test giver to explain a question, the test giver is instructed to repeat the question and not give further explanation. Giving a response that is consistent with that of all other test givers is a means of assuring reliability; however, it may negatively impact validity, as the results may not be an accurate description of the participant's intelligence. The argument for reliability is that, if the purpose of our research is to compare the sample results in a longitudinal manner, we want the protocol for gathering the results to be precisely the same; but no two protocol are precisely the same. Efforts to achieve objective reliability must always be weighed in relation to the potential for enhanced validity.

One of my students, a member of the Choctaw tribe, wanted to conduct research on the role of art in the Trail of Tears trauma. The ethical dilemma in this research protocol had to do with the balance of emphasis between reliability and validity. The fact that this student was a member of the tribe that was the subject of the research inquiry might certainly impact the data gathering procedure. One approach, in favor of reliability, would suggest that the person conducting the inquiry, gathering the data, should have no connection whatsoever to those individuals from whom the data is being gathered. From this standpoint, my student should not have been the researcher. She might contaminate the data. The other perspective is that, from a validity standpoint, my student had a much greater opportunity of gathering data that represented the authentic views of the research participants. Her access to information was greatly enhanced because she is a member of this tribe and because her ancestors were among those who traveled on the Trail of Tears. Even beyond this, it is probable that her own connection to these individuals from whom she was gathering data facilitated her understanding of their responses in a manner that allow clarity and precision in follow-up questions and depth as well as degree of data obtained, which would allow for a greater probability of validity of the data generated. Ethnography is a primary means of data gathering in the field of anthropology, a field committed to the study of the human experience. I encouraged my student to pursue her research study.

When we conduct research from a basis of fear of contamination, striving for the myth of objectivity, are we creating an ethical dilemma in terms of a sense of false confidence that we can have in the validity of the data? When conducting research on understanding and facilitating change in the human experience, is our being enamored with statistical significance an ethical issue? We associate statistical significance with approximations of truth, when it is simply a probability formula.

The relationship between researcher and participant is an ethical variable in research that can impact the validity of the data, the participants, and the public. I believe that ethics in research is best served by requiring researchers to address the impact of their bias and their relationship with the research participants as the perspective from which the results are viewed. I suggest that it would be unethical to suggest that results are valid whenever we have "no relationship" with the participants.

MY ETHICAL DILEMMA

How could I determine whether a community mural making project would pose a scope of practice issue?

As an art therapist, I have served as a member of the Institutional Review Board (IRB) at the university where I work. One proposed research study involved using both the creation of a mural and the image of the completed mural as a means of developing collaboration and cohesion in a community where there had been community unrest. Members of two different gangs that are active in the neighborhood surrounding the site of the proposed mural would be creating the mural. I was enthusiastic about the project until I realized that neither the researcher nor any of the facilitators or consultants in the proposed project was an art therapist.

How would you respond?

For the writer's response, see Appendix B, page 401.

Relationship with the Image

Although the image created by the participant is a central component of the art therapy process, little has been written about ethical issues related to research focused upon the creation of the image and the image, itself, as a way of knowing. There is growing literature that looks at the image form a reductionistic perspective (e.g., defining formal elements, measuring size, line quality, use of space). While there is value in reducing the image to the absence or presence of some of these variables, the accumulation of these variables does not address the gestalt of the image. Furthermore, it is this gestalt that we consider to be a critical tenet of art therapy. From a research perspective, how would the creation of the image and the image, itself, constitute data?

The creation of the image in art therapy is a negotiation between internal conscious and/or unconscious material and external variables such as intention, skill, and a myriad contextual variables. Art therapy theory includes the idea that it is this negotiation process that is the primary therapeutic component; other theories suggest that understanding the internal material represented in the external image is the primary component of the therapeutic process. How one might go about determining the internal material that might be represented by the external image raises research-based ethical issues of validity and reliability.

Ethics and Evidence

The field of art therapy has been generally unsuccessful in developing protocols for establishing the validity of a method of identifying, organizing, and communicating data generated by the images produced in art therapy other than through reductionistic procedures; however, the latter are limited in their ability to capture the essence of the image as a whole unit. *Is it ethical to abandon research efforts to measure evidence of the therapeutic meaningfulness of the image as data? Is it ethical to suggest that this process cannot be translated into evidence or to suggest that one must be an artist to understand? Is it ethical to conduct a business agreement with the public if we cannot clearly explain what we are doing and how it will impact them? Is it ethical to implement that contract with a vulnerable population when we cannot produce research evidence of how it works?*

The appropriate answer to these questions is *yes*. It is ethical to continue the contract with vulnerable populations for art therapy services. The issue is not that we do not have evidence that image is a way of knowing; we do have evidence related to the meaningfulness of images and that evidence is the basis of our implementing art therapy strategies in the way that we do. The problem is not that we do not have evidence; the problem is that there is a considerable gap in what is the required language and definition of evidence as implemented in the practice model as compared to that required by the research model. We *know*, however, we have been unable, thus far, to translate that knowledge into the accepted language of science.

Concluding Thoughts Regarding Research and Dual Relationships

When we do research with a client in protocol where the focus of the research is not established best practices, there is a risk of conflict. An example would be having a client in a control group for purposes of research when you could actually be rendering services to that client. It would be unethical to render services in a manner that would not be in the best interest of the client for research purposes alone. While this seems obvious, there are instances in research where the protocol may, for example, create anxiety in the clients for the purposes of measuring that anxiety in a controlled environment. This would be unethical when working with clients, unless the provoking of anxiety and the subsequent controlled intervention were therapeutically indicated for that client at that time. It is generally unethical to conduct research with clients when there is a risk for the relationship to shift from therapist/client to therapist/subject. However, as mentioned earlier, it is efficacious and even ethically indicated to conduct research with clients when the focus of that research is the impact of the therapeutic process upon that client.

When there is a dual role issue, such as the researcher also being the mentor or educator of potential participants, our responsibility goes beyond ensuring informed consent to considering whether the power differential between us might be exerting some unacknowledged influence upon the relationship. In summary, ethics is critical in defining the scope and responsibility of the art therapist and in protecting the public. That responsibility includes not only endeavoring to ferret out instances when our work would benefit from greater clarity (such as when we are fulfilling dual roles), but also committing ourselves to the deliberate, well-considered exploration of art as a way of knowing and art as evidence.

REFLECTIVE ART EXPERIENCES & DISCUSSION QUESTIONS

1. Create two landscapes: one from the perspective of the artist; the other from the perspective of the scientist. Then integrate the above art pieces into a single landscape.
2. When is bias a detriment and when is it an advantage in inquiry?
3. What is the art therapist/researcher's responsibility in using art-based methods of inquiry?

References

Langer, S.K. (1942). *Philosophy in a new key: A study in the symbolism of reason, rite, and art.* London: Pelican Books.

Langer, S.K. (1953). *Feeling and form: A theory of art.* New York: Charles Scribner's Sons.

Moore, T. (1994). *Care of the soul: A guide for cultivating depth and sacredness in everyday life.* New York: HarperPerennial.

28

HOVERING BETWEEN ART EDUCATION AND "ART THERAPY"

The Ethical Perspective of a Ghanaian Art Educator

Mavis Osei

Indigenous "Art Therapy" in Ghana

Art is infused into the very fabric of Ghanaian society. Visual forms of art include pottery (pots and earthenware bowls traditionally known as *asanka*), sculpture (*akuaba* or wooden dolls), stools, and linguist staffs (when an Asante ruler is seeking counsel, the imagery on the staff is used by the *okyeame*, a high-ranking advisor, to convey Asante proverbs regarding power and institutional responsibilities), textiles (mainly the rich and colorful *kente* from the Ashanti region, but also the *fuugu* from northern Ghana, as well as wax prints), beadwork, and scarification. Performing arts include rituals, music, incantations, drumming, and dancing.

In Ghana, there are traditional priests and priestesses (also known as traditional therapists) who employ art making and creativity to enhance the social and emotional well-being of their clients. They are perhaps akin to western art therapists, but are especially similar to the *shamans* or native healers who use colorful sand paintings for healing in southwestern America. For example, until very recently, a woman who was considered to be barren would meet with the traditional priest and undergo rituals and incantations amid music, drumming, and dancing. Afterward, she would be given a sculptured piece called *akuaba*, a wooden doll consecrated by the priest, who would invoke the help of his deity to induce pregnancy in the user. These dolls can have special names and are accorded special power which may or may not have to do with childbirth (Pyne, Osei, & Adu-Agyem, 2013). The woman would be encouraged to role play with the doll as a mother, with the hope that she would have a child of her own. Most of the time, this worked! Is this not art therapy, since the traditional therapist enhanced the client's emotional and social well-being by aiding her transformation (from a state of barrenness to the state of motherhood) through employing the arts? Although the client did not make art, the therapist used art forms. Wouldn't her care for the wooden doll—feeding, clothing, and carrying it on her back like a real baby—qualify as creativity?

Art Therapy in Ghana

It was not until the mid-1990s that art therapy was introduced to Ghana, in the form of two courses. The individual who was responsible for this feat was my mentor and PhD supervisor, Alhaji Professor Yakubu Seidu Peligah, Professor of Art Therapy and Art Education and a past Dean, Faculty of Creative Arts and Technology, of Kumasi Technical University (formerly Kumasi Polytechnic). He was the first person to study art therapy formally, during his doctoral studies at the University of Central England (formerly Birmingham Polytechnic) from 1991–1994. Upon his return from England in 1995, he introduced art therapy to the then Department of Art Education (now Educational Innovations) at the Kwame Nkrumah University of Science and Technology (KNUST) in Kumasi, the commercial, industrial, and cultural capital of the Ashanti Region of Ghana (Peligah, 1999). Since art educators work with children with special needs, perhaps the art therapy component of the art education curriculum reflected the realization that skills in both areas are needed (Packard & Anderson, 1976). Through a Fulbright Scholarship, Mr. Joseph Amenowode studied art therapy at the Pratt Institute in New York City, earning a Master of Professional Studies degree in Art Therapy in 1997 before becoming a doctoral candidate of Professor Peligah. He later left to pursue a political career and served as Minister of the Volta Region (one of the ten regions of the Republic of Ghana) from 2009 to 2012.

Under Professor Peligah's tutelage, I—like a countless number of students—was able to get a taste of art therapy while pursuing a degree in Art Education. A myriad research studies were taking place in mental health and school settings during this period. Glime (1995) used art therapeutically and worked successfully with discharged psychiatric patients in Kumasi, while Gombilla (1997) used art beneficially with mentally ill individuals in Tamale. In 2004, Acquaye evaluated the role of art in psychiatric institutions in Ghana. Obu (2010) worked with discharged mental patients in Kumasi, introducing skill development while using textiles to help the patients enhance their sense of self-esteem. I supervised Arhin (2013), who used drawings in teaching mathematics, improving the performance of 62 pupils at a primary school where the pupils had previously had a low level of performance in mathematics. I also supervised Saah (2017), an MPhil student who developed a teaching model based upon art therapy for autistic learners, and Aba-Afari (2017), a PhD student in Ghana, who used art to bring psychological relief to traumatized victims of human trafficking. A thesis by Koomson (2017) focused upon using art with female prisoners and Koney's thesis (2017) assessed how art therapy is used in a care center.

A Chance Encounter with Art Therapy

In 2000, I was an undergraduate at KNUST. Being a painter, I was in the studio when Professor Peligah, who is also a trained artist, stopped by. We chatted about my painting and my love for children, interests which later were reflected in both my BA thesis and my PhD dissertation. This was when he mentioned that there was actually a course that could combine my love of art and my concern for children's well-being by enabling me to use art to help children and adults in different settings. The course was in Art Therapy.

Several years later, I enrolled in the Master's degree program in Art Education at KNUST. My aim was to become a teacher with a knowledge of art therapy that would enable me to help my students. As a result of my performance during my first year of study, Professor Peligah, who was head of the department, encouraged me to apply for a PhD scholarship at the university that was aimed at recruiting young scholars for lectureship positions. My dissertation centered on using art to assess children's temperament, in order to enhance their learning; when a teacher knows and understands a child's personality, it is easier for him or her to tailor lessons to suit the child and, eventually, make learning more pleasurable for the child (Enti, 2008). Positive emotions have been found to enhance learning, while the opposite is true of negative emotions (Vail, 2001). I was the proud recipient of the "Silver Award in the Humanities" from the Ghana Academy of Arts and Sciences for my PhD dissertation entitled, "The Influence of Temperament on the Artwork of Children." Professor Peligah left to head another institution in 2006 and, in 2009, I stepped into his shoes.

My Own Ethical Struggles with Art Therapy

During an Art Education class, everyone seemed listless. It was in the middle of the semester and many assignments were due; the students were worried that they hadn't done enough. It was clear to me that they were experiencing academic stress. I stopped the lecture and asked everyone to draw anything that they wanted to draw. With a sense of glee, they delved into the drawing exercise. When we discussed their drawings, the themes that arose were amazing.

Almost all of the students portrayed what was keeping them from concentrating upon the lecture, such as being homesick and worrying that their assignments were piling up.

The mood change that I witnessed as these students talked about their drawings was such a priceless gift that I later wrote about it (Osei, 2013). As the students stepped out of class that day, I could see that they were better prepared for the next class; indeed, research has shown that positive emotions enhance learning (Vail, 2001). I was not sure whether I was acting as an art educator or an art therapist, but the goal was to enhance the students' emotional well-being. My ethical dilemma was that, although I was not clinically trained to use art diagnostically, there were times when, having seen their drawings over a period of time, I was able to deduce that certain students were struggling emotionally and I found ways to counsel them, since they would not go to the school counselor even when I asked them to go. For the most part, I was successful with these students, but I always wondered about my role; the line between being an art educator and having some knowledge in art therapy seemed so blurred. Hmmm!

Teaching Art Therapy

Within the Art Education Department, I teach classes in Art Therapy at both the undergraduate and the postgraduate level. During the first semester, undergraduates learn about the theories and techniques of art therapy in the "Introduction to Art Therapy." In "Practicum in Art Therapy," during the second semester, they put to use (mainly in schools) what they learnt in the previous semester. The postgraduate courses are fashioned after the undergraduate courses, but are in more depth. Most past and current of the students in the postgraduate classes are teachers in high schools, colleges, or universities; a few of them are heads of departments at their institutions. Several students have backgrounds in the military or in police work.

An Art Educator/"Art Therapist" Dilemma

At the time I am writing this chapter, there are no Master's degree programs in Ghana for training art therapists in accordance with the standards of the American Art Therapy Association. Hence, when our students, who are mainly teachers, graduate, many seem to believe that—because they have experienced two semesters of art therapy—they are equipped, to a certain degree, to offer art therapy services, particularly in their classrooms or in school settings. This is where the art education/art therapy dichotomy arises. Although the degree that these individuals have obtained is a Master's in Art Education, if these students took art therapy courses as electives, their dissertations would be written about *art therapy*, rather than art education. *So are they art educators or art therapists?* Because many have been able to see indications of learning disabilities and/or emotional struggles in their students' drawings, probably the art educator becomes a kind of "therapist" in the classroom when the need arises.

MY ETHICAL DILEMMA

Opportunities to use art "therapeutically"

If, in a country with no full-fledged academic art therapy training program, an art educator has taken the art therapy courses available, would it be more—or less—ethical to ignore opportunities to use art "therapeutically"?

How would you respond?

For the writer's response, see Appendix B, page 425.

Art Therapy and Ghana: The Future

My quest to become a trained art therapist did not end after receiving my PhD in 2008. I joined the American Art Therapy Association (AATA) to keep up with research that was going on in art therapy, through the journals I received and, at AATA's 2015 annual conference in Minneapolis, Minnesota, I presented my research proposal at the AATA Research Committee's "Research Round Table." In 2016, after competing with several thousand applicants, I received a Fulbright scholarship to study Clinical Art Therapy here in New York. Finally! I am hopeful that this will give me the tools to establish a one-year Creative Art Therapy training program in Ghana—the plans for which I had written up prior to receiving the scholarship.

Talwar, Iyer, and Doby-Copeland (2004) observed that "the cultural identity of art therapy lies in its EuroAmerican roots" (p. 44). In order to make art therapy culturally relevant to the people of my country, I want to focus especially upon multicultural competencies and ways in which to use art—including the indigenous arts—therapeutically within the Ghanaian context. As mentioned earlier, Ghanaian forms of art go far beyond the painting and drawing which are most prominent in western art-based assessments and therapeutic interventions. Moreover, many Ghanaians are not "fond of" traditional forms of therapy. Thus, an eclectic approach that draws from different theories and styles, including community art therapy, might suit the Ghanaian community, since it can be a participatory practice aimed at strengthening the capacity for social action and change (Jacobs, 2002), while allowing for the exploration of the wide variety of art forms that are an intrinsic part of Ghanaian culture. As I pursue my dream, I expect to have many more questions, but isn't persistence—and creativity—part of what art therapists bring to their work?

REFLECTIVE ART EXPERIENCES & DISCUSSION QUESTIONS

1. Using an African proverb of your choice (perhaps one that has to do with an identity crisis), create a motif to be used for a cloth.
2. Using any pottery technique, create and decorate two pots. One should depict how you perceive yourself; the other, people's perception of you.
3. Envision yourself developing an art therapy training program for the people of Ghana. How would you tailor a specific course to their particular social and cultural needs?
4. Based upon the author's description of the wide variety of art forms in Ghanaian society, develop an art therapy intervention that would be based upon visual and/or performing arts that are an inherent part of the culture.

References

Aba-Afari, S. (2017). Art therapy as an intervention to mitigate traumatic effects upon victims of human trafficking: A case of Kumasi metropolis. Unpublished doctoral dissertation. Kwame Nkrumah University of Science and Technology (KNUST), Department of Educational Innovations, Kumasi, Ghana.

Acquaye, R. (2004). Evaluation of art therapy practices in psychiatric institutions in Ghana. Unpublished master's thesis. KNUST, Kumasi, Ghana.

Arhin, E.L., & Osei, M. (2013). Children's mathematics performance and drawing activities: A constructive correlation. *Journal of Education and Practice*, 4(9), 28–34.

Enti, M. (2008). The influence of temperament on the artwork of children. Unpublished doctoral dissertation. KNUST, Kumasi, Ghana.

Glime, O. (1995). The impact of therapeutic art in the rehabilitation of discharged psychiatric patients in Ghana: A case study of the Kumasi Cheshire Home. Unpublished doctoral thesis. KNUST, Kumasi, Ghana.

Gombilla, E. (1997). Art of the insane: A special study in Tamale. Unpublished master's thesis. KNUST, Kumasi, Ghana.

Jacobs, J.A. (2002). Drawing is a catharsis for children. *National Undergraduate Research Clearinghouse*, 5. Retrieved from www.clearinghouse.net/volume/

Koney, J.N.A. (2017). An evaluative study of art therapy in the management of trauma in children at the Touch a Life Care Center, Kumasi. Unpublished master's thesis. KNUST, Kumasi, Ghana.

Koomson, E. (2017). Art therapy for stress management among prison inmates: A case of Kumasi female prison. Unpublished master's thesis. KNUST, Kumasi, Ghana.

Obu, P. (2010). The response of discharged mental patients (inmates) to selected art activities in textiles at the Kumasi Cheshire Home. Unpublished master's thesis. KNUST, Kumasi, Ghana.

Osei, M. (2013, November). Relieving stress: The art factor. Paper presented at the 6th International Conference on Education, Research and Innovation, Seville, Spain.

Packard, S., & Anderson, F. (1976). A shared identity crisis: Art education and art therapy. *Art Therapy: Journal of the American Art Therapy Association*, 16(7), 21–28.

Peligah, Y.S. (1999). What is art therapy? *Journal of the University of Science and Technology, Kumasi*, 19(1–3), 39–46.

Pyne, S., Osei, M. & Adu-Agyem, J. (2013). The use of indigenous arts in the therapeutic practices of traditional priests and priestesses of Asante, Ghana. *International Journal of Innovative Research & Development,* 2(11), 464–474.

Saah, G.E. (2017). Art therapy in special needs education: A case of autism at New Horizon Special School in Accra. Unpublished master's thesis. KNUST, Kumasi, Ghana.

Talwar, S., Iyer, J., & Doby-Copeland, C. (2004). The invisible veil: Changing paradigms in the art therapy profession. *Art Therapy: Journal of the American Art Therapy Association*, 21(1), 44–48.

Tyng, C.M., Amin, H.U., Saad, M.N.M, & Malik, A.S. (2017). The influences of emotion on learning and memory. *Frontiers in Psychology*, 8, 1454.

Vail, P.L. (2001). The role of emotions in learning. Retrieved from www.greatschools.net/cgibin/showarticle/2369

29

IT'S NOT ALL ACADEMIC

Addressing Non-academic Ethical Issues That Arise in Art Therapy Education

Mary Roberts

But I Just Got Here!

During my first two months as the Program Director of a graduate art therapy program, I received an alarming email from a faculty member: "I have a student in my class who disclosed his substance use in his journal assignment. What should I do?"

It was as if a bright spotlight had illuminated an ethical dilemma for me. Immediately, I was barraged by questions: *As Program Director, what is my role regarding student substance use? What are the boundaries in educational assignments? How will I determine if this student is ready for an internship with patients? What is our institution's policy regarding students who are in need of support due to mental illness or other problems? Is this cause for dismissal from the program? Should it be cause for dismissal from the program? How do my beliefs as an art therapist intersect with my values and goals as an educator and with the policies and procedures that are in place? How do I support this faculty member, while also supporting the student, and uphold the academic standards of the program and the institution? How much of the situation is confidential and what can be shared with the faculty, the student affairs office, or other university officials?*

What Did I Do?

I felt the need to investigate the substance use disclosed in the course assignment, the relationship between the faculty member and the student, the relevant policies and procedures, the resources available for students, and the options for intervention. I asked the faculty member to email me all of the student's work pertaining to the disclosure, as well as the course assignment in the syllabus. It was important for me to understand the boundaries of the assignment; being new to the program, I had not yet reviewed every syllabus and course assignment.

I then turned to the "Responsibilities to Art Therapy Students and Supervisees" section of the American Art Therapy Association's (AATA's) *Ethical Principles for Art Therapists*:

Art therapists do not require students or supervisees to disclose personal infor-mation in course or program-related activities…except when (a) the program or training facility has clearly identified this requirement in its admissions and program materials, or (b) the information is necessary to evaluate or obtain assistance for students whose personal problems could reasonably be judged to be preventing them from performing their training or professional related activities in a competent manner or whose personal problems could reasonably be judged to pose a threat to the students, their clients, or others.

American Art Therapy Association, 2013, Principle 8.5

The course description and assignments provided students with freedom of choice in responding to "Action Exercises," one of which was described as follows:

Identify a substance you are willing not to ingest or an activity you are willing not to participate in for the next two weeks of class … You will not be graded on whether or not you were able to refrain from the substance or activity, but rather on the depth of your responses, reflective skills, and self-understanding.

By instructor report, historically most students had selected to abstain from substances such as sugar or caffeine, rather than alcohol or drugs. The student's written response to the assignment documented his decision to abstain from alcohol and described his struggles to meet this goal, indicating that he had experienced relapses from abstin-ence, each becoming more severe.

I asked that I be sent any correspondence the faculty member had had with the student so that I could evaluate the professionalism of the relationship, based upon University policy regarding the teacher/learner relationship and principle 8.2 of AATA's ethics code:

Art therapists are aware of their influential position with respect to students and supervisees, and they avoid exploiting the trust and dependency of such persons. Art therapists, therefore, do not engage in a therapeutic relationship with their students or supervisees.

As an educator, I struggled with ethical boundaries in evaluating the non-academic behaviors of the student. It was difficult to turn off my clinical ability to assess the content of his paper as indicating a problem with addiction. I decided to consult with the Associate Dean of Student Affairs to assist in the evaluation of my concerns, thereby enabling me to proceed to the next step, with institutional support. After evaluating the student's response to the assignment, the Associate Dean agreed that the content of the student's paper met a level of concern that warranted intervention. As the student planned to enroll in an internship the following semester, we also spoke about patient care. The Dean and I determined that there was sufficient concern to interview the student, to make a referral for substance use/addictions treatment, and to draw up a Student Impairment Plan.

Although the student readily acknowledged that his journal responses to the assignment were accurate, he became anxious and disgruntled once he understood that I had concerns for his well-being and patient safety. I was concerned about not embarrassing the student or disclosing the student's struggles, yet, being new to the program, I thought it best for his faculty advisor to be aware of the student's problems. The Council for the Advancement of Standards in Higher Education's ethics code (2006) states, "We maintain confidentiality of interactions, student records, and information related to legal and private matters" (principle V). Therefore, I asked the student specifically if I could share information with his faculty advisor; he consented. This gave him access to the support of a faculty member whom he knew, while engaging in an action plan process with the institution and with me.

The Student Affairs Office did intervene, to help place the student on a Student Impairment Plan, which required the student to have a third party mental health and substance use/addiction evaluation. The evaluation led to a recommendation for treatment and a "fit for work" evaluation. This evaluation resulted in a recommendation that the student engage in addiction treatment, attend Alcoholics Anonymous meetings, and refrain from enrolling in classes or internship during a Medical Leave of Absence, until it was determined that he was "fit for work."

It took a month to coordinate and officially enact the Student Impairment Plan. The student actively engaged in both the plan and treatment over the course of a semester, successfully completed another "fit for work" assessment, and transitioned back into the program with continued participation in treatment and AA while completing academic requirements and internship. The plan included the student signing consent for disclosure between his substance use treatment provider and the university. Thus, I was able to consult with the treatment provider to ensure that the student was attending and engaged, as well as to reassure faculty that the student was on track and safe with patients, without disclosing any information to the faculty. Ultimately, the student was successful in managing his addiction, treatment, academic, and non-academic challenges and successfully graduated from the program.

When Educators Are Also (Art) Therapists

But My Other Hat Is All Broken In

In small higher education programs, often faculty have multiple roles with students, such as instructor, advisor, capstone/thesis chair, art therapy supervisor, or administrator. The intersection of these roles can easily give rise to ethical dilemmas. It is also worth keeping in mind that art therapy education is practice oriented; moreover, usually the faculty of art therapy programs have moved from clinical practice to higher education—often without having received training in education. When students present with mental health issues that impact their academic and non-academic performance, art therapy faculty members can face ethical dilemmas regarding how, when, and whether to apply their clinical knowledge—as opposed to educational policies and procedures—to the situation at hand. At times, the "decision" might not even be conscious.

MY ETHICAL DILEMMA

How should I respond when I hear: "He seems to be doing well, considering his emotional state"?

A student who you believe is struggling with mental health issues appears to be experiencing a great deal of difficulty in completing an assignment which will account for a large percentage of his grade in your course. The paper is due in a week.

How would you respond?

For the writer's response, see Appendix B, page 430.

When confronted by ethical dilemmas, I have often called upon my training in Administration and the Supervision of Educators. I believe that it is crucial for art therapy educators to be trained not only in best practices in art therapy, but also in best practices in education, as well as to familiarize themselves with laws that pertain to education (e.g., students' rights). Distinguishing our dual professional identity from our singular educator identity with students is crucial to ensuring compliance with AATA's ethical principle 8.2 (presented earlier in this chapter).

But I'm an Art Therapist—How Can I Possibly Grade Student Artwork?

Art therapy faculty members often express difficulty in evaluating the artwork of art therapy students. If, as art therapists, we regard all artistic creations as being of value, how, then, can we attach grades to them? Our program addressed the ethical issue of evaluating student artwork by creating a rubric that captures competencies that are not based upon aesthetics or artistic talent, but upon clarity of conceptualization in artwork and level of investment; quality of artwork; display and presentation; and clarity of written commentary. The degree of the student's competence in each area is presented in developmental, growth-oriented language: *advanced, proficient, developing, emerging*, and *inadequate* (see Figure 29.1). Art therapy students who rush through their art making or approach the assignment with minimal investment typically do not have clarity in conceptualizing their artwork, which becomes evident in its presentation and in the written commentary. Art therapy students who take risks, display self-awareness, creatively apply learning and skills (evident in the resulting art piece and written commentary), and invest in visualizing learning are evaluated as having proficient or advanced competency. Using this rubric promotes the ethical treatment of student artwork, as well as greater objectivity in evaluating it, while maintaining the valued practice of using art to reveal, reflect upon, and integrate various aspects of the learning process.

Student: _____

Instructor: _____

Art Project Rubric

Art Project Rubric Competencies	10-9.4 Advanced	9.3-8.4 Proficient-Adequate	8.3-7.4 Developing	7.3-1 Emerging	0 Inade-quate	Total	%
(60%) Clarity of Conceptual-ization in Artwork/Level of Personal Investment:	Exceptional skill and investment in exploration (insert topic of assignment), insight gained, and ability to express this in a creative and concise manner. Originality and creativity are considered here. Individual openness and self-awareness. Conceptualization and personal investment are the primary goals of the project.	Above average investment in exploration of processes and materials, insight gained, and ability to express this in a creative and concise manner. Evidence of critical thought.	Average personal investment and exploration.	Barely average grasp of directions and concepts. Poor investment in personal exploration. Rushed, not thoughtful approach to project.	Did not complete.		
(20%) Quality of Artwork:	Exceptional skill and investment in the use of media with regard to craftsmanship, choice of materials, and aesthetics. Unique, original artwork. Evidence of investment and time.	Above average craftsmanship; appropriate choice of materials and aesthetics.	Average craftsmanship and choice of materials.	Little to no investment, below average craftsmanship.	Did not complete.		
(10%) Display and Presentation:	Artwork is exhibited in a unique and exceptional way to impact the viewer. Professional offering for view and explanation, including the presenter's verbal commentary and presentation behavior.	Above average and thought out presentation of artwork. Above average level of professionalism in verbal and non-verbal presentation of artwork.	Average and predictable display. Some areas may lack clarity, but overall presentation is effective.	Brief verbal presentation with unclear messages. Little evidence of planning and practice. Intention is unclear.	Did not complete.		
(10%) Clarity of Written Commentary:	Thorough explanations or interpretations used to illustrate, clarify or convey the meaning of the artwork and/or the art making process that led to its creation. The viewer should be able to understand the meaning of the artwork by viewing it and reading the commentary. References have been cited. The writing is edited to be grammatically correct and error free.	Viewer/reader has an understanding of concept and intention. Few questions may remain. Few to no errors in writing.	Viewer/reader has a general idea of the meaning/intention of the artwork. Some questions may remain. Some errors in writing.	Unclear messages in writing. Viewer has many questions as to the meaning of the artwork and intention. Many distracting errors in writing.	Did not complete.		

Total Points Earned:

Total Deductions:

Total Points:

•Feedback to student:

Created by: Mary Roberts, EdS, LPC, ATR-BC (2013); Cheryl Shiflett, PhD, LPC, ATR-BC (2014); edited by: Matthew Bernier, MCAT, ATR-BC (2015)

FIGURE 29.1 *Art Project Rubric.*

Collaboration, Communication, Consensus

Since best practices in education call for an education team to have a collective mission, vision, and core values which drive program education practices, policies, and procedures impacting both faculty and students (Dufour, Dufour, Eaker, & Many, 2010), shortly after being hired, I facilitated a faculty retreat in which we collectively revised our mission and vision statements and identified our core values (integrity, creativity, self-awareness, humanity, collaboration, and depth). Our program is based upon social constructivist, experiential, and growth-oriented education practices (McAuliffe & Eriksen, 2011; Dweck, 2008). We believe that, through an organizational culture (Gorton, Alston, & Snowden, 2007) of growth-oriented experiences and meaning-making within a social context, we can cultivate the artist-therapist identity and competencies. The importance of collaboration among faculty members and administrators in this process cannot be overly emphasized—nor can the importance of the regularly scheduled faculty meetings that provide the opportunity for such collaboration, as participants raise issues, air concerns, explore options, and work to reach consensus.

Boundary setting with students, particularly challenged students, can pose ethical issues for faculty. When a student's performance falls below expectations, it can feel natural to adopt a therapeutic perspective, trying to gain a better understanding of the student's situation. Doing so can result in the underreporting—or the withholding—of concerns from the Program Director and other faculty. Sharing this information with "the boss" can feel like tattling or exposing one's inadequacy as a teacher, but concerns cannot be addressed, monitored, or laid to rest unless they are aired. Consider the following scenarios.

MY ETHICAL DILEMMA

A student failed her initial courses; no action plan had been initiated. How should I proceed?

During her first semester coursework, a student repeatedly does poorly on written assignments. Although general concern about the student's writing is raised, no clear, detailed accounts of the student's below average performance on summative and formative assessments is offered. When she fails these fundamental courses, the student is unable to progress to the next semester, which involves working with clients.

How would you respond?

For the writer's response, see Appendix B, page 431.

MY ETHICAL DILEMMA

What should be done when a student who is in good academic standing exhibits a lack of investment in her internship?

A student who was in good academic standing, based upon course grades, exhibited a lack of investment in her internship and a lack of empathy for the clients assigned to her, missing days of her internship without letting her supervisors or the faculty know, and documenting work late or not at all. Many weeks later, the student claimed that her mental illness was impacting her ability to meet expectations.

How would you respond?

For the writer's response, see Appendix B, page 431.

OUR ETHICAL DILEMMA

How do we allow an individual with a mental illness to become an art therapist? How do we disallow an individual with a mental illness to become an art therapist?

A student openly disclosed her struggles with mental illness, a condition that seemed to sap her energy, cause her to struggle to attain only surface-level engagement in coursework, and participate only minimally at her internship. She made no progress during a semester of thesis work. Faculty members struggled with this ethical dilemma.

How would you respond?

For the writer's response, see Appendix B, page 432.

Conclusion

Structuring our weekly faculty meetings to include a discussion of the performance of each of our students has enabled us to provide increased challenge for those who are excelling and additional support for those who are struggling. Action plans and mechanisms for monitoring progress are documented in faculty meeting minutes. Care is taken to ensure that the policies and procedures described in the Student

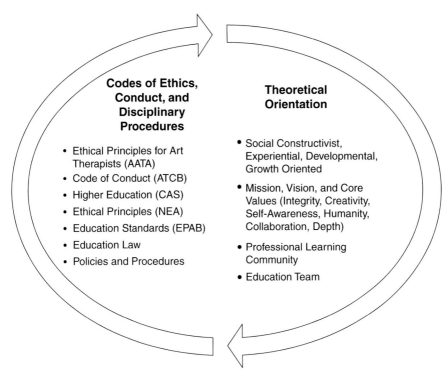

FIGURE 29.2 *Our Program's Ethical Lens.*

Handbook reflect the roles, responsibilities, and ethical boundaries of both faculty and students. Every art therapy program is a work in progress and every ethical dilemma that presents itself provides an opportunity for program improvement. Developing ethical principles for art therapy educators is a logical next step. Only by looking carefully at each situation through an ethical lens can an art therapy program meet its ethical responsibility to students, to clients, and to the profession.

REFLECTIVE ART EXPERIENCES & DISCUSSION QUESTIONS

Create an image of your artist/therapist/educator identity.

a. Describe the formal elements of the art image.
b. Describe the space, form, and balance of the symbolic representation of artist, therapist, and educator.
c. How does this representation bring insight into your areas of focus and your professional development needs?

d. How do your beliefs as an art therapist intersect with your values and goals as an educator and with the policies and procedures that are in place where you work?

Create a visual representation of a challenged student.

a. What does the image reveal about your unintentional biases toward challenged students?
b. What does the image reveal about the values of your art therapist self regarding challenged students?
c. What does the image reveal about your affective responses to challenged students?
d. What is your role with, and what are your ethical responsibilities to, challenged students?

References

American Art Therapy Association (2013). Ethical principles for art therapists. Retrieved from: www.arttherapy.org/upload/ethicalprinciples.pdf

Council for the Advancement of Standards in Higher Education (2006). *CAS* Statement of Shared Ethical Principles. Retrieved from: http://cas.membershipsoftware.org/files/CASethicsstatement.pdf

DuFour, R., DuFour, R., Eaker, R., & Many, T. (2010). *Learning by doing: A handbook for professional learning communities at work* (2nd ed.). Bloomington, IN: Solution Tree Press.

Dweck, C. (2008). *Mindset: The new psychology of success*. New York: Random House.

Gorton, R., Alston, J.A., Snowden, P. (2007). *School leadership and administration: Important concepts, case studies, and simulations* (7th ed.). Boston, MA: McGraw-Hill.

Graduate Art Therapy and Counseling Program (2016). *Student handbook*. Norfolk, VA: Eastern Virginia Medical School.

McAuliffe, G., & Eriksen, K. (Eds). (2011). *Handbook of counselor preparation: Constructivist, developmental, and experiential approaches*. Los Angeles, CA: Sage.

30

TESTIFYING ON THE TERMINATION OF PARENTAL RIGHTS

Art Therapy and Case Management in an Early Intervention Program

Cheryl Doby-Copeland

When an Art Therapist Isn't Called an Art Therapist

Despite having over 40 years of experience as an art therapist, there have been many times when I have had to remind myself of my preferred clinical identity. My experience is consistent with that described by Gussak and Orr (2005), in that I have seldom held the professional title of art therapist. It wasn't until I began working for an urban behavioral health system that I encountered an institutional posture that simultaneously endorsed the benefits of art therapy while suggesting that social workers are the standard for independent clinical practice, as well as program management. In spite of this, I have been able to maintain my identity as an art therapist while endeavoring to advance my professional career. Fortunately, years of personal values clarification, cultural competence training, experience as Chairperson of the Ethics Committee of the American Art Therapy Association (AATA), and training in reflective supervision have furnished me with a solid foundation from which to address the ethical dilemmas I face daily.

I have provided art therapy to several populations, including chronically institutionalized adult/geriatric patients with schizophrenia and adolescents in a maximum-security juvenile detention facility. My family art therapy experience began in a community-based clinic where half of my hours were devoted to providing art therapy to children in schools or in their homes. Currently, I am a founding member of a community-based early intervention program, providing art and play therapy to families with children under eight years old who present with behaviors that are consistent with ADHD, ODD, mood disorders, attachment disorders, anxiety, depression, or autism spectrum disorders. In addition to maintaining my clinical caseload and providing case management, I am a clinical program coordinator of the child psychiatrists triage team, I train/supervise staff in Child Parent Psychotherapy (CPP) for families with children exposed to trauma, and I supervise the clinic front desk staff.

Putting Aspirational Values into Practice

From the moment a client enters our clinic, I encourage the front desk staff to greet clients in a welcoming and empathic manner, conveying positive regard and a person-centered approach to treatment. I find that I'm frequently the one who reminds staff and administrators of the need for informed consent—not just when we begin treatment, but when we video tape clients, offer them new evidence-based treatments, interview them for newspaper articles, invite them to speak at conferences, involve students/interns in providing mental health services/supervision, or, of course, want to use clients' artwork in my teaching. Orienting families that are unfamiliar with, suspicious of, or unmotivated to participate in mental health services in general and art therapy in particular, is almost a daily task for me. I consciously work to convey not only *nonmaleficence*, but also the *beneficence*, *justice*, and respect for *autonomy* that all clients have a right to expect (AATA, 2013). As a government-run mental health service, we are required to provide, with *fidelity*, evidence-based interventions to children with presenting problems such as social-emotional disorders, exposure to domestic/community violence, grief/loss, neglect, sexual/physical/emotional abuse, and placement in foster care. Personally, I value offering art therapy and case management services with fidelity to my clients, thereby working with integrity and *creativity*, and ensuring my honesty and faithfulness to the therapeutic relationship (AATA, 2013).

Fulfilling the Roles of Case Manager and Art Therapist

Frequently Encountered Ethical Issues

Fidelity versus client choice. I learned several models of case management when I was trained in Psychiatric Rehabilitation early in my career. The clinical case management model, which closely resembles my therapeutic approach, includes several activities that guide the effective case manager, such as connecting with clients, planning for services, linking clients to services, and advocating for service improvements (Anthony, Cohen, & Farkas, 1990). I am involved in each of these activities with every client on my caseload. It is humbling to work with those who bring their children to our clinic: parents who feel as if they have failed as caregivers; grandparents who are trying to raise grandchildren because their own children have been murdered, incarcerated, neglectful, or abusive; or foster parents who want to adopt their charges, are being court ordered to come, or are risking a monthly state stipend unless they come. Using a strength-based approach, I endeavor to determine the benevolent intent of each guardian with whom I work. An example follows.

MY ETHICAL DILEMMA

When fidelity and client choice conflict, how do I proceed?

I have frequently experienced an ethical dilemma when told by a guardian that he or she has explained to the young child in his or her care that their parent is "away in college" instead of telling the child the truth: that the parent is incarcerated.

How would you respond?

For the writer's response, see Appendix B, page 404.

Physical closeness. In therapy, all of my encounters are cross-cultural. Therefore, I endeavor to determine how I can support the development of trust in me as a clinician that will, in turn, support the child and family as they work to achieve their treatment goals. Connecting with clients often raises ethical dilemmas related to issues of physical closeness, such as when children hug me, hold my hand, or try to touch my jewelry, versus when adult male guardians hug me spontaneously or as a method of greeting me. Although the need for physical closeness can stem from inadequate social skills, unsatisfying relationships, and poor boundaries, each instance must be viewed individually with an understanding of the client's culture, presenting problem, and rationale for the need to touch the therapist (Furman, 2013). The action of a three-year-old child who runs to greet me with a big hug carries a different meaning than that of a 50-year-old father who attempts to hug me. When a five-year-old child with impulse control issues spontaneously reaches for my hand instead of running down the hallway, this suggests increased self-regulation and is, therefore, encouraged. My clinical supervision has allowed me to discuss the therapeutic value of using touch in therapy in order to avoid misinterpretation (Furman, 2013).

When the intake process is over and therapy begins, I explain the use of art making as a therapeutic intervention to the parents of my young clients, often to hear parents say, *"My child can draw pictures at home!"* So, in addition to being able to explain art therapy to other professionals, it is important to be able to explain art therapy to parents, child welfare workers, guardians *ad litem*, and family court judges. Since explaining the utility of art therapy to families that are not used to receiving mental health services can be challenging, I often engage them in an art making activity to help them grasp its usefulness in addressing their treatment goals. Art-making tasks such as mandalas, family art evaluations, bird's nest drawings, and bilateral scribbling have all yielded great success in introducing families with young children to art therapy.

Gift giving and receiving. When I worked at a community-based family therapy clinic, the agency practice of giving holiday gifts to clients created an ethical dilemma, as the clients' siblings weren't included in the gift exchange; eventually this practice was suspended. Gift giving takes on complex forms, from children who bring gifts to me after their vacations to my giving gifts such as completion of therapy certificates or journals to honor clients' accomplishments (Furman, 2013). Many of my African American clients have given me gifts, from a small flower vase to a ceramic mask. I tend to accept these gifts as they symbolize a cultural practice of showing appreciation; however, I am also mindful of my agency's $10 limit on the value of a gift (Furman, 2013).

Complex Ethical Decision Making

Kapitan (2008) states that, "In any complex ethical decision-making process … the first step is to recognize the moral dimension at stake" (p. 155). As a case manager and therapist, I must advocate not only for services for my clients, but also—in cases where the child is no longer in the custody of the parent(s)—for a permanency placement that is in the best interest of the child.

Over the course of my career, I have been subpoenaed several times. In one instance, the guardian's attorney who subpoenaed me provided 60 questions to help me prepare. The questions focused upon the primary purpose of my testimony; my eligibility to qualify as an expert witness; the therapeutic services that I provided to the child, including a description of my observations of the interactions between the child and the prospective adoptive parent; the child's diagnosis; and the results of any psychological testing or other assessments administered. On another occasion, I was subpoenaed by the attorney of a pre-adoptive parent. When I indicated that the child and the pre-adoptive parent had attended fewer than half of our scheduled clinical appointments within two years, the attorney decided not to call me to testify.

MY ETHICAL DILEMMA

How should I respond when subpoenaed to testify on the termination of the parental rights?

Monae was 26 months old when she was referred to our clinic due to exposure to parental domestic violence, substance use, and maternal neglect. She was smearing feces, pulling out her hair, and acting aggressively toward her one-year-old sister (e.g., pushing her, taking her toys, and pulling out her hair). After their father punched a hole in the wall and both parents tested positive for PCP at the time, the home was deemed unsafe for the two young children and they were removed from their parents' care.

Because the permanency goal for the two girls was reunification with one or both parents, the family was provided with family therapy, which the parents attended consistently despite no longer living as a couple. The mother complied with court requirements that she receive substance use screenings and obtain adequate housing and employment. Both parents were very attuned to their children and actively participated in the child-centered play therapy and art therapy that were used to address parent/child relationships. In fact, they needed on-going support to allow Monae to lead the play, as they were eager to play with the toys and to direct the art-making activities. Observing themes in Monae's play and art was particularly important, as her articulation problems made her speech difficult to understand.

Unfortunately, events in the lives of both parents caused them to relapse and to be arrested; eventually mother lost her job and housing. The child welfare agency requires that children placed in care have a permanency arrangement within 18–24 months. In Monae's case, over two years passed as the agency and I tried to support mother through her relapse to get the services she needed in the hope that she could be reunited with her children. Despite this, mother and father relapsed again and the mother was rearrested. Given these events, the permanency plan changed from reunification to adoption by the foster mother, and the mother's attorney subpoenaed me to testify in court about the family therapy. I found myself in an ethical dilemma. As Monae's therapist, I was committed to advocate for what was in her best interest. Monae's mother anticipated that I would testify against the termination of her parental rights and I knew that the termination of those rights would be devastating, placing her tenuous recovery in jeopardy. Although the father indicated his willingness to be the girls' guardian, he was unemployed and without adequate housing. I anticipated being asked under oath if I felt that parental rights should be terminated.

How would you respond?

For the writer's response, see Appendix B, page 404.

Concluding Thoughts: The Process of Ethical Decision Making

Each time I am subpoenaed to testify in court as an expert witness in art therapy, I anticipate that my clinical interventions will be called into question. Reflective supervision (Heffron & Murch, 2010)—which is my approach to training staff and interns—promotes the uncovering of the meaning of the client's, the therapist's, and the supervisor's behaviors, as a guide to developing interventions. Discussions during my own reflective supervision sessions considered the implications of my clinical interventions, the choice of actions/words/responses during court testimony, my understanding of the cultural and contextual aspects of the work, and how my art psychotherapy approaches and other related experiences inform my work. Besides benefitting from the clinical supervision of two experienced colleagues, I learned in one of the best ethics trainings I have attended that ethical decision-making derives from being intentional in my actions and having moral principles, sound clinical knowledge, and the courage of my convictions (Jobes, 2011). Jobes's "Pillars of Ethical Practice" also includes acknowledging my ethical responsibility to all family members in a case, continually obtaining informed consent, maintaining thorough and concurrent documentation, documenting my professional consultation, and developing the professional backbone to act in the best interest of my clients.

On the day of my testimony, one of many things I reminded myself of was the following: "I know what I know and I know what I don't know. Neither the judge nor any of the attorneys knows what I know. Therefore, I testify with confidence."

REFLECTIVE ART EXPERIENCES & DISCUSSION QUESTIONS

1. Being asked by a guardian to support the perpetuation of an untruthful explanation of the whereabouts of a parent can cause an ethical dilemma for the therapist.

a. Draw what feelings this situation brings up for you.
b. What strengths, resources, and treatment goals could be identified in the situation described above?

2. Envision having a family therapy session with your client and her parents after your court testimony appeared to support the termination of their parental rights and the adoption of the child by her foster parent. Draw your role as an advocate for the well-being of your client, keeping in mind how various possibilities/events might change over time.
3. Consider how your role as an advocate for the best interests of the child could place you at odds with the parents' desire for reunification. What might you say to the parents to minimize a disruption of the therapeutic bond you have formed with them throughout the course of treatment?

References

American Art Therapy Association (2013). *Ethical principles for art therapists*. Alexandria, VA: Author.

Anthony, W., Cohen, M., & Farkas, M. (1990). *Psychiatric Rehabilitation*. Boston, MA: Boston University Sargent College of Allied Health Professions.

Furman, L.R. (2013). *Ethics in art therapy: Challenging topics for a complex modality*. London: Jessica Kingsley.

Gussak, D.E., & Orr, P. (2005). Ethical responsibilities: Preparing students for the real art therapy world. *Art Therapy: Journal of the American Art Therapy Association*, 22(2), 101–104.

Heffron, M.C., & Murch, T. (2010). *Reflective supervision and leadership in infant and early childhood programs*. Washington, DC: Zero to Three National Center for Infants and Toddlers.

Jobes, D.A. (2011, February). Contemporary ethics and risk management. Ethics training conducted at St. Elizabeths Hospital, Washington, DC.

Kapitan, L. (2008). Moral courage, ethical choice: Taking responsibility for change. *Art Therapy: Journal of the American Art Therapy Association*, 25(4), 154–155.

31

THE ART THERAPIST/ART TEACHER

Practicing Ethically in Treatment Settings and School Settings

Barbara Mandel

Epiphany

Browsing through my college library, I came across a book by an author I had never heard of, about a field I knew nothing about: *Art as Therapy with Children* by Edith Kramer (1971). It was a life-changing experience. I knew immediately that I had discovered my future profession. My devotion to the improvement of people's lives through creativity, which had found expression in my work as an art teacher, now had a name—*art therapy*. I would return to teaching but, before long, entered an art therapy graduate program and began my career as an art therapist. This chapter compares the roles of art therapist and art educator and presents ethical issues that arise in the two professions.

Commonalities and Differences

The art therapist must provide an environment where unconscious fears and fantasies can be expressed free of censorship and must guide the creative process, not direct it. This requires specified time limits, spatial boundaries, developmentally appropriate art supplies, and a commitment to confidentiality (breached only when there is evidence of abuse, suicidality, or an imminent intention to harm others). Consistent rules limiting physical contact and providing for the safe use of materials must be respected. Self-disclosure is used judiciously. With these guidelines in place, the art therapist can assist the client in activating the transformative, healing power of art and the creative potential that resides in each one of us.

Similarly, the art teacher ensures that the classroom is safe and supportive and conveys the message that individuality is respected and that there can be many solutions to problems. Materials are developmentally appropriate and clear expectations and rules govern their use. Respect for the teacher, each student, and every work of art is emphasized. Goals and ethical practices in the classroom are very different from those in the clinical setting, however. There are fewer choices. The art teacher chooses the media, designs the projects, teaches skills, and guides the process towards an aesthetically pleasing final product. Exhibiting artwork (allowed in art therapy only under carefully prescribed conditions) is very important, celebrating the students' identities as artists. Gifts may be accepted from students, especially during holidays and times of transition. Touch is used selectively, such as when saying goodbye at the end of the year. Self-disclosure occurs, but only with a clear purpose (e.g., showing students my artwork as a source of inspiration and sharing a common interest in movies, sports, and music, to foster positive relationships). Assessments, including grades that evaluate craftsmanship, creativity, risk-taking, completion of work, and respect for peers, adults, materials, and the work space, are common practice.

Art Therapy

For 15 years I worked as an art therapist at a residential treatment center for severely emotionally disturbed children and adolescents with histories of psychosis, aggression, and abuse. The average stay was one to two years, so my work was long-term. Clients were referred to me by their primary therapists; after conducting art therapy evaluations, I would determine if they were likely to benefit from art therapy and, if so, whether to see them individually or in one of several groups I developed.

Art Therapy/Puppetry Group

My art therapy groups often incorporated elements of dramatic play. Puppetry enables socially isolated children to present dilemmas and try out new solutions to them. Forbidden wishes and impulses can be safely discharged. I led a year-long puppetry therapy group for four 10-year-old boys. Jack, intermittently psychotic and preoccupied with death, was a victim of extreme family dysfunction and suspected physical abuse; his "*wizard*" puppet allowed him to express morbid fantasies, while providing momentary relief from feelings of powerlessness. John, who suffered from Gilles de la Tourette syndrome, created a "*bandit*" puppet with a taped-over mouth, his attempt to gain control over impulses. Gary, a victim of abandonment, created a marionette. As he manipulated the strings, he practiced mastering fear of rejection by taking control of the comings and goings of his puppet. Stanley, a withdrawn, socially isolated child who related through whining and crying, made a "telephone" puppet that reflected a desire to connect with other group members, as well as an attempt to overcome fear of interpersonal contact.

Thematic Art Therapy Groups

For slightly older boys, more capable of conceptual reasoning and socialization, I designed thematic groups. Although the time and focused attention I gave to designing and preparing these groups (e.g., decorating the spaces, collecting truck-loads of art materials) probably stemmed from my role as an art teacher, the way in which I took each group member's individual needs, strengths, and emotional/social/cognitive goals into consideration during every step of these therapeutic journeys reflected my training as an art therapist.

"Space Journey" group. In preparing for the "Space Journey" group, an ethical issue arose regarding the selection of art materials that would be offered to the boys.

MY ETHICAL DILEMMA

What factors should be taken into consideration when providing art materials for clients' use? What happens when those factors conflict with each other (e.g., when the duty to create a safe space conflicts with supporting industry, choice, and a sense of autonomy)?

Had the boys with whom I worked been able to live at home, society would have provided for the tasks of latency—development of social skills, growth of a sense of autonomy and independence, experiences in mastery—through participation in activities such as clubs, camps, music or dance lessons. The invitation to embark on a "Space Journey" was meant to allow them to give expression to these developmentally appropriate needs. I could provide them with the usual art therapy materials, such as pastels, paints, or clay, or I could offer them found art materials and carpentry tools that would promote creative problem-solving. What I had in mind was to ask staff members to bring in old appliances that were not in working order—egg beaters, blenders, fans, radios, record players, tape recorders, toasters, hair driers, vacuum cleaners—and then to equip the boys with screwdrivers, wrenches, and pliers and invite them to disassemble the appliances and repurpose the found objects into helmets. The process could involve some minimal risk, but appropriate precautions could be taken.

How would you respond?

For the writer's response, see Appendix B, page 418.

The "Space Journey" involved the creation of planets out of wooden cheese wheels, rocket ships out of cardboard tubes, and space helmets out of large ice cream containers (see Figure 31.1). The individual planets represented the boys' social isolation, while their individually crafted rocket ships (which could land on planets only with the permission of their "owners") expressed a need for improved interpersonal communication. The space journey culminated in shared experiences with costumes, intergalactic passports, and space food. With the room darkened, strings of fairy lights sparkling like stars, and "Flight of the Valkyries" playing in the background, I assumed the role of reporter, interviewing each space traveler about customs, habits, and concerns on his planet.

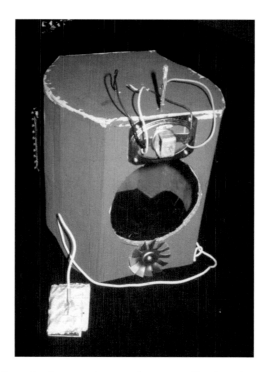

FIGURE 31.1 Helmet for the space journey (note use of hardware).

"Capturing the Magic Stone," a board game group. Board games were another effective vehicle for working with latency-age boys. Games encourage impulse control, adherence to rules, and persistence, while requiring problem solving, cooperation, and compromise. "Capturing the Magic Stone" was a board game I invented which symbolized life's journey through obstacles in search of rewards. After creating cardboard "heraldry shields" (armor) for themselves, the boys jointly constructed a castle, symbolizing the security that can be attained by working together. A "friendship chalice" contained scrolls on which the "knights" had signed their names, pledging to follow the "Code of Honor" (group rules). "Wizard cards" asked group members trivia questions that they had to answer correctly to move a step toward the castle; landing on a space labeled "Obstacle" required them to play a trust game before advancing. A knight might have to limbo through a hoop strung with gummy worms (snakes) or jump from one cushion to another (stepping stones) without landing on a square of red carpet (the lava pit). The object of the game was to capture the magic stone and return it to the castle, which symbolized the development of skills needed to face obstacles and gain control over life situations.

Baseball group. Spring was the perfect time to introduce a baseball-themed group. After drawing a large baseball diamond on the floor of the art therapy studio, group members created life-sized figures out of cardboard (clad in painted baseball uniforms), standing on an armature that could be moved from base to base (see Figure 31.2). The

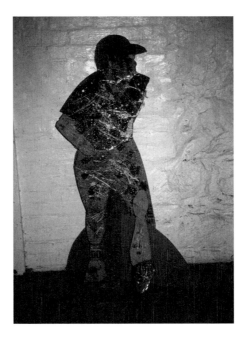

FIGURE 31.2 Life-sized baseball board game piece.

boys designed baseball cards with their photos on the front and personal stats on the back and constructed baseball stadiums out of boxes. A post-game press conference and banquet were held at the end of the group as a vehicle for sharing progress and saying goodbye. Once again, I played the role of reporter/interviewer, asking questions and presenting awards.

While in residential treatment, the boys were missing another important aspect of latency-age development: participation in team sports. The goals of the baseball group were to help the boys handle healthful competition while improving their ability to cooperate and work as a team. On a symbolic level, the baseball theme represented the boys' progress in therapy (their movement from base to base) and the ultimate goal of returning to their home bases.

Art Education

When, after 15 years practicing art therapy, I returned to art education, I wondered whether I could find the same degree of satisfaction in a school setting, where art was more about pleasure than pain, more about enrichment than survival. I soon came to appreciate that both art therapy and art teaching provide children with an outlet for the expression of emotion and a path for the attainment of self-esteem. While teaching is more directive and more concerned with technical instruction, the creation of art, in and of itself, can be therapeutic. As an art therapist working as an art teacher in the classroom, I continued to pay attention to children's social and emotional needs and to offer open-ended projects that encouraged self-expression, reflection, and group cooperation. For example, while studying Latin America, third graders created *retablos*, portable altars that originated in Mexico. *Retablos* portray scenes of people and objects, contained in small boxes. Boxes are the perfect medium for holding and releasing hidden thoughts and feelings, useful in both therapeutic and school settings. At the residential treatment center, I had observed that art therapy clients often chose the box structure as a preferred mode of expression, meeting their needs for privacy, boundaries, safe release, and the working through of trauma.

Self-portraits and themes such as "windows" and "mirrors" were introduced to encourage reflection among adolescents. Carly's portrait of a girl gazing into a mirror, surrounded by cobwebs, symbolized her "desire to be someone else." The cobwebs represented "days when you feel there is no hope for the future." The mirror represented "another world, one that has laughter, hope, and warmth, and maybe even a different version of yourself." As natural as it might have felt to respond to Carly as an art therapist would, I refrained from probing for deeper content or explanations; as an art teacher, I never played the role of therapist, but reported my concerns to the school counselor. My art therapy training and experience made itself known in other ways, however. When asked to jury student art shows, enter student artwork in competitions, or facilitate the sale of student artwork, for example, I declined.

In addition to self-exploration, adolescents need to feel that their education is meaningful and useful, to believe that they can foster change and contribute to the welfare of others, not only locally, but also globally. Global competence was also addressed on the elementary school level.

MY ETHICAL DILEMMA

Are uneven cultural exchanges ethical?

Ethical dilemmas related to the creation of art are not confined to treatment settings. During a multicultural art exchange, first graders painted a mural of DC monuments amid cherry blossoms for a school in Guatemala and sent it with cards they'd written in Spanish. In return, the Guatemalan children sent us *bolsitas*, small, carefully stitched bags, a project that took them many months to complete. Both groups shared colorful traditions, but the *bolsitas* required far more work. I feared that the Guatemalan children had given away prized possessions and wasn't sure whether we should accept their precious *bolsitas*.

How would you respond?

For the writer's response, see Appendix B, page 418.

Conclusion

Edith Kramer describes her art therapy approach as "distinct from psychotherapy. Its healing potentialities depend on the psychological processes that are activated in creative work" (1971, p. 25). "The art therapist makes himself the ally of the child's creative venture, lending both technical assistance and emotional support" (Kramer, 1971, p. 34). For art therapists and art educators alike, teaching skills leads to our ultimate goal—making inner worlds visible. Over the years I have conveyed many of the same messages and used many of the same techniques with both art therapy clients and art students. While art therapy is more process-oriented and focused upon treatment and art education is more product-oriented and concerned with design principles, both disciplines deal with the power of art to communicate and express one's innermost feelings. Both professions must adhere to ethical principles of consistency, safety, and respect for the individual. How lucky I was that day to find Kramer's book in my college library stacks—and luckier still when the professor of my class in "Art Therapy with Children" turned out to be Edith Kramer, herself! Having begun her career as an art teacher, Edith Kramer really was a role model for bridging the gap between art education and art therapy.

REFLECTIVE ART EXPERIENCES & DISCUSSION QUESTIONS

1. Imagine that you are creating a *batik* with hot melted wax; using chemicals to develop photographs in a darkroom; creating an assemblage with hot glue; printmaking with gouges; constructing a clay sculpture with knives and needle tools; or scoring cardboard with an Exacto knife. Picture yourself using spray paint, paint thinners, or fixatives. Create artwork that expresses the level of comfort that you, personally, feel when using materials that might cause a cut or a burn or expose you to fumes (even if they are non-toxic).
2. How do your own feelings about using potentially hazardous or risky materials influence your choice of materials for your clients? Under what circumstances would you offer any of these less traditional art materials? What precautions would you take to ensure safety?

References

Ginott, H. (2003). *Between parent and child* (Rev. ed.). New York: Three Rivers Press.
Kramer, E. (1971). *Art as therapy with children*. New York: Schocken Books.

Scope of Practice

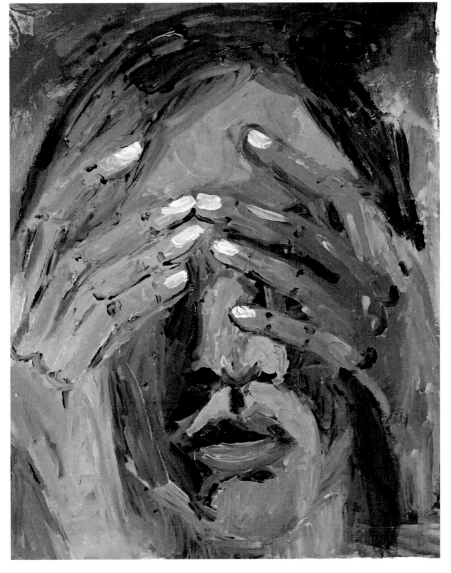

Hannah Wittman *(see color insert)*

32

ADAPTING THE INSTINCTUAL TRAUMA RESPONSE MODEL TO MEET THE NEEDS OF CLIENTS IN UKRAINE

Ethical Considerations

Iryna Natalushko

As an art therapist and trauma therapist (certified in the use of the Instinctual Trauma Response Model) in Ukraine, my home, I work with adults whose trauma histories vary from a single instance to repeated or chronic traumatization, from prenatal and preverbal to very recent traumatic experiences. My clients are affected by a variety of post-traumatic consequences, as well as by the thwarting of their potential.

Trauma in Ukrainian History and Culture

People in Ukraine have survived collective historical, recent, and ongoing traumatic experiences, such as the world wars and the Holocaust, the artificial famine of the 1930s, the economic crisis and poverty of the late 20th and early 21st centuries, the violence and shootings at the Maidan protests in 2014, and the ongoing military conflict in eastern Ukraine. These collective traumatic experiences can be compounded by individual ones, such as the shocking normalization of sexual abuse, openly acknowledged—perhaps for the first time—in the social media campaign that began in Ukraine during the summer of 2016 (#IAmNotAfraidToSay).

As the legacy of trauma travels through generations, it is reflected in how people feel about themselves and others, how they parent, discipline, teach, and more. Meanwhile, they have adapted in order to carry on with their lives. Trauma therapy services are not always accessible to, or utilized by, many who could benefit from them. Historically, psychiatry was misused, to politically oppress; few therapists have had an opportunity to receive quality training in trauma-focused interventions; and many clients are financially vulnerable and, thus, unable to afford therapeutic services when prioritized against other needs.

The Instinctual Trauma Response Model

My understanding of how trauma is experienced and results in post-traumatic consequences, and how the latter can be released, is grounded in two models. One is neuropsychiatrist Daniel Siegel's understanding of mental health and the therapeutic process as integration (Siegel, 2012). The other is a neuroscience-based approach developed by my teachers, art therapist Linda Gantt and psychiatrist Louis Tinnin (Gantt & Tinnin, 2009; Tinnin & Gantt, 2013). Supported by an outcome study with clients with post-traumatic stress disorder and dissociative disorders (Gantt & Tinnin, 2007), it has been used in a range of settings with populations affected by traumatic experiences.

The Instinctual Trauma Response (ITR) model procedures are embedded in a phase-oriented treatment where thorough assessment, trauma screening, psycho-education, and grounding/resourcing as practiced skills (as well as stabilization if needed) precede trauma processing. When target preverbal and other clinically significant trauma are identified, the client and the therapist use:

1. *guided imagery* (optional), *graphic narrative*, and *graphic narrative representation* to safely access, integrate, and give closure to trauma memory, and
2. *externalized dialogue* to reverse traumatic dissociation and victim mythology and to address other post-traumatic consequences or symptoms.

The ITR model also provides tools for continued self-care and reintegration into life (with support if needed) after trauma is processed (Tinnin & Gantt, 2013).

Is it ethical to try to modify parts of a well-conceived, well-constructed, and well-researched treatment model in which every part plays a crucial role—a model that was intended to be used as a unit? This chapter presents my experience in adapting parts of the ITR model and certain aspects of their application to meet the needs of my clients in Ukraine, given the resources available to them, to me, and to our working context, highlighting the ethical issues that arose in doing so. To prevent conveying even the illusion that I am providing instruction in the use of the ITR model, rather than attempting to summarize the model's goals, tasks, and treatment phases, I have chosen to focus only upon those parts of the ITR model that are relevant to the cases that illustrate the adaptations I made. Readers who are interested in knowing more about the model should consult Tinnin and Gantt's *The Instinctual Trauma Response and Dual-Brain Dynamics: A Guide for Trauma Therapy* (2013). Readers who are interested in learning to apply the model should contact the ITR Training Institute (http://helpfortrauma.com/training) to be trained and become certified in its use. Although I will be illustrating ways in which I have adapted parts and aspects of the ITR to meet the needs of my clients, readers are cautioned that it is inadvisable to do likewise without the training necessary both to understand the intended use of the ITR model and to anticipate the various ways in which someone might react to it, as not doing so could result in unintended consequences for the client.

Taking Trauma History and Adapting the Model Flow to a Single Session

Taking and Externalizing Trauma History

An important part of using the ITR model is taking a thorough trauma history. One way for clients to externalize their trauma history is to draw a *life line* along which to plot traumatic events, indicating the time frame when each took place (Tinnin & Gantt, 2013). My experience is that using the *life line* engages clients as partners in therapy from the start; gives a sense of trauma categories, types, and developmental stages at which they took place; and allows for the discussion of other relevant contexts in which trauma occurred, to help assess impact and clarify stressors. By visualizing the "big picture," the *life line* helps us to focus, first, upon the most significant trauma. Taking a complete trauma history can take one hour to several hours, in the case of complex and multiple traumas or when clients need assistance in recognizing traumatic experiences that might be impacting them; in regulating the related states that come up during screening, or in determining how much detail is sufficient, safe, and helpful to put into words at this stage. In Ukraine, however, I routinely see individuals impacted by complex trauma histories that overlap with their responses to ongoing stressors and who expect, or hope for, a tangible therapeutic outcome within the one to several hours available. Often, this is due to the very limited time and resources of individuals and helping organizations; to client expectations that are based upon little experience with therapy; or to living within a stressful personal and collective context in which immediate needs trump continued therapy.

Although the cases illustrate adaptations to *the flow of steps in therapy, the timing and the scope of taking and externalizing trauma history,* they also include *creating a graphic narrative.*

Creating a Graphic Narrative

When working to process a targeted traumatic experience, the client creates *a graphic narrative*—a series of drawings—to help organize elements of the nonverbal trauma memory into a story with a beginning, a middle, and an end (before; fight/flight; freeze; altered state; automatic obedience; self-repair; after). Integrated into a narrative that includes all aspects of the experience, it is represented (narrated) by the therapist for the client to process, giving closure to the traumatic memory (Tinnin & Gantt, 2013).

The composites of cases and contexts that follow, carefully constructed to reflect the realities and necessities of my work, omit some session details in order to zoom in on adaptations I made to the ITR model, why they were needed, and what ethical considerations arose in deciding to use them.

Case 1—Inga

Inga, a 32-year-old single woman, came to see me a week after she had watched a news broadcast that showed a bus filled with civilians exploding in eastern Ukraine. When she arrived she was agitated and unfocused. It was her second time seeing a therapist; the first was a single session with another professional. She seemed nervous and uncertain how to explain what brought her, though open to connect and follow suggestions. I led Inga through a grounding exercise that engaged her breathing and her five senses, after which she seemed calmer and ready to talk about why she had come. She said that she had been watching news accounts of the explosion repeatedly for a week and was becoming unusually tired. Her friends said that she did not look like herself and recommended that she consult a therapist.

From talking with Inga on the phone to schedule the session, I knew that we would have two hours together that day and that she did not plan on multiple sessions. As she began to share her response to watching the news in more detail, speaking rapidly, I decided to dispense with the complete trauma screening and, instead, asked if she would draw what had happened as a story with a beginning, a middle, and an end—as though she were an observer (the directive for creating *a graphic narrative*). As she spoke and created images on paper using markers, I helped her to recognize the instinctual trauma responses in her experience. The story line went from the time she was going through her life routine, to her instinctual trauma response to seeing the news accounts, to the self-repair evident in her coming to the session and becoming grounded. I invited her to hear me represent the experience to her and she listened carefully. Afterward, she added a safe "after drawing" to her narrative which showed her in session with me after I had represented the experience back to her. Immediately, her focus shifted to talking about plans she had for that evening, as though the traumatic experience had lost its prior significance. Her body looked more relaxed, connected, and grounded.

During the final quarter of the two-hour session, I invited Inga to draw a *life line* on a separate sheet of paper, noting her age, and to include the experience that brought her in that day. Then I invited her to think of other events or experiences at any time in her life that reminded her either of the bus explosion, as an event, or the way that it made her feel. She immediately drew several other single and repeated experiences and spoke of physically and emotionally abusive disciplinary practices in her family while she was growing up. She said that she was surprised by the connection and that it added clarity to why the ongoing military conflict was affecting her "this much" (since she had no family or friends who were directly involved or were in danger). I checked to see that she was grounded, shared some psycho-educational information regarding the potential impact of trauma and the therapeutic shifts that were possible after more extended therapy, and recommended a full screening and processing of earlier traumas. I summarized what we did in session and answered her questions about how and why the process worked. Inga said that she would consider seeing a therapist to integrate those memories at a later time, thanked me, and left the room.

Having assessed Inga's state when she came into the room and knowing how little time we had, my priority was to help Inga become grounded and to process the experience that had brought her to therapy. I did not want to potentially overwhelm her by eliciting a complete trauma history when she was coping with a recent event and our time together was too short to provide her with a thorough screening and assessment. After helping her to process her response to the news broadcast, however, I chose to use the opportunity to check for traumatic experiences that might have contributed to the current stressor and to lay groundwork that would encourage her to process earlier trauma memories when time and resources became available. Did I feel conflicted about how to prioritize Inga's needs? I did. There are risks to fragmented screening or to no screening at all (e.g., missing important history or failing to uncover risks), as well as to devoting all the time to screening and failing to help alleviate the ongoing stress.

Case 2—Dima

In his first session, a 46-year-old man named Dima shared that, although he had moved away from a conflict-affected area in eastern Ukraine a year before, he felt that the experience there was still impacting him and he was hoping for relief. He had seen another therapist and was aware of his trauma history, parts of which he had worked to integrate during irregular sessions over the previous year, whenever he had resources. He told me that he came to me to work on just the military conflict-related events that he had not gotten a chance to process before, events that he believed were affecting his ability to find employment in the city. He hoped that greater mental clarity would enable him to navigate job interviews and probationary periods of employment successfully. Since, before his appointment, I had explained that it can take several hours to process—or begin to process—an experience such as the one he had had, Dima had committed to working with me for a single 4-hour intensive session.

After discussing his previous trauma history, I asked Dima to draw a partial *life line* that extended from just before the first signs of the military conflict to the present. The *life line* he drew included the following: seeing armed men in his hometown during the beginning of the military conflict; hearing repeated explosions over time; experiencing the danger and the stress of getting out of the conflict area several months after the conflict began; searching for resources and a home in a new city; worrying about the potential loss of his abandoned apartment; feeling anxious about extended family members who were attached to their homes and refused to move; experiencing a sense of shock from the apparent normalcy of life in the city, while people in parts of eastern Ukraine were still in danger and lacked basic resources.

When asked which of the events or situations he thought affected him most, Dima said, without hesitation, that his uncle, to whom he had been close while growing up, refused to leave the conflict area or the apartment in which he had spent most of his life, and Dima was afraid for his uncle's safety, as well as his physical and mental health. Now that we had a target to work with, I invited Dima to create *a graphic narrative*, using markers on paper. He was very engaged in creating the drawings and explained how the events had unfolded. When I encouraged him to use the ITR handout to identify the instinctive traumatic responses in his artwork, he was able to recognize all them in the ways in which he had responded to his concerns about the potential danger to his uncle. In the process of doing this, Dima realized that the area in which his uncle lived had become much safer in the past three months; thus, a reasonably safe "after" image could be added to his drawings.

After I narrated this experience for Dima to hear, I asked him to look, again, at the partial *life line* of conflict-related events and to notice how he experienced it at that moment. He took some time to look at the events he had depicted, then said that that entire timeline felt much less intense to him. I observed a greater sense of calm and presence in his affect and his posture.

At times, clients have experienced a series of recent overlapping stressors (individual events or prolonged contexts) that vary in the degree of closure and impact, but are not able to engage in therapy for the optimal number of hours. Dima's situation illustrates that well. Given his recent stressors and their intensity in his life, my observations and his account of his state and functioning, as well as his openness to working with earlier traumas, I suggested that we use a brief *life line* to zoom in on a period of time and then choose a target to focus upon, with the goal of bringing about tangible, though partial, relief. Would it be enough? Perhaps not, but, as with all my clients, I provided him with psycho-educational information and encouragement to process all clinically significant trauma as soon as resources became available.

MY ETHICAL DILEMMA

Only one session for complex needs

If I anticipate that I will have only one session with a client who has complex needs, including a trauma history, what, ethically, should I try to accomplish?

How would you respond?

For the writer's response, see Appendix B, page 424.

Concluding Thoughts

In the face of great need, where does one draw a line between protocol and compromise? When does compromise dilute our original intention to the extent that the outcome is harmful, rather than helpful? I do not have answers to these questions, but as I continue my work in Ukraine, these questions remain with me.

REFLECTIVE ART EXPERIENCES & DISCUSSION QUESTIONS

1. Think of a time when an effective therapeutic approach in which you had been trained did not fit the existing treatment context or the resources that were available to you, your client, or the organization. How would you go about adapting what you had learned, in an ethical way?
2. As you recall that experience, notice any parts of you that feel conflicted about making adaptations. Become aware of these parts of you as *sensations*, *emotions*, *thoughts*, or *attitudes*, and notice how you experience them in or

around your body. Using art materials, make an image that includes each of those parts. Dialogue with them in writing to get to know them and identify their concerns or their intentions and, perhaps, address those concerns.
3. Return to your memory of the work setting that was not conducive to using the treatment approach in which you were trained. Notice how you feel now about adapting that approach, in an ethical way. Reflect upon your process through discussion or journaling.

References

Gantt, L.M., & Tinnin, L.W. (2007). Intensive trauma therapy for PTSD and dissociation: An outcome study. *The Arts in Psychotherapy*, 34(1), pp. 69–80.

Gantt, L.M., & Tinnin, L.W. (2009). Support for a neurobiological view of trauma with implications for art therapy. *The Arts in Psychotherapy*, 36(3), pp. 148–153.

Siegel, D.J. (2012). *The developing mind: How relationships and the brain interact to shape who we are* (2nd ed.). New York: Guilford Press.

Tinnin, L.W., & Gantt, L.M. (2013). *The instinctual trauma response and dual-brain dynamics: A guide for trauma therapy*. Morgantown, WV: Gargoyle Press.

33

APPS, TELEHEALTH, AND ART THERAPY

Online Treatment and Ethical Issues for the Digital Age

Ellen G. Horovitz

Although the term *telehealth* can encompass a variety of communication techniques, including telephone, email, text, and remote monitoring, *telemedicine* includes the provision of mental health diagnostic, therapeutic, or management services via real-time, interactive video-conferencing and/or the use of apps prior to and in between sessions to measure change over time and the efficacy of any kind of therapeutic treatment. Research on telemedicine indicates that

- telemedicine has more than 50 years of history in providing medical care to patients via technology in distant and remote locations;
- the provision of behavioral health care is one of the earliest healthcare specialties offered by telemedicine (in fact, psychiatry and other behavioral health services are the most frequent type of telemedicine, second only to radiology);
- recent improvements in the cost and quality of technology have made deployment possible for the routine practice of medicine; and
- the empirical base of telemental health consistently shows that diagnostic accuracy and treatment efficacy is equivalent to face-to-face (F2F) for most populations and settings (Fishkind & Cuyler, 2013; Grady, Myers, & Nelson, 2009; Yellowlees, Shore, & Roberts, 2010).

In this chapter, I illustrate the use of three apps:

1. the DASS-21 (Depression Anxiety Depression Scale), a measurement of depression, anxiety, and stress;
2. pre-session summaries (questions posed to clients before each session); and
3. Paper 53, an App that can be used to draw, paint, and communicate in and between sessions.

A case presentation illustrates the use of these tools to track the efficacy of treatment. First, it is important to understand the ethical guidelines necessary to operate within a telehealth system.

Ethical Guidelines for Providing Mental Health Care via Telemedicine

Constructing a practice that incorporates telemedicine may be new to some, but done properly it can be a safe and effective way in which to improve access for clients and provide practitioners with options that can increase efficiency and flexibility. Although there are many telehealth companies, it is important to choose one that is HIPAA compliant, provides the necessary technology, offers management assistance, and provides customer support. Although I refer to the features of Breakthrough (which no longer covers individual practitioners) and iCouch in this chapter, I urge those of you who are interested in learning more about launching a telemedicine practice to decide which features you need and then to compare what various telehealth companies have to offer.

Laws and regulations that establish the ground rules for tele-psychiatry/clinical practice follow the same standards of care used in face-to-face contact. For example, the professional must:

- Hold a state license for the location in which he or she dwells and services are delivered.
- Consider features such as adequate soundproofing; freedom from interruption or disturbance by others; secured access to files or electronic medical records; password-protected computers with up-to-date anti-virus protection; and secure e-health communication.
- Obtain a signed, informed, "Consent for Treatment" that describes delivery of services via telemedicine (some telehealth companies provide this form); provide "HIPAA Notice of Privacy Practices;" establish doctor/patient relationship: examination, medical history, make referrals as necessary; determine and advise patient of procedure for managing emergencies, including availability of emergency services in the community (nearby Emergency Department, Crisis Stabilization Services).
- Ensure that lighting, camera, and audio feedback are working prior to sessions. Echoing and ambient sounds are generally eliminated when both clinician and patient wear headphones.
- Provide treatment planning, risk-management, assessment, and re-assessment.

Regarding the latter, prior to each session (via Breakthrough), the patient fills out a pre-session summary that is sent to the practitioner before the session begins. This offers the clinician a snapshot of how the patient is feeling and allows the therapist to zero in on areas of immediate concern. Figure 33.1 shows the pre-session questions that were posed and the responses that were provided before a patient's first and sixth

Pre-session Summary, Session 1

How often in the past two weeks did you...

Feel unhappy or sad?	**Very Often**
Have little or no energy?	**Very Often**
Feel tense or nervous?	**Very Often**
Feel hopeless about the future?	**Sometimes**
Have problems with sleep (too much or too little)?	**Often**
Think about harming yourself?	**Rarely**
Feel unproductive at work or other daily activities?	**Very Often**
Have a hard time paying attention?	**Very Often**
Have a hard time getting along with family or friends?	**Often**
Feel lonely?	**Very Often**
Have someone express concern about your alcohol or drug use?	**Never**
Have five or more drinks of alcohol at one time?	**Never**
Have a problem at work, school or home because of drug or alcohol use?	**Never**

Pre-session Summary, Session 6

How often in the past two weeks did you...

Feel unhappy or sad?	**Sometimes**
Have little or no energy?	**Rarely**
Feel tense or nervous?	**Sometimes**
Feel hopeless about the future?	**Rarely**
Have problems with sleep (too much or too little)?	**Rarely**
Think about harming yourself?	**Never**
Feel unproductive at work or other daily activities?	**Rarely**
Have a hard time paying attention?	**Rarely**
Have a hard time getting along with family or friends?	**Rarely**
Feel lonely?	**Sometimes**
Have someone express concern about your alcohol or drug use?	**Never**
Have five or more drinks of alcohol at one time?	**Never**
Have a problem at work, school or home because of drug or alcohol use?	**Never**

FIGURE 33.1 Preliminary questions answered before sessions 1 and 6 (Breakthrough format).

sessions. By comparing the two, one can see that the patient's mood and overall mental health improved between sessions 1 and 6.

Breakthrough's capability to graph results over time allows a practitioner to monitor a patient's progress visually (see www.breakthrough.com/for-providers for more information). I sometimes share results with my patients, so that they may track their own progress. Figure 33.2 shows the progress made by the patient, above, between sessions 1 and 6.

Advantages of Telehealth Applications

- From the privacy of your own home office, you can offer clients appointments at virtually any time that's convenient for them---even when you, or they, are traveling or when there's a need for an emergency therapy session.
- Sophisticated messaging systems send you an email as soon as clients message you and allow you to confirm upcoming appointments and check-in or recap salient points with clients between sessions.
- Files may be shared between—and even during—sessions, allowing both the client and the practitioner to view artwork and discuss it during the session. This can approximate real time discussion without the visual interference of holding up the artwork, which can block the facial expression of the client or practitioner.
- For a flat fee per session, some telehealth companies will handle billing and deal with insurance companies.

Ethical Challenges of Working Online

There are distinct disadvantages of working at a distance; those that have affected my practice include:

Providing support from a distance. When a client becomes visibly upset or begins to cry, I cannot offer her tissues or a gentle touch on the hand or shoulder to provide reassurance.

Having a restricted view of the client. Talking about certain topics (such as part sexual abuse) may cause extreme agitation; if the patient is framed from the chest up, however, one may miss nonverbal cues (such as nervous twitching or foot tapping) that would be obvious in a F2F session. Unless we ask, we may never see the whole person. With a patient who had an eating disorder, sexual abuse issues, and PTSD, being able to address her whole body was an important part of our treatment, so I would ask her to back up from the camera when we did *pranayama*/yoga breath exercises so I could see how her entire body responded to the directive.

Not being able to offer art materials during sessions. At times, I send materials (by post) to my patient's home ahead of a session; then, I can use an

How often in the <u>past two weeks</u> did you...

Feel unhappy or sad?

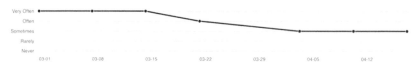

Have little or no energy?

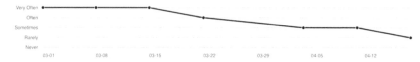

Feel tense or nervous?

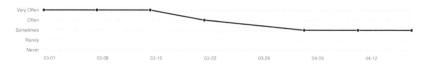

Feel hopeless about the future?

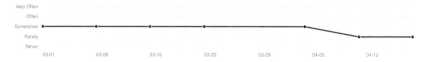

Have problems with sleep (too much or too little)?

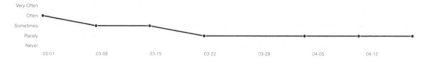

Think about harming yourself?

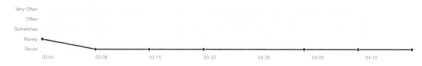

FIGURE 33.2 Pre-session summary graph exported as a PDF (Breakthrough format).

Feel unproductive at work or other daily activities?

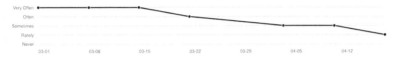

Have a hard time paying attention?

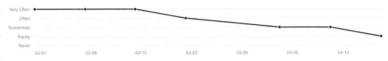

Have a hard time getting along with family or friends?

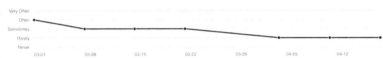

Feel lonely?

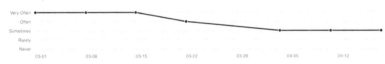

Have someone express concern about your alcohol or drug use?

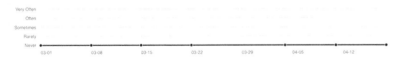

Have five or more drinks of alcohol at one time?

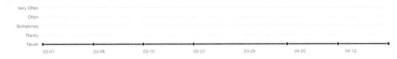

Have a problem at work, school or home because of drug or alcohol use?

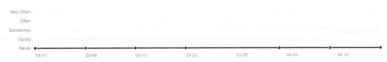

FIGURE 33.2 (Continued)

App such as Paper 53 to conduct the session. (For other apps, see *Digital Art Therapy: Material, Methods and Applications* [Garner, 2016].) To see the patient actually create artwork, Splashtop's 360Mirroring program allows client and therapist to share the desktop and draw together using their own apps.

The lack of ready supervision for online work. For the practitioner seeking supervision or support, it can be pretty lonely out there. I have had to rely upon meeting with peers who have little idea what it is like to operate in a telehealth world. A supervision site on the iCouch platform allows telehealth providers to see each other in real time and discuss such issues.

So, let's look briefly at a case, to get a glimmer of how apps can enhance treatment online.

Apps, Session Summaries, and Counter-transference

When I am going to work with patients in person, I ask them to complete and return a health form to me prior to our first meeting. (A sample form may be found in the Appendix, Horovitz & Elgelid, 2015.) The iCouch telehealth platform allows me to send documents through their Papers system. Figure 33.3 shows the information that I received prior to the client's initial video session when using Breakthrough's platform.

I also asked my client to fill out the DASS (Depression Anxiety Scale) online. Her response, which indicated mild anxiety, moderate depression, and extremely severe stress, would serve as a barometer against which to measure progress or regression in therapy (Figure 33.4).

How often in the <u>past two weeks</u> did you...

Feel unhappy or sad?	**Often**
Have little or no energy?	**Sometimes**
Feel tense or nervous?	**Often**
Feel hopeless about the future?	**Sometimes**
Have problems with sleep (too much or too little)?	**Very Often**
Think about harming yourself?	**Never**
Feel unproductive at work or other daily activities?	**Never**
Have a hard time paying attention?	**Often**
Have a hard time getting along with family or friends?	**Sometimes**
Feel lonely?	**Sometimes**
Have someone express concern about your alcohol or drug use?	**Never**
Have five or more drinks of alcohol at one time?	**Rarely**
Have a problem at work, school or home because of drug or alcohol use?	**Rarely**

FIGURE 33.3 My client's answers to pre-session questions (Breakthrough format).

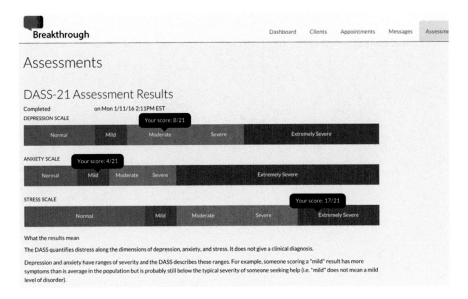

Breakthrough Dashboard Clients Appointments Messages Assessme

Assessments

DASS-21 Assessment Results

Completed   on Mon 1/11/16 2:11PM EST

DEPRESSION SCALE

Your score: 8/21

| Normal | Mild | Moderate | Severe | Extremely Severe |

ANXIETY SCALE

Your score: 4/21

| Normal | Mild | Moderate | Severe | Extremely Severe |

STRESS SCALE

Your score: 17/21

| Normal | Mild | Moderate | Severe | Extremely Severe |

What the results mean

The DASS quantifies distress along the dimensions of depression, anxiety, and stress. It does not give a clinical diagnosis.

Depression and anxiety have ranges of severity and the DASS describes these ranges. For example, someone scoring a "mild" result has more symptoms than is average in the population but is probably still below the typical severity of someone seeking help (i.e. "mild" does not mean a mild level of disorder).

FIGURE 33.4 My client's DASS results.

I was able to learn something about my client's family makeup and her culture. The Genogram Analytics App (Horovitz, 2014) allows one to create a genogram and to add to it as information unfolds during sessions. I can send the genogram to a client in a PDF or jpeg format through the messaging or Paper system (via iCouch), enabling the client to make corrections and/or additions in between sessions. This allows the dialogue between client and therapist to continue between sessions, further cementing the therapeutic alliance despite the lack of face-to-face (F2F) in-person—as opposed to video—contact.

So, by our first session, I already knew quite a bit about my client. During our initial F2F video session, I learned that she and her boyfriend had been together four years, living together for two. Both traveled four days a week due to their jobs, spending only weekends together. Culturally, they were very different and, while she attempted to learn his primary language, Spanish, he refused to speak it with her and pointedly dismissed her desire to become more knowledgeable about, and attuned to, his culture. She had attended 11 weddings in the past year and, although he had mentioned having children someday, he studiously avoided the topic of marriage. She was 29.

I empathized with her desire to move things to the next level but felt it was important to explore some deeper issues. She was having difficulty sleeping, so, through the messaging app, I sent her an MP3 Yoga Nidra with my voice to play on her audio device, so she could fall asleep more easily. I also suggested that she practice breathing exercises and ease into the conversation with her boyfriend by talking with him about some of the issues which had surfaced. Through the messaging service, I also sent her a recap of the highlights of the session, as well as a homework assignment to be done before our next session, using the Paper 53 App. The directive was to trace her hands and then to map out her goals by writing, on the left hand, where she was at present and, on the right hand, where she wanted to be in the future (Figure 33.5).

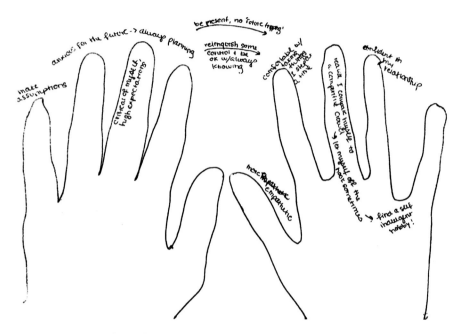

FIGURE 33.5 My client's homework regarding goals (using Paper 53 app).

MY ETHICAL DILEMMA

How do I deal with counter-transference in telehealth?

During the fifth session, I became aware of strong counter-transference when my client mentioned that therapy was considered a symbol of status, due to its lack of affordability to "others." She joked that she knew the name of her high school girlfriend's therapist because her friend had talked about her therapist so often. I wondered whether my name was being bandied about the way the name of her girlfriend's therapist's was. This gave me pause, as suddenly I had a vision of my client viewing me as an acquisition, as something to adorn her, like a Gucci bag. I was becoming increasingly uncomfortable with this perception of myself.

How would you respond?

For the writer's response, see Appendix B, page 411.

One day, my client messaged me that her boyfriend had received a job offer that would necessitate moving abroad. She had resisted talking with him about how it affected her because she believed that discussion would not alter his decision. She ended by writing that she was going to try "not to focus on it because I feel somewhat at a loss." I scheduled an emergency video session with her that night, during which to discuss options and ways in which she could not only broach her feelings but also let him know how *sad* she was. As it turned out, her fears were allayed when they talked. He had *not* planned to take the position without talking to her and involving her in the decision-making process. Moreover, the offer was just in the preliminary stages. Part of their miscommunication had occurred because (a) the information about the offer had all been communicated by text and (b) they did not talk over the phone during the four days a week when they were away on business. Ironically, since their reliance upon digital messaging had caused the miscommunication between them, I suggested that they might want to consider FaceTime, Skype, or *some* means of visual communication during their work week.

By Session 10, things were improving and they were moving into a new apartment together. After our session, I message-recapped the following:

1. Have a conversation about your joint finances, leading to more transparency and protection of one another. (Tell your boyfriend that this nudge came from me.)
2. Don't forego that Friday night event because of two officious souls. This will give you an opportunity to turn on your heel, walk away, and socialize with people you *truly* care about.
3. Try to turn a blind eye to people who flaunt their engagements.

In sum, my client had surmounted the original reasons for reaching out for therapy. While more sessions clearly could have been beneficial, therapy ended shortly after that point; she was better equipped to deal effectively with the issues that had plagued her. I heard from her a year later, conducted one couple's session, and shortly thereafter worked with her for another six months when their relationship dissolved.

Conclusion

While telehealth might not yet be a part of your therapist toolbox, it is clearly part of the digital future. So, what does the future hold? Practice guidelines for telemedicine are important to ensure the effective and safe delivery of quality healthcare. Existing practice guidelines have been well received by the telemedicine community and are being adopted by numerous practices. Some state medical boards have incorporated in their regulations the practice guidelines of the American Telemedicine Association, by stating that *physicians must practice telemedicine in compliance with standards endorsed by the ATA* (Krupinski, Antoniotti, & Burdick, 2010; Krupinski & Bernard, 2014). We will need to develop telehealth guidelines for the field of Art Therapy. Although this is needed to help convince payers and legislators that telemedicine is just another way to provide effective patient care and, thus, should be reimbursed in the same manner that other medical interventions are, it is also a means by which to ensure that, as the world becomes increasingly digital, ethical principles regarding the ways in which we practice don't lag behind.

REFLECTIVE ART EXPERIENCES & DISCUSSION QUESTIONS

1. Envision an opportunity to share your desktop with the patient. (This can be done through the Mirroring 360 app—see www.mirroring360.com.) Using a simple drawing or painting application such as Paper 53, Studio Artist, or Corel Painter 11, share your desktop with your patient. Start the evening's conversation with a blank desktop and spend 15 minutes working on artwork together, then do the rest of the session face-to-face (via video feed), discussing the experience with your patient.
2. How did it feel to create artwork together, even though you were experiencing it via video?
3. Ask your patient to bring a photograph of him- or herself (with others—possibly family or the person whom the patient is discussing in therapy). Take turns discussing what is going on in the photo (e.g., by asking the patient, "If you had to write a caption for this picture, what would it say?"). What did you learn from this experience? Discuss how the two of you saw the photograph differently and what information that yielded.

References

Fishkind, A., & Cuyler, R. (2013). Telepsychiatry. In L.S. Lun (Ed.), *Behavioral emergencies: A handbook for emergency physicians*. New York: Cambridge University Press.

Garner, R.L. (Ed.) (2016). *Digital art therapy: Material, methods, and applications*. Philadelphia, PA: Jessica Kingsley.

Grady, B., Myers, K., & Nelson, E. (2009). Evidence-based practice for telemental health. *American Telemedicine Association*, July. Retrieved from www.americantelemed.org/docs/default-source/standards/evidence-based-practice-for-telemental-health.pdf?sfvrsn=4

Horovitz, E.G., & Eksten, S. L. (Eds.) (2009). *The art therapists' primer: A clinical guide to writing assessment, diagnosis, and treatment*. Springfield, IL: Charles C. Thomas.

Horovitz, E.G. (Ed.) (2014). *The art therapists' primer: A clinical guide to writing assessment, diagnosis, and treatment* (2nd ed.). Springfield, IL: Charles C Thomas.

Horovitz, E.G., & Elgelid, S. (2015). *Yoga therapy: Theory and practice*. New York: Routledge.

Icouch. Retrieved from www.capterra.com/p/142270/iCouch/

Krupinski, E.A., & Bernard, J. (2014). Review: Standards and guidelines in telemedicine and telehealth. *Healthcare, 2,* 74–93.

Krupinski, E.A, Antoniotti, N., & Burdick, A. (2010). Standards and guidelines development in the American Telemedicine Association. In A. Moumtzoglou & A. Kastania (Eds.), *E-health systems quality and reliability: Models and standards* (pp. 703–732). Hershey, NY: Medical Information Reference.

Yellowlees, P., Shore, J., & Roberts, L. (2010). Practice guidelines for videoconferencing-based telemental health. *Telemedicine and e-Health,* (16)10, 1074–1089.

34

A SAFE SPACE, STANDARDS, AND "GUT FEELINGS"

Ethics and Cultural Diversity in Art Therapy Training Groups

Diane Waller

For many years I have conducted art psychotherapy training workshops in several European countries, most of which were unfamiliar with the models of art therapy and group work used in the UK and USA. From 1980 to 1987, I trained psychiatrists and mental health nurses at the Medical Academy in Sofia, Bulgaria, a program that was an off-shoot of a World Health Organization-funded project to establish new psychosocial interventions in the Bulgarian National Health Service. My co-facilitators were psychologists with an interest in the arts and the aim of changing the prevailing medicalized approach to mental health and bringing new insights into conditions such as alcoholism and drug addiction. They have continued to develop art therapy services, despite difficult financial conditions in Bulgaria.

Another long-term project, from 1992 to 2004, was to assist in developing two postgraduate training programs in art therapy in Switzerland that achieved validation through the University of London when they were offered independently at university level. Similar projects took place in Budapest, Leeuwarden, Berlin, and Bologna. Training workshops were conducted in the former Yugoslavia until they were halted by the civil war. Between 1984 and 2004, I visited Italy several times a year to provide intensive art therapy training to staff from Italy, Spain, South America, and Southeast Asia as part of a United Nations-sponsored initiative for the treatment of substance abuse and the training of staff to work in this field.

Standards of Proficiency, Conduct, Training, and Ethics

Following a long campaign to persuade the British Department of Health to support it, in 1997, by means of an Act of Parliament, arts therapy became one of the 16 professions in the UK (including psychology and social work) regulated by the Health and Care Professions Council. As such, it received title protection and became subject to the legally enforceable standards of Proficiency, Conduct and Competence, Training and Education set by the HCPC.

Having established a postgraduate training program in art therapy at Goldsmiths, University of London in the 1970s and been a major player in achieving recognition for art therapy in the National Health Service (NHS), I was used to working with clear, practical ethical standards when I began to work abroad in the early 1980s. Looking back, I am now astonished by the huge differences in understanding *even the term art therapy* that existed within both Eastern and Western European countries, but such was my enthusiasm for the work that I put aside thoughts of any drawbacks that I might encounter in delivering it. Producing a book about the European development of art therapy (Waller, 1998) was one way of getting my head around such differences and coming to terms with the reality of helping colleagues to deliver suitable training programs within socio-cultural contexts that were so varied. Having witnessed training programs in related professions that were an example of cultural and academic colonialism—in that the language, culture, politics, and customs of the host country were ignored—I was committed to providing training that would be culturally sensitive and not dominated by UK thinking about psychotherapy and psychoanalysis, which—along with a firm foundation in art and design—provided much of the theoretical basis of training in the UK. Attempting to do so raised questions such as: *How does one go about honoring differences yet upholding ethical standards? Whose ethical standards are being upheld? To what extent are ethical standards intimately related to the cultural context?* Although the ethical challenges that I have selected to discuss are based upon work that took place many years ago in Italy, similar issues have been encountered elsewhere.

Boundary Issues: Space and Participants

Redrawing Boundaries

Art therapists have worked in dining rooms, corridors, boiler rooms, and huts. In the old psychiatric hospitals, art therapists often had large studios secluded from the rest of the hospital, where the staff sent "difficult patients." Nowadays, art therapists may have to adapt spaces that are less than ideal, but, thanks to health and safety standards, we can ask that basic requirements, such as room for everyone to move around in comfort, privacy, and access to water, be provided.

Early in my career as an art therapist/group psychotherapist, I accepted an offer to run a week-long experiential workshop for staff at a university medical centre while I was on holiday in Italy. The very enthusiastic head psychiatrist was keen to introduce new treatments to his service and had heard one of my talks in which I outlined the possible benefits of art therapy to people with psychosis. Given the rather small room available, I said that it would be possible to work with a group of eight; fourteen people arrived that morning, some from great distances. It was impossible to set up tables, so the group suggested using the walls, covering them with paper, and even the floor! They also opened the window very wide, enabling people to climb outside onto the grass—extending the boundaries even further!

I did not interview participants beforehand, as I would have now. Thus, I discovered that there were family members in the group and that most people were well known to each other socially as well as through work. I, also, did not have time to explore whether there would be difficulties for participants in terms of hierarchy, given that there were senior consultants as well as very junior doctors present. On that first day, I faced so many challenges that I had to work out quite quickly whether they were ethically problematic or whether my aim of working within the cultural context—one in which all were welcomed—should prevail. I decided that it was possible to maintain boundaries, provided that we addressed some of the issues as a group. For participants who had a strong background in psychiatry and mental health but none in psychoanalysis, presenting the above as any kind of challenge or as posing a potential risk to the group was difficult, but they accepted my reasoning and agreed to discuss openly any problems that arose. We had a lively, often hilarious week which included engaging in spontaneous role plays, making a film, and creating large group images that were carried out of the room, through the window, and onto the grass. I did insist upon carefully processing all work done and discussing group dynamics with a very receptive but also highly argumentative group.

The ethical challenges were: I did not interview potential members of the group beforehand, as they were staff from the center or colleagues of the chief; therefore, I did not provide them with information on what they might expect from an art therapy group. I did not insist upon maintaining the group at 8 people but went along with the participants' desire not to leave anyone out. I allowed extension of the boundaries, even permitting climbing through a window, which, although close to floor level, nevertheless posed risks. Because I did not know the participants, I did not address adequately the impact of working with family members, friends, or colleagues (including those who had supervisory authority over others).

Even in retrospect, I feel that it was more important to go with the participants' wish to include everyone who came; denying the participation of people who had traveled long distances to experience art therapy would have infringed upon the strong sense of hospitality that was offered to colleagues from hospitals in other parts of the country. By ensuring the safety of participants at all times and enlisting the resources of this group of experienced professionals, I believe that ethical standards were maintained.

Breaking Boundaries

Despite sending careful instructions as to the resources required, when I arrived in Southern Italy to run a week-long art therapy workshop, I found that the room I had been given had school desks lined up in rows and no access to water or places to store materials. Not wishing to give up or to accept a nearly impossible location, I explored the centre and all its out buildings in search of something better. Having discovered and managed to negotiate to use a very large attic space, I observed that it had a wide balcony outside on which there was a tap used to water the plants that had been placed there. This was ideal for the purposes of an art therapy workshop and I decided that the balcony could form part of the boundary for the workshop space.

Upon arrival, I was informed that there would be 16 participants in the group instead of the 12 expected. Although not too happy about this, I agreed, as the director of the institution reassured me that he had met all the group members and that each had expressed a commitment to stay for the entire week. Nevertheless, on the basis of previous experience, I decided to interview everyone the day before the workshop began, to advise them about the nature of the experience to follow. Most were staff from neighboring mental health centers who had heard about art therapy from colleagues who had participated in earlier workshops I had run.

Before I began the interviews, a woman whom I shall call Marta arrived, sat down at the table where I was having a coffee, and asked if I would look at her paintings and give her my impression. Alarm bells rang. She was very intense and demanding. I politely told her that it would not be appropriate to do this and explained my role as art therapist and facilitator of the forthcoming workshop. She could not see what the problem was and became angry, telling me that she had brought her paintings specifically so that I could look at them and advise her. I spent some time trying to convince her that I was not being dismissive of her or her paintings but was staying within my assigned role. I started to worry about whether Marta would be suitable for the workshop as she did not seem to understand how a group process would work but, instead, had sought a one-to-one relationship with me. I suggested that the workshop might not be to her liking and that perhaps she would prefer to find an individual art therapist, but she scornfully declined my suggestion. I had a really strong feeling that I should have insisted and not accepted her into the group, but was torn because she had been recommended by the center management. As it turned out, my "gut feeling" was correct.

It quickly became apparent that Marta had experienced some traumatic event and that she had difficulty in relating to others in the group, all of whom happened to be female. She came across as angry and dismissive of others' efforts, refusing to hear the group's feedback and constantly asking me directly to comment on her own work. A crisis arose after she had been working in a small group of three women. To clarify my instructions about boundaries, I had informed the group that the attic room and the balcony would be available to them only during workshop hours; I would unlock the room at 8:00 every morning when we arrived, but it would be closed during breaks and locked again at 5:00 when we finished. Everyone appeared to understand that the room was a special place that would be available only for the workshop. This was important as strong feelings are aroused during an interactive art therapy group and people need to feel that the space is safe, containing, and restricted to the group. They seemed to understand that nobody else would be entering the space during the week or until the group had ended and the artwork had been taken away. Imagine my shock, then, when—upon unlocking the room on the fourth day—I noticed that several significant changes had been made to a sculpture that had been created by the small group of which Marta was a part. When the participants arrived, there was a furious exchange among the three, who accused each other of changing—indeed, violating—their images. Everyone in the group became involved, with Marta at the center of some very aggressive attention which had been building in the days before the incident.

Asking the group to form a circle, I said that this constituted a "disturbance" that had to be processed; in theme-centered interaction, a disturbance is a serious issue that always takes precedence over other issues. There was much grumbling, many angry comments directed towards Marta and me, and a general reluctance to discuss the matter. Someone shouted, "She's been unfriendly all week and doesn't want to be here, throw her out!"—a sentiment echoed by others. Upon examining the sculpture—which had been formed as a result of the three women attaching their individually designed pieces—we saw that the base on which the sculpture was placed had been repainted in a dark color; a small doll that had been given to Marta as a "peace offering" by one of the women had been crushed underneath a large stone; and red paint had been splattered, like blood, over the whole area. The art seemed to contain a strong sense of violent rage, as if a murder had been committed. On a previous day, Marta had destroyed a box by angrily stabbing and cutting it to bits with scissors. Witnessing this made me shiver and suspect that Marta had been working out some deeply traumatic events which she could not speak about. I had a dilemma.

MY ETHICAL DILEMMA

Is it ethical to maintain in a group someone who seems to need the group but has violated its boundaries and behaved aggressively, albeit symbolically?

I pointed out to the group that the boundaries of the workshop had been violated and that one of the rules of the group (not to damage the work of others or oneself) had been broken, and that we had to work out why this had happened and what to do next. The two women in Marta's group were becoming increasingly furious. The chorus of "Throw her out!" was getting stronger.

Trying to think about the basics of group interactive art therapy ethics and group management, I knew that this was scapegoating and that I could not dismiss Marta unless she posed an immediate physical risk to herself or others, but what to do? She had behaved aggressively, albeit symbolically through painting and the abuse of a doll. *Would it be worse to ask her to leave, thus confirming the feeling she must have had of being excluded? Was her action symbolic of some serious abuse, probably sexual abuse, being acted out? Did she pose a physical or psychological threat to other group members? Would staying in the group be damaging to her?* She had, on all occasions, declined when invited to speak about her work, saying that it spoke for itself, refusing to comment further or to hear feedback.

How would you respond?

For the writer's response, see Appendix B, page 440.

Conclusion

Writing up these experiences has taken me back into the settings in which they occurred. I experienced the same rapid heartbeat and somewhat sick feelings, along with a real worry that I had made serious mistakes or was about to do so. It was only by pausing, reflecting, going back to the theoretical underpinnings of group interactive art therapy (Waller, 2014), and trusting the resources of the group that I got through. In real time, decisions often have to be made quickly and, even in situations where physical violence might occur, it is essential not to panic and to trust the process. Sounds easy, but it isn't. By having a thorough understanding of why we need boundaries, why the space has to be safe, and why we must be vigilant in ensuring that no harm comes to our participants, we can manage these ethical dilemmas in the best way we know.

Despite the very different social and cultural contexts in which we might work, those fundamentals seem, to me, to be relevant—and, moreover, helpful—in enabling us to maintain a place where strong emotions can be contained.

REFLECTIVE ART EXPERIENCES & DISCUSSION QUESTIONS

1. The following can be a time limited exercise so that, say, five couples in a supervision group of ten can make and present their objects to the group and the group can respond:
2. Work with a partner to spontaneously construct an object which reflects an ethical dilemma that you have confronted or are facing now. Allow your partner to help by sharing your feelings with him or her as you are making it. Then change places, enabling your partner to create an object which reflects an ethical dilemma that he or she has encountered. Afterward, share the process with the whole group and have the group respond by constructing a safe environment for all the objects.
3. Share one of the most stressful clinical experiences you've had and what you learned from it.
4. Describe an instance when—despite all other factors to the contrary—a "gut feeling" about how to address an ethical issue turned out to be correct. How do you determine how much weight should be given to your "gut feelings"?

References

Waller, D. (2014). *Group interactive art therapy: Its use in training and treatment* (2nd ed.). Hove: Routledge.

Waller, D. (1998). *Towards a European art therapy: Creating a profession.* Buckingham: Open University Press.

35

BUT WHO REALLY *IS* ON FIRST?

Art Therapy as Collaborative Treatment for Trauma Disorders

Tally Tripp

Art therapists often work collaboratively with other mental health professionals to expand or enhance treatment options for their patients. However, identifying the benefits of adding adjunctive therapeutic modalities to trauma treatment must be carefully coordinated with all involved to ensure an integrated and effective outcome and, perhaps most importantly, to ensure that no unintended ethical consequences result from such treatment plan decisions.

In my 35 years of experience, I have worked in tandem with dozens of other mental health professions including psychiatrists, social workers, psychologists, family counselors, and others who have referred patients to me for trauma treatment. The reasons for including art therapy in their treatment plans vary, but in general there are three principle reasons for accessing this modality:

1. when a patient has had a positive experience with art therapy during hospitalization;
2. when a patient displays an interest and/or talent in art making;
3. when a therapist has reached an impasse with a patient and language is no longer an effective way to communicate; that is, when "words are not enough."

Benefits of Art Therapy as an Adjunctive Approach for Trauma Treatment

The use of experiential and expressive therapies for the management of symptoms and resolution of trauma is now heartily embraced by researchers, academics, and clinicians who study and treat trauma. Art therapy, eye movement desensitization and reprocessing (EMDR), trauma-sensitive Yoga, mindfulness, neurofeedback, somatic therapies, acupuncture, and a variety of other experiential and holistic approaches are increasingly recognized as best practices.

Art therapy is in a unique position to provide rapid access to traumatic memories and facilitate the healing process because it provides direct access to implicit, emotional states that can be easily avoided in therapies that rely on verbalization alone (Tripp, 2007, 2016). My experience as a trauma therapist confirms a belief that effective treatment is "not about the story" (J. Fisher, personal communication, October 29, 2015; Tripp and Beauregard, 2013–2014), but rather about dealing with the lasting imprints of traumatic experiences that are ever present, dramatically affecting the individual's life and world view (van der Kolk, McFarlane, & Weisaeth, 1996; van der Kolk, 2014).

While it might be easy to identify the *benefits* of adding adjunctive modalities such as art therapy to trauma treatment, therapists face complexities, pitfalls, and ethical dilemmas when shifting from individual therapy to a model that may include collaboration with other practitioners. From my perspective, there are a few essential questions that should be part of any collaborative treatment decision process:

- Why is the referral being made and what are the precise expectations or goals of the work? Are they realistic?
- How frequently—weekly, monthly, or as needed—will the "adjunctive" sessions be provided? How does the frequency impact the sessions and how will this be addressed when moving between therapies?
- What are the unique aspects of each approach? How does one support or influence the flow, pace, or intensity of the other?
- What are the roles and boundaries among members of the treatment team? How often do therapists share information? How is transference and countertransference managed? What happens when two therapists have different responses to the same clinical situation?

Clearly, each of the potential concerns embodied in the questions above can positively or negatively influence the overall therapeutic frame. Ultimately, the benefit of collaborative therapy must be weighed against the potential pitfalls, along with at least one significant caveat; that is, treating trauma requires years of specialized training and experience. As such, a collaborative team approach is often the best choice to provide the best care. What follows are some cases that illustrate both the potential benefits and challenges of using art therapy as an adjunctive treatment approach.

A Case for Collaboration

Martina, a client diagnosed with Dissociative Identity Disorder (DID), implored her psychiatrist to "find her an art therapist." The request was due to Martina's positive response to a regime of weekly art therapy during an inpatient hospitalization. She believed art therapy provided something different that facilitated healing and resolution of her trauma and dissociation in a way that verbal therapy did not. So, in her on-going outpatient work, Martina attended both art therapy, with me, and verbal therapy, with her psychiatrist. She, and her system of dissociated "parts," valued *both approaches* simultaneously and strongly felt she needed to work with both therapists to have a positive outcome. In essence, the art therapy provided access to younger, less verbal parts holding implicit memories of childhood trauma, while the verbal sessions allowed her to explore the imagery verbally and gain further insight. It was fascinating to note that the art facilitated communication not only within her system of dissociated parts, but also between her two therapists.

Because the therapists communicated regularly and consistently about the work, splitting these therapies worked seamlessly. So well, in fact, that we often wondered if our work together actually increased Martina's—and her parts'—ability to resolve the trauma and integrate her alter personalities. While this experience is an example of an "ideal" collaborative treatment outcome, most often these collaborations are far more difficult to manage and are rife with ethical dilemmas.

The Initial Consult: Why are we working together?

Art therapy is a wonderful tool for clients who appear to be "shut down" and unable to access or connect with traumatic memories through rational thought or language. Making art with an art therapist can accelerate the pace of traditional verbal treatment by bringing the richness of unconscious imagery into the room. But no matter the situation, it is important to determine the goals for the use of art therapy and to carefully consider its potential impact on the overall treatment plan.

Potential Potholes on the Road to Collaboration

You Say Goodbye and I Say Hello

A therapist referred a client to me after realizing her client's unresolved childhood trauma was standing in the way of their progress. Despite providing years of "supportive" counseling to the client, this therapist did not feel equipped to work with her trauma. I agreed to provide the client a few exploratory sessions before I recommended adjunctive art therapy as a plan. While the art therapy progressed smoothly, it soon became evident that the primary therapist had reduced the frequency of sessions with her client. When I contacted the therapist, she admitted feeling ineffective in contrast to art therapy's more dynamic approach. She suggested I continue treating the patient alone. This change brought up abandonment issues for the client and a feeling of being "dumped" for me; both of these issues had to be resolved before anything could progress.

How Many, How Often, How Well?

It is not unusual to use a "team" approach to treat trauma-related disorders. For example, trauma focused cognitive behavioral therapy (CBT) can help with changing thoughts and dysfunctional beliefs. Neurofeedback and somatic therapies can be useful for self-regulation and affect management. Art therapy is especially effective for facilitating creative expression and communication. However, do not assume that "more is better." Even with good skills and adequate communication, not all clients benefit from all approaches.

A female anorexic client with whom I worked was also being seen by a psychologist, a psychiatrist, a nutritionist, a life coach, and a mentor. Despite this intensive outpatient model, her "team" was surprised to learn that she required hospitalization when several of us took vacation during the same week. Clearly, the treatment had become so compartmentalized and fragmented that the client was unable to recognize or make use of her own internal resources. After the hospital stay, the team decided to decrease the number of adjunctive modalities to facilitate more self- agency on the client's part. Ultimately, the client became more assertive and self-reliant and was able to better manage other disruptions and breaks in her routine.

Art Envy: What to Do When a Non-Art Therapist Provides Art Materials

Art therapists may be the recipient of "art envy" when a collaborating verbal therapist tries to bring art making into a psychotherapy session. This may be in response to the well-intentioned request of a client who assumes that any of her providers can provide art therapy. However, when untrained therapists integrate art making in their sessions, it is not uncommon for problems to arise.

I provided art therapy in an outpatient clinic in collaboration with a primary care verbal therapist. When we began art therapy sessions the client was nearly mute, silenced by a long-standing history of malicious physical and sexual abuse at the hand of a relative. The client had been struggling with severe anxiety and chronic dissociation, and we hoped art therapy would provide a new language and way to communicate. Indeed, this client made great progress accessing and expressing difficult feelings, working with clay and watercolor. The problem occurred when she began accessing more intense feelings, particularly rage and shame surrounding significant traumas that had been dissociated from conscious awareness.

Since my role was "adjunctive," it was the primary therapist's role to provide emergency case management and stabilization. However, accessing these memories resulted in the client becoming dysregulated and suicidal and as a result she frequently called or emailed me in crisis between sessions. It was only when the client emailed me a graphic image she had created in her recent *verbal* session that I learned that the primary therapist had begun using art! The artwork had triggered a traumatic response in the client, while the therapist had unknowingly crossed a professional and ethical boundary by working outside of her expertise. It was then necessary for me to have a heart-to-heart talk with the therapist and later with the client to clarify how a non-art therapist might use art. Finding a way to discuss this without (a) alienating the therapist and (b) shaming the client was not easy. The other therapist and I also sought out consultation from a recognized trauma expert and this helped us get our treatment planning better aligned.

Occasionally in collaborative treatment, art therapy will completely replace a primary verbal therapy for a specific number of sessions. Shifting the primary focus between verbal and art therapy can present interesting challenges. It is not unusual for a client to discover that art brings completely new information to the surface and this causes tension when negotiating a return to the original therapist. It is important to be clear about the role of each therapist and not to overstep prescribed boundaries.

MY ETHICAL DILEMMA

What can I take away from hearing, "I asked you to help me remodel the kitchen, not renovate the entire house!"?

Ellen was a 30-year-old single female who had struggled with lifelong depression and anxiety related to an extensive childhood trauma history. She was raised in a chaotic and unsafe household. Her parents were both verbally and physically abusive with one another and Ellen was often a pawn in their battles. Ellen was never able to develop a sense of safety in relationships and was isolative, anxious and insecure. While she expressed a longing for intimacy in her life, she avoided dating and spent most nights at home smoking pot and watching TV.

Ellen had been in traditional psychotherapy for several years but the treatment had reached its limit and even reinforced keeping feelings at bay. Like most trauma survivors, Ellen was fearful of experiencing feelings even though she was aware that her underlying problems were interfering with her happiness. Having been recently rejected in a relationship, art therapy was recommended to help her access her emotions and "jump start" the verbal therapy.

Verbal therapy was suspended for 10 weeks while I worked with Ellen. Both the referring psychologist and I assured her that we would communicate regularly regarding her progress. We did not want to replicate the dysfunctional parenting style of her parents by splitting loyalties and expecting her to navigate both therapies simultaneously. The arrangement would also allow the client to whole-heartedly commit to the art therapy for a specified period.

Even in her initial art-making session, tears came to Ellen's eyes when I asked her to create a loose scribble and develop an image from within (Figure 35.1). She drew an "unsteady" red figure that appears to be both moving forward and falling backwards, as if trying to balance. The metaphor was an apt self-portrait and we discussed the way she seemed unsure of her path, as if she had one foot in the present and the other in the past.

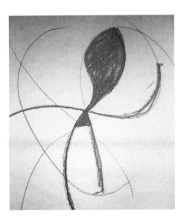

FIGURE 35.1 An unsteady self-portrait.

Understanding this conundrum was important and highlighted a concern: was Ellen ready to feel her feelings in the present and deal with her traumatic past? This picture foreshadowed themes from her trauma history that had largely been avoided in the verbal psychotherapy. Was this the path she wanted to take?

Within the first month of art therapy, some extremely disturbing memories emerged in rapid succession. In one heavily sketched pastel picture, Ellen depicted a figure laying down on her back with her chest being crushed by a lead weight. She described this memory of going to sleep as a child, fearful and sad, wanting to tear her heart out of her chest and wishing she could die. Ellen experienced this crushing as a literal sensation in her body, sobbing as she was flooded with emotion.

Ellen hoped to use art therapy to "move through" her problems; to get some relief and to gain understanding about her difficulty with relationships. However, she made it clear she did not wish to re-visit these distressing emotional childhood memories. Yet, the art she produced continually took us back to the implicit memories of her traumatic past.

How would you respond?

For the writer's response, see Appendix B, page 438.

Summary Recommendations

If you are at a point at which you are thinking about working collaboratively to treat trauma disorders, you might consider the following:

- *Contracting.* Establishing a verbal contract that delineates client and therapist's roles and expectations will prevent problems. Ask the referring therapist: "How do you see the art therapy affecting your continued work with your client?"
- *Education.* It is important to clearly convey that art therapy is more than making pretty pictures and that the art can be triggering and result in regression. I often tell the therapists and clients that art therapy may change the course of treatment.
- *Communication.* Therapists should communicate regularly with one another for continuity and seek consultation when necessary. The art therapist can encourage the client to take photos of the art and share the images with the verbal therapist to promote continued discourse that may help with communication and understanding.
- *Professional boundaries.* Collaboratively engaged therapists must take precautions not to push ahead too quickly or overstep the boundaries of their work Therapists must create a plan to find a complementary pace.
- *Flexibility* is key when blending several modalities into a client's treatment. Regardless of the number of modalities, an individualized approach based on the

unique needs of the individual is crucial. And, most importantly, whenever you are working with an individual with a trauma disorder—whether you are collaborating with other therapists or serving as sole practitioner—

- *Emotional regulation.* While it is necessary to visit a traumatic memory to revise it, the dysregulated client will not be able to do the work without a safe base. A foundation for trauma work must include developing tools for grounding and stabilization.

REFLECTIVE ART EXPERIENCES & DISCUSSION QUESTIONS

1. Describe an instance when you felt that the goals of your client's various treaters collided/competed with each other. How did this impact you and how did it impact the overall treatment? How was the situation handled? How do you wish it had been handled?
2. Describe an instance when, looking back, you believe that you could have been more supportive of a client's autonomy. What do you think prevented you from doing so at the time?
3. Draw a picture of yourself, as a sole practitioner, in relationship with your client.
4. Draw yourself in relationship with your client and each of the client's other therapists and/or team members. Draw a second picture, reflecting any changes you might wish to make to the image/the relationships. Discuss both drawings.

References

Tripp, T. (2007). A short-term approach to processing trauma: Art therapy and bilateral stimulation. *Art Therapy: Journal of the American Art Therapy Association*, 24(4), 176–183.

Tripp, T. (2016). A body-based bilateral art protocol for reprocessing trauma. In J. King (Ed.), *Art therapy, trauma and neuroscience: Theoretical and practical perspectives* (pp. 173–194). New York: Routledge.

Tripp, T., & Beauregard, J. (2013–2014). It's not about the story: Using art, yoga and the body in trauma treatment. Workshops presented at Integrative Psychotherapy Institute, Washington, DC.

van der Kolk, B. A. (2014). *The body keeps the score: Brain, mind and body in the healing of trauma.* New York: Viking Penguin.

van der Kolk, B. A., McFarlane, L., & Weisaeth, A. C. (Eds.) (1996). *Traumatic stress: The overwhelming experience on mind, body, and society.* New York: Guilford Press.

36

ETHICAL CONCERNS WHEN APPLYING DRAWING TO PROMOTE MEMORY

Research Conducted in Iceland

Unnur Ottarsdottir

There are approximately 20 art therapists in Iceland, about half of whom are practicing at the time of writing. The history of art therapy as a profession in Iceland spans about four decades. The Icelandic Art Therapy Association, along with its regulations and code of ethics, was formed in 1998. As there is no graduate art therapy education program in Iceland, all Icelandic art therapists have acquired their education abroad; most have a MA degree and one has a PhD degree. Art therapists in Iceland have sought recognition from the state in the form of licensure but have not yet succeeded. They are free, however, to open a private practice without any restriction from the government.

Although the lack of governmental restrictions in setting up an art therapy private practice and the small number of art therapists in Iceland creates fertile ground from which new ideas and methods can emerge, it takes time, trial and error, and careful thinking to form boundaries around the new methods. In the meantime, ethical concerns may arise.

Art Educational Therapy

My experience when working with children as a teacher and an art therapist in a preschool, secondary schools, and a high school, is the background of the study introduced in this chapter. The motivation for conducting the research was originally derived from when I worked as an art therapist and at the same time as a special education teacher, in schools in Iceland, observing the effect of applying art making for children's coursework learning and emotional well-being. The subject of this chapter relates to a period when I worked at an Icelandic school as an art therapist, a special education teacher, and a researcher conducting PhD research (Ottarsdottir, 2005, 2010a, 2010b). The five children who took part in the research had experienced stress and/or trauma and had specific learning difficulties. The children received art educational therapy (AET) (Ottarsdottir, 2010a), whereby the learning of school subjects is integrated into art therapy with the aim of facilitating emotional well-being and coursework learning. I developed AET through the research and its theoretical framework is composed of theories derived from art therapy and educational psychotherapy (Best, 2014). An important aspect of AET is the interplay between words and images, which is called *writing-images* (Ottarsdottir, 2010b). In AET, children are free to choose the way in which they prefer to work, in terms of art making, coursework learning, and verbal expression.

One of the ethically sensitive aspects of AET involves memorising through drawing. Specifically, there is a concern that when the memory drawings are made within an educational context, the process may bring up emotionally laden material related to memories of personal experiences while strong enough emotional containment necessary to process and integrate those feelings may be unavailable.

A Case Study: Lisa

Five children between the ages of 11 and 14 participated in the research, with the informed consent of their parents. Altogether, they received 123 therapeutic sessions. The case study research method was used in order to study, in depth, the educational and therapeutic processes of each child. The grounded theory research method was applied for the data analysis. This chapter presents part of the case study of one of the children, Lisa, in relation to memory drawing.

Lisa, age 11, attended 41 sessions, twice weekly. Sessions included (a) spontaneous art making, (b) coursework integrated into art therapy through art making, (c) direct teaching, and (d), integration of all of the above. Lisa was free to choose the method, subject matter, coursework, and materials to work with.

Although born in Norway, the family moved to Iceland when Lisa was one year old and moved frequently during the next five years. When she was six years old, she packed all her things into bags, saying that she wanted to move back to her previous home.

When Lisa was one year old, she was admitted to a hospital for a week because of diarrhea. A heart condition was discovered the following year and from then on she was regularly monitored by her doctor. As a young child, Lisa was frequently ill with stomach pains and ear infections. After her tonsils were removed, at age six, she became healthier, but, at eleven, she often complained of stomach pains and headaches. She seemed to have a fear of doctors.

Because both of Lisa's parents worked long hours, leaving the house early and returning late, Lisa was on her own after school, from mid-afternoon until early evening. Lisa rarely completed her homework before her mother came home, even though she gave her money to finish it before she returned. According to her mother, Lisa was "lazy." Occasionally, the mother assisted Lisa with her homework until 12:30 at night. Lisa, who became easily irritated doing her homework, sometimes crumpled up her assignments and told her mother, "Leave me alone!" Her mother did not understand Lisa's mathematics homework and her father, who had finished his compulsory schooling at 15, was unable to help Lisa with her coursework.

Lisa was an early talker and her reading progressed normally. The year before beginning therapy, she began to have trouble with most subjects, but primarily mathematics and history—which involve remembering facts—rather than reading. She enjoyed art lessons and knitting at school, and was happy to attend the AET sessions.

When she began therapy, Lisa was pale and withdrawn, spoke in a low, breathless voice; her movements were unsure and hesitant. Although she seemed willing to make contact, she was rather passive. She answered questions monosyllabically and made no attempt to initiate conversation. Initially, she resisted doing, and talking about, her coursework; as time passed, she became more willing to study—eagerly placing her books on the table at the beginning of sessions, requesting assistance. Lisa's teacher reported that, during the first six months of therapy, Lisa was doing much better at school. As therapy drew towards its end, however, she no longer wanted to study during sessions and her teacher complained about Lisa's behavior having reverted to a pre-therapy stage. After Lisa expressed her feelings about our imminent separation, she once again became eager to learn, which indicated that separation anxiety, loneliness, and lack of contact interfered with her ability and/or willingness to study.

Lisa brought coursework for various subjects to the AET sessions and learning in these areas was integrated as much as possible into the art making. Lisa had trouble understanding and remembering the information in her geography text. In one of the sessions she chose a section about the main industry in Norway to read aloud and I explained any difficult words, following which she drew a boatload of people working at an oil platform, which looks insecurely grounded (see Figure 36.1). Her choice of Norway indicates that, on some level, she may have been working with emotional material related to an early experience.

Lisa found learning poetry by heart difficult. In another session, she chose to work with a poem about a man who had severe arthritis and had trouble writing. Since Lisa often wished to draw with me—a choice that I suspect was linked to her loneliness—I suggested that each of us write down a line of the poem and illustrate it (see Figure 36.2). I wrote the first line of the poem and, at the end of the line, drew an image that would convey the meaning of the line. The line said that the man's hands became stiff when he was writing and I drew an open book with dots on it. Lisa wrote the second line, which said that the man's weapon (his pen) was loose in his hand, and then she drew a man dropping his weapon. We took turns in this way until we completed the poem. At the bottom of the page, Lisa drew a man who was sick and alone in a cave, which may have symbolized her own loneliness and health problems. When Lisa attempted to recite the poem without looking at the lines and had difficulty doing so, I asked, "If you imagine the drawing in your mind, can you then remember?" She was able to recall the text using this method. The images, first drawn and then visualized, appeared to serve as a bridge from the poem to her memory.

When the grades that Lisa had received before starting therapy, during therapy, and after completing therapy were compared, it showed that all of her grades had improved during the course of AET and the two terms following it. The Child Behaviour Checklist completed by Lisa's mother before the initiation of AET and after its completion indicated that Lisa complained less frequently about physical pain, demonstrated less anxiety, and was more social following therapy. The Attention Deficit/Hyperactivity Disorder Rating Scale-IV completed by her mother indicated

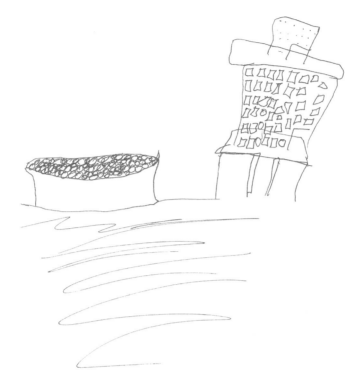

FIGURE 36.1 Oil platform and a boatload of people working there.

better concentration following therapy. Her overall IQ score showed a seven-point rise after the completion of AET.

A few months into the therapy time, which was early in the year 2000, I had witnessed, in the case studies, various instances where drawing seemed to facilitate memory of coursework, such as in the case of Lisa when she was to memorise the poem (Figure 36.2). In order to study more systematically the effects of drawing upon memory, I conducted a quantitative research with 134 children, ages nine to fourteen. The research showed that, nine weeks after the initial memorisation, the median amount of recalled drawings was five times higher than for written words (Ottarsdottir, 2018).

Ethical Concerns

Is it only good news that drawing generally facilitates long term memory much more than writing? From an art therapeutic point of view, the answer involves careful thinking about complex ethical questions and concerns regarding the emotional and cognitive well-being of our students and clients.

In the instances when Lisa chose coursework subjects to draw about, the topics seemed to reflect a personal connection and sensitive emotional material. If her

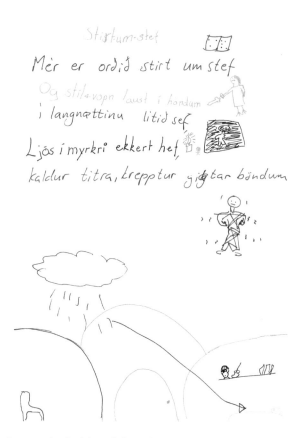

FIGURE 36.2 A man who is sick and alone in a cave.

decision to focus upon Norway, where she was born (Figure 36.1), related to early pre-verbal experiences (being ill in hospital, moving between places), it would underline the importance of memory drawing being done within an environment which is able to provide strong therapeutic containment and safety. Likewise, Lisa's decision to focus upon someone who was sick, alone, and having difficulty writing could have symbolized her own specific learning difficulties, her isolation, and her illnesses, which included a heart condition that resulted in continual medical monitoring and hospital visits. Thus, the case study indicated that while Lisa was using drawing as a means by which to mem-orise educational material, the process seems to have tapped into emotions that could relate to unconscious and possibly pre-verbal memories associated with the subjects she chose to draw. The therapeutic relationship provided both connection and contain-ment, which was important for her emotional and academic progress, as the setback in her studying that occurred when the therapy was coming to an end was reversed when she was able to address, in therapy, emotions related to the upcoming separation.

According to art therapy theories, drawing can tap into emotions, personal experiences, and the unconscious. Because of this, it is possible that (a) a person who is drawing an image in response to a particular word might bring to the meaning of that drawing (word) connections that come from a deeper source within him- or herself than when writing that word, and (b) the process of factual content hooking up with personal meaning through drawing might enable the individual to memorize coursework content more easily than through writing. Because drawing can tap into personal meaning more than writing, therapy may be needed for individuals who make memory drawings if they are vulnerable, have had a lot of difficult experiences, and/or lack support.

In 1973, Paivio and Csapo published the results of research they had conducted comparing short-term memory recall of pictures versus words; in one experiment, they found that drawings were remembered more easily than words (Paivio & Csapo, 1973). Wammes, Meade, and Fernandes (2016) conducted quantitative memory drawing research that, in some ways, was similar to the quantitative memory drawing research I had conducted in 2000 (mentioned earlier in this chapter), comparing memorisation of words and drawings. They found that drawings were better remembered than written words in the short term. They posited that drawing creates a cohesive memory trace through integrating visual, motor, and semantic information. There is no mention of the researchers taking into consideration the potential emotional involvement in the drawing process.

In my opinion, an important addition to the explanation put forth by Wammes, Meade, and Fernandes (2016) as to why drawing facilitates memory is that drawing can facilitate a connection to personally meaningful experiences and emotions—a key premise of art therapy.

MY ETHICAL DILEMMA

How can I prepare professionals to provide strong enough emotional containment for clients and students who make memory drawings?

Memory drawings may tap into sensitive emotional material, which might cause further difficulties for vulnerable children, particularly if the drawings are facilitated by a non-therapist, in that emotional containment may not be available to help such children process and integrate their feelings.

How would you respond?

For the writer's response, see Appendix B, page 425.

Conclusion

As we saw in the case of Lisa, art therapy can provide a safe space for vulnerable children to process and integrate emotions that might emerge during the memory drawing process. Through observing the children with whom I have worked, I have become increasingly aware of the importance of forming boundaries around the new method of memory drawing, partly in the form of introducing art therapeutic theories and methods to the person who holds the space where memory drawings are made. This includes educating professionals about memory drawing in relation to art therapy theories and methods, in order for them to better understand the symbolic expression included in the children's drawings, and, thus, become more able to emotionally contain, understand, and/or recognize vulnerable children who may need referral to therapy.

REFLECTIVE ART EXPERIENCES & DISCUSSION QUESTIONS

1. Think of a school subject with which you had difficulty when you were a child. Draw a picture that relates to that subject. Be aware of your thoughts and feelings when you draw. What kind of setting and relationship do you think would serve you best in memorizing the school subject and processing and integrating the emotions evoked in the drawing process?
2. Discuss the advantages and disadvantages of conducting memory drawing research in an educational setting.
3. What would you do if you were teaching a class of 25 children who were making memory drawings for educational purposes and you observed that a child was making an image that contained emotionally sensitive material?

References

Best, R. (2014). Educational psychotherapy: An approach to working with children whose learning is impeded by emotional problems. *Support for Learning*, 29(3), 201–216.

Ottarsdottir, U. (2005). *Art therapy in education: For children with specific learning difficulties who have experienced stress and/or trauma.* Unpublished doctoral dissertation. University of Hertfordshire, Hatfield.

Ottarsdottir, U. (2010a). Art therapy in education for children with specific learning difficulties who have experienced stress and/or trauma. In V. Karkou (Ed.), *Arts therapies in schools: Research and practice* (pp. 145–160). London: Jessica Kingsley.

Ottarsdottir, U. (2010b). Writing-images. *Art Therapy: Journal of the American Art Therapy Association*, 27(1), 32–39.

Ottarsdottir, U. (2018). Processing emotions and memorising coursework through memory drawing. *ATOL: Art Therapy OnLine*, 9(1). Retrieved from http://journals.gold.ac.uk/index.php/atol/article/view/486/pdf

Paivio, A., & Csapo, K. (1973). Picture superiority in free recall: Imagery or dual coding? *Cognitive Psychology*, 5(2), 176–206.

Wammes, J.D., Meade, M.E., & Fernandes, M.A. (2016). The drawing effect: Evidence for reliable and robust memory benefits in free recall. *The Quarterly Journal of Experimental Psychology*, 69(9), 1752–1776.

37

MY FIRST YEAR AS AN ART THERAPIST IN INDIA

Ethical, Cultural, Logistical, and Supervisory Issues

Sangeeta Prasad

In 1987, after completing a master's degree in art therapy in the United States, I was excited to return to India to work in the kindergarten and primary school that had been founded in 1965 by my mother, who served as its principal until the school closed 50 years later. Having worked there as a kindergarten teacher, I knew the teachers very well and they, too, were looking forward to my bringing art therapy to the school. Special education had not yet been established in India and very few schools catered to children with intellectual disabilities. Mental health was not yet considered to be something that needed to be addressed within a school setting, so counselors were not a part of school staff. Since this school included several children with special needs, the teachers were looking for help with how to reach them.

I soon realized that there were many issues to be considered—ethical, cultural, logistical, supervisory—and there was no art therapy association, art therapy training program, or ethics code for art therapists in India. Indeed, I was aware of no other art therapists in the country. In this chapter, I share some of the ethical challenges I faced and describe how I addressed them. Although these reflections are from many years ago, I find art therapists grapple with these issues today, especially as they introduce art therapy to new cultures or new environments. I present my approach not as the only way—or the best way—to handle these situations, but as a way of generating ideas that could be of use to art therapists who find themselves in similar situations. Following the discussion of each issue, relevant standards from the American Art Therapy Association's (AATA's) *Ethical Principles for Art Therapists* (2013) or the (American) Art Therapy Credentials Board's *Code of Ethics, Conduct, and Disciplinary Procedures* (2018) are presented. The ATCB did not exist at the time about which I'm writing.

Ethical Challenges

1. Did my training provide me with the skills to work with a population which has such a wide range of special needs?
Upon my arrival at the school, the list I was given of those who needed art therapy included children who had been diagnosed by pediatricians as having autism, Down's syndrome, cerebral palsy, and attention deficit disorder (ADD), usually with hyper-activity (ADHD). My first question was whether I was qualified to work with children who had these conditions. My internships had been in a special education setting with emotionally disturbed children and at an inpatient psychiatric hospital for adults. Both art therapy programs were psychodynamically oriented. Would that approach work with these children, within this setting? What were the various art therapy approaches I would need to use in order to work successfully with them?

The first thing I did was to learn more about each child's condition. I visited schools, talked with other professionals, and, since there were no art therapy books available in India, wrote to the director of the art therapy program I'd attended in the US, asking for material on these topics. In response, she sent me an entire collection of art therapy journals donated by professionals in the field—an amazing resource to help me learn the different approaches that art therapists used in working with chil-dren who had developmental disabilities! I decided to employ a developmental, art-as-therapy approach with the children who had autism and other intellectual disabilities.

> 1.2.3 Art therapists shall assess, treat, or advise only in those cases in which they are competent as determined by their education, training, and experience.
>
> *ATCB, 2018*

2. Since (pre-Internet) I could not avail myself of additional education or training in art therapy in India, how could I develop my competence as an art therapist as I continued to expand my experience?
Since art therapy supervision was not available, I had to rely upon other forms of help. I contacted several psychologists and social workers in the city and formed a small peer discussion group, so that we could learn from one another. This gave me an opportunity to talk to people with a clinical background about some of the issues I was facing. When I later returned to the US and applied to become a Registered Art Therapist (ATR) with AATA, I reviewed the work I had done in India and gained insight into what had and had not worked. Today, of course, one may reach out through the Internet to art therapists around the world for supervision, consultation, or mentoring.

3. Since there was no record keeping in schools in India, other than report cards and notes tracking educational progress—information that was usu-ally conveyed to parents verbally—should I keep written records of my therapeutic work? If so, what standards or model should I follow?
As I collected family histories and teachers' concerns, I wondered whether I should create records for each child. Who would see these records? Our school staff? Parents? Staff at other educational programs the children would attend after leaving this school?

Was there a process whereby information was exchanged among mental health and school professionals? I came to realize that, in schools in India, most information was conveyed verbally and parents or other professionals did not request or receive written reports. In consultation with management, it was decided that I would keep personal notes and, if a parent or another professional requested information, I would respond verbally or in writing about the progress of the child, given the parent's consent. No records would be maintained in the school.

Over the years, record keeping has been introduced into many special education schools in India.

I like to think that, if I had continued to work there, I would have researched the laws or regulations followed by other professionals in the field of mental health and set up a formal record keeping system. Though hindsight is 20/20, I can't emphasize enough how important it is for us to step back, periodically, to see if the solutions and compromises we developed in the course of integrating into a new working environment align with our own professional ethical standards, such as the one that follows.

2.7 Art therapists must maintain records that:

2.7.1 Are in compliance with federal, provincial, state, and local regulations and any licensure requirements governing the provision of art therapy services for the location in which the art therapy services are provided.

2.7.2 Are in compliance with the standards, policies, and requirements at the art therapist's place of employment.

ATCB, 2018

4. To what extent could I—or should I—transfer the education and experience I learned from one culture to another culture?

Although art is part of everyday life, religion, and social interaction in India, it was not part of the curriculum in most schools. There were no art teachers with a degree in art education; most were either trained or self-taught artists, and art classes involved learning drawing, painting, and sculpting skills, as well as copying art and coloring pre-drawn images. Parents and children alike expected this activity to result in attractive (if conventional) art products. The appearance of *rangoli* designs (floor drawings also called *kolams*), postcard-like images (triangular mountains, a sunrise, and a stream), and religious icons (figurative renderings of Ganesha or other deities) were part of the culture's art expression.

My art therapy training in the West provided me with a very different perspective concerning education, disabilities, and art, and I wondered if the creation of the kind of artwork described above might meet a need that was similar to that met by the stereotypic superheroes and cartoon characters found in the artwork of children in the West. I had to learn to see these images from a cultural standpoint. Should I encourage creative thinking within the framework of existing art forms? How does this culture view creativity and how does this view fit into the value system of the culture? If people are told what to do in an art class and need to follow the instructor's directions, what role does creative thinking play within this environment? Should I encourage creative thinking or skill building? What contributes to the development of self-esteem?

I found myself encouraging the children to elaborate upon the images or designs that they chose to make. For example, if a child were to draw a picture of Ganesha, the Elephant God, I might ask him or her, "What does Ganesha like to wear (or to eat or to do)?" I recall one child adding an umbrella to the traditional Ganesha form that was always made. And with changes, often came stories… I also began to use the kinds of local art materials and processes that were available in India. Chalk on a black-top table—or on a cement floor—was an excellent way for children to express their ideas without feeling inhibited. After all, this was familiar to them. At 6 a.m. each day in southern India, their mother, or the maid, would draw a 10" square *kolam* in white chalk powder on the walkway outside their front door, as a way of welcoming the good spirits into the house. The next morning, this *kolam* would be erased so a new one could take its place. Art did not have to be permanent. This practice exemplified the importance of focusing upon the process, rather than the product (a maxim of art therapy), and reusing space or materials minimized costs.

Observing that most children were uncomfortable with the large sheets of paper and large spaces I had become used to in the US, I soon realized that small sheets of paper, newspaper, brown paper bags, and recycled paper were more acceptable to them. I found that mixing powdered paint, rather than using expensive tempera paint, resulted in a freer use of the medium, because the children no longer worried that they were "wasting paint" when they were working. In an effort to help children to distinguish between art therapy and art class, I conducted art therapy sessions individually or in small groups in a separate room. Desk space was at a premium whenever I taught an art expression class. Since classrooms were open to the outside, though, it was easy for the children to go out to collect found objects (such as flowers, leaves, and stones) for use in their art making. I also made my own clay. Local products were easily available and a much better choice than the more expensive imported art materials.

> 7.2 Art therapists take reasonable steps to ensure that they are sensitive to differences that exist among cultures. They strive in their attempts to learn about the belief systems of people in any given cultural group in order to provide culturally relevant interventions and treatment.
>
> *AATA, 2013*

The concepts of confidentiality and informed consent. I liked the informality of the verbal exchange of information that was standard in educational settings in India, yet I worried about the lack of confidentiality. How was I to maintain confidentiality in a setting in which so many people were interacting with the child—not only teachers, but also van drivers, the maids who accompanied some of the children to school, and extended family members? Rather than having a discussion with parents about the potential benefits of art therapy for their children, should I have obtained formal, written "permission to treat" from them? Should I have asked parents to sign a "release of information" form to photograph artwork and the children who created it? How did the parents regard therapy, counseling, and art? Did they understand that, in art therapy, the art is a means of self-expression and, therefore, one may feel a need to keep it private, unlike in an art class, where one may be proud to display the art product? Had I not done a sufficient job of explaining what art therapy is—or was I introducing Western concepts into a culture that did not regard privacy in the same way and, in fact, might perceive it as *foreign* and, perhaps, completely unnecessary?

MY ETHICAL DILEMMA

Boundaries of confidentiality and consent

Is it necessary to institute, in a more informal cultural environment, the strict boundaries regarding confidentiality and informed consent that are such an important feature of therapeutic work in the US?

How would you respond?

For the writer's response, see Appendix B, page 428.

Conclusion

As I write this chapter, 30 years after most of the events I've described took place, I know of five art therapists—and three expressive arts therapy certificate-level programs—in India. Not only has interest been expressed in the development of an Indian art therapy association, but a newsletter has been created, illustrating ways in which others have introduced art therapy within their environments, as well as describing ways in which art therapists have been able to obtain the training, support, and resources necessary to help the field grow.

In order to provide a forum for the exchange of questions, ideas, and information regarding the development of art therapy in India, as well as to provide mentoring to young art therapists working there, in 2015, I set up the "Indian Art Therapy Discussion Forum" on the Internet. As an art therapist who has deep ties with India but now lives and works in the United States, I hope that the forum helps to bridge the information divide and provides a place where art therapists working in India may raise their questions. I remember an art therapist who shared with me her experience at a boys' rehabilitation center at a mental health facility in India. She had conducted art therapy there for a month and felt that the boys were being mistreated and abused by the staff. What could or should she have done? Situations such as this pose unique ethical challenges within a cultural context. What may seem unethical in one culture may be the norm in another. As Bruce Moon (2015) so beautifully put it, "Each art therapist must decide how the principles in the ethics documents apply to the particular problem he or she is facing. This can be difficult, sometimes confusing, and sometimes frightening work" (p. xi).

REFLECTIVE ART EXPERIENCES & DISCUSSION QUESTIONS

1. When you work in an environment, culture, or setting where art therapy is new, what are some of the ethical issues you must consider before you begin your work there?
2. Using materials with which you are unfamiliar, create a piece that represents your role in the new environment.
3. How would you go about integrating your cultural experience, education, and ethical practices within a new setting?
4. Working on paper or with three-dimensional materials, create a symbol to represent yourself. On another sheet of paper or with another mound of clay or the like, represent the new environment. Consider where you would place yourself in the new environment and what changes or adaptations you would need to make (to yourself, to the environment) to ensure a "good fit."

References

American Art Therapy Association (2013). *Ethical principles for art therapists.* Alexandria, VA: Author.

Art Therapy Credentials Board (2018). *Code of ethics, conduct, and disciplinary procedures.* Greensboro, NC: Author.

Moon, B. L. (2015). *Ethical issues in art therapy* (3rd ed.). Springfield, IL: Charles C. Thomas.

38

THE MINI ART THERAPEUTIC SESSION PROGRAM IN A SCHOOL SETTING IN JAPAN

Yuriko Ichiki and Mercedes Ballbé ter Maat

> *Speech is silver, silence is golden.*
> *Out of the mouth comes evil.*
> *Nails seen out of the ground must be nailed down.*

Proverbs such as these are characteristic of traditional Japanese egalitarianism, which was the cultural norm when I left Kyoto in the mid-1980s to pursue a master's degree in Art Therapy in the United States. Upon returning to Japan, I earned a doctorate in Clinical Psychology and worked in a variety of settings, such as a mental health hospital, a nursing home, and a children's center for therapy and assessment. As a university professor, I now teach school psychology and applied clinical psychology to education majors. As a school counselor, I also work in public schools with children and their parents, consulting with teachers as needed. One of my challenges—the one I am sharing in this narrative—is how therapeutic art interventions can be incorporated into the Japanese educational system in an ethical, safe, and nonthreatening way.

During the past 20 years, Japan has seen a transformation in the type of psychological support provided to students. School counselors were first introduced in junior high schools and then in elementary schools in Japan in 1995, something that would not have been possible had it not been for the work of Kawai, a clinical psychologist who said that school counseling was a step towards "a discovery of individuality in school" (2000, p. 91). Indeed, the phrase "to develop students' individuality" appears in the Ministry of Education's General Policies Regarding Curriculum Formation (1998, p. 1), implying that schools were to attend to the students' social and personal needs, as well as their academic needs. In 2006, school counselors started to be assigned to all junior high schools. Teachers are being trained to carry out developmentally appropriate, psycho-educational programs in their classrooms on topics such as social-skill training, assertiveness training, and decision-making skills. These programs aim to foster healthful interpersonal relationships and to prevent school-related problems such as school refusal, bullying, and delinquency.

I saw this change as an opportunity to introduce art therapy interventions into the school setting. Since limited attempts had been made to use art as a non-verbal medium for facilitating expression of psychological needs in schools (Okada, 2009), I developed the "Mini Art Therapeutic Session Program" (MATSP) in an effort to help Japanese children to express their feelings more comfortably. Since the number of school psychologists and, certainly, art therapists in Japanese schools is quite limited (their positions being itinerant in nature), I believed that teachers with the right attitude, knowledge, and training could carry out this program successfully. After all, the classroom teacher is the person who is most familiar with the students and the person in school whom students seem to trust. Below, I discuss the program in detail and the ethical dilemmas that arose during its implementation.

The Mini Art Therapeutic Session Program

While I was working as a school counselor at an elementary school, a fourth-grade teacher approached me with a concern about the students in her class: "[They] don't seem to be curious." Having worked as a teacher for many years, she said that she had never had a class that she had understood less, in terms of her ability to assess how they felt. She was concerned that they were not sharing their thoughts, feelings, and ideas. I thought that art would be the perfect medium to help students learn more about their emotions and how to express them and that the Mini Art Therapeutic Session Project (MATSP) could help teachers to understand their students better. The teachers had already been asking their students to summarize their day by jotting down a sentence describing what had happened and how they felt. I proposed using the MATSP as an alternative to this "one-line journal" task.

My proposal that the MATSP be used in the classroom as a way in which to help students express their thoughts and feelings through the art therapy method was accepted by the teacher and the school administrators. In summary:

- the art activity would be brief (no more than 5–10 minutes long), so that it could easily be integrated into the daily school schedule;
- the topic would be relatively simple, so that students and teacher could readily understand its purpose and meaning; and
- the procedure would be followed consistently.

I suggested using simple art supplies, such as crayons, colored pencils, and small sheets of paper (half the size of a standard sheet of copier paper). The first technique I proposed was a *mandala* drawing, because the opportunity to draw inside, as well as outside, a circle can give an indication of the students' ways of experiencing their inner and outer worlds. I called these drawings "Feeling Pictures for the Day" because the task was oriented toward the expression of feelings. I added a step to the art task, which, translated from Japanese, is *twittering*. *Twittering* is simply adding a couple of words or a title to a drawing, thereby helping teachers to understand the drawing more easily and challenging students to explore words associated with feeling states. Although students initially wanted more time to complete the mini art therapeutic drawings, they gradually became used to the format and were able to finish the task within the given time frame.

Before the MATSP began, students were taught the procedure and the purpose of the activity. The MATSP consisted of the undirected use of colors, lines, and shapes during a 5–10 minute period once or twice a week at the end of the school day, for the purpose of expressing feelings about the day or anything else that came to mind. Upon completion of the drawings, students would glue them onto their individual files and give them to the teacher. It was emphasized that during and after the MATSP, there would be no talking or teasing.

Help

Monthly, I met with teachers, the school nurse, and (via Skype) an art therapist in the United States (the co-author of this chapter) to talk about the mini art therapeutic sessions and to look at the students' drawings. On one occasion, a teacher showed us a scribble drawing created in black crayon, entitled *Help*. The teacher had not asked the student to talk about his drawing or to clarify the type of help he needed before she had dismissed the class for the day. Over the next few days, she had watched the student closely but reported no significant change in behavior or reason to worry; the student was thought to be "fine," as he did not draw similar pictures in subsequent mini art therapeutic sessions.

Because I had anticipated that teachers would see artwork that could raise concern because of its content, I had advised them, in these circumstances, not to overreact or to ask students about the meaning of their work in front of the other students, in order to respect their privacy. I had explained that their facial expressions, verbal comments, or reactions to the students' artwork could influence future drawings, *twittering*, or the students' willingness to talk about their drawings for fear of negative reprisal, embarrassment, or dishonor.

When I followed up with this teacher, she mentioned that, just before the child drew the *Help* picture, she had witnessed him and his friend fighting; she concluded that he must have felt "miserable" because of the fight. The teacher made a conscious decision not to respond verbally to the student about his drawing or to the word "Help," but, instead, intuitively smiled at him, hoping that her smile would soothe him. As I listened to the teacher, I was convinced that she had done the right thing. Yet … what if the teacher had not witnessed the fight? What if she had been unable to interpret the visual cues that seemed so obvious to me (i.e., that the student was asking for help)? When she asked what she could do if this were to happen again in the future, I suggested that she continue to watch the student carefully.

MY FIRST ETHICAL DILEMMA

Training teachers or other non-art therapists

Is it ethical to train teachers or other non-art therapists to use art in psycho-education ways?

How would you respond?

For the writer's response, see Appendix B, page 413.

MY SECOND ETHICAL DILEMMA

Incorporating MATSP

What would be the most ethical way in which to incorporate the MATSP into Japanese schools?

How would you respond?

For the writer's response, see Appendix B, page 413.

Ownership of the Art

Another issue involves the final product of the MATSP, the artwork that is glued to each student's individual educational file. At the end of the school year, I struggled to decide whether the artwork created during the MATSP should be returned to the students or kept as part of their educational files. Although the American Art Therapy Association's *Ethical Principles for Art Therapists* (2013) states that "Art therapists obtain written informed consent from clients or, when applicable, legal guardians, in order to keep client artwork" (Principle 4.2), in Japanese schools, creating art is considered to be an educational task (much like homework, short essays, and tests) and, as such, it may or may not be returned to the student, at the discretion of the teacher.

MY THIRD ETHICAL DILEMMA

To whom does the artwork belong?

Does the artwork belong to the student artist or the educational system in which it was created?

How would you respond?

For the writer's response, see Appendix B, page 414.

The Question of Consent

My previous dilemma led to another, more far-reaching one. The "one-line journal" teachers did not inform or explain this activity to the parents; teachers did not inform the parents of, or explain this activity to, the parents. The MATSP became a substitute for the "one-line journal." Should the teachers have abruptly changed the practice of not informing the parents? Was it the responsibility of the teacher or the school to tell parents about the MATSP prior to its implementation? Should the parents have had to consent to their students' participation in it?

Let's pretend that the baffling, black crayon scribble drawing with the word "Help" was brought home by the student. How would his parents react? I would assume that they might be confused as to the meaning of such a drawing/activity. On one occasion, a parent asked a teacher about the MATSP, because she had heard about it from her daughter. The parent was concerned that her child was creating feeling pictures because she was misbehaving at school. The teacher gladly told the parent how her daughter was performing, socially and academically, while emphasizing the value of communicating feelings via the mini art therapeutic drawings. Although this kind of parent-teacher communication can be extremely effective, teachers would need to learn what and how to share sensitive information with parents, and parents would need to be trusted to receive sensitive information in a way that would not result in potential harm, embarrassment, or dishonor to the students.

MY FOURTH ETHICAL DILEMMA

Should the parents decide?

Should parents have the right to decide if their children should participate in the MATSP through an informed consent process or is the MATSP part of the required educational school curriculum and, thus, not subject to parental consent?

How would you respond?

For the writer's response, see Appendix B, page 414.

MY FIFTH ETHICAL DILEMMA

Confidentiality rights of minors

What are the rights of minors (students), with regard to confidentiality, in deliberations between parents and school personnel (teachers, nurses, counselors)?

How would you respond?

For the writer's response, see Appendix B, page 414.

Concluding Thoughts

Although I introduced the Mini Art Therapeutic Session Program as a psycho-educational activity within the school setting, using art for emotional understanding caused concerns that signaled ethical dilemmas. Should I have offered this project in the way that I did?

Even though the MATSP was not administered within a therapeutic framework or as a therapeutic tool (it was a psycho-educational activity), art can sometimes convey messages and elicit confidences. In a school setting, art can reveal personal information that is then held by a teacher who may lack the professional training to assess problems and provide needed psychological support. In weighing the usefulness of the MATSP against the possible challenges inherent in untrained professionals being privy to students' calls for "Help" but unequipped to provide that help, should I, as a school counselor and art therapist, continue to offer the MATSP for use in Japanese schools?

Would the resolutions to the aforementioned ethical dilemmas, found in the Appendix, enable an appropriate balance to be maintained between adopting the MATSP in a Japanese school and respecting the privacy of students' personal information, while recognizing parental rights? Would offering emotional support to those in need by training the teachers be the answer? What would you want to be done if you were the teacher, the parent, or the child?

REFLECTIVE ART EXPERIENCES & DISCUSSION QUESTIONS

1. Think about the teacher who seemed to understand you best. Draw the relationship between the two of you.
2. How would you help teachers to better understand their students through the artwork they make in class?
3. Where would you draw the fine line between children's artwork that, clinically, you believe should be shared with other professionals and artwork whose message you feel that you should *hold*? What would be the best way to tell others (e.g., professionals, parents) about artwork that is worrisome?

References

American Art Therapy Association (2013). *Ethical principles for art therapists.* Alexandria, VA: Author.

Kawai, H. (2000). *Nihon Bunka no yukue.* Tokyo, Japan: Iwanami Gendaibunko.

Ministry of Education (1998). *General policies regarding curriculum formulation.* Tokyo, Japan: Author.

Okada, T. (2009). Psycho-educational approach with application of psychotherapy in elementary school: Trial and results of the technique picture drawing play. *Japanese Arts Therapy Journal,* 40(1), 43–45.

39

TRAVELING WITHOUT MY GPS

Creating the First 100% Online Art Therapy Master's Degree Program

Penelope Orr

Why the Need for an Online Master's Degree Program in Art Therapy?

As an art therapist for more than 25 years, two of my long-term concerns about the profession have been the lack of diversity among its clinicians and the lack of ready access to its training programs. I am worried that there aren't more persons with disabilities, more persons with gender differences, more persons of color, and more persons of various religions. The American Art Therapy Association (AATA) membership survey (2013) shows that 93% of its members are female and 87.8% are Caucasian. The survey does not ask about other diverse factors. My concern stems from my observation, over the years, of the differences between art therapists and many of those who are receiving art therapy services.

My discomfort with the lack of easy access to educational programs arose while I was a member of the Art Therapy Credentials Board (ATCB). In talking with people who wanted to become art therapists, I discovered that many were unable to do so because they couldn't take time away from their jobs, couldn't leave their families, or couldn't afford the costs of an art therapy education. I came to the conclusion that our field needed an accessible, cost-effective art therapy program that would not require students to move or to travel extensively. The journey that I have taken, in an effort to expand access to study in art therapy, has been long and circuitous. I found myself working without a GPS to guide me, as the online education environment was new territory for the field of art therapy.

Preparing to Meet the Need

In 2008, I made the difficult decision to move from a renowned graduate art therapy program to the graduate art education department of a state university which had no art therapy program, because the latter was supportive of the development of the kind of program I envisioned and was known for its low tuition, making it affordable for my future students. Because I felt that this program would need to be available online in order to be accessible to all students who wanted to become art therapists, I ran into my first set of ethical dilemmas:

- Could therapeutic interaction skills be taught well online?
- How would art-making interactions be taught online?
- Would distance supervision be adequate to produce good art therapists?
- Would an online program provide the support needed by students learning to become practitioners?

Ethically, I believe that all Master's in Art Therapy programs are responsible for making sure that students get a strong education in the content areas, therapeutic skills, art skills, and art therapy skills, and that they graduate well-prepared to be good art therapists. I reviewed the ATCB *Code of Professional Practice* to uncover any ethical issues that I had not yet considered. I felt that I didn't have enough information to understand fully whether online art therapy education was ethical or even possible. Since there were no studies on these issues at that time, I chose to move slowly and carefully towards this goal, to ensure that I comprehended all aspects of the endeavor. I wanted to make sure that I could create a program that would meet AATA's educational requirements; would be ethically responsible to students and supervisees (ATCB, 2011); and would produce art therapists who embodied the ethical standards of professional competence and integrity.

Developing a "Pilot Program"

In 2009, I decided that I would begin by working with an art education colleague to develop a 100% online master's degree program in art education, because such programs already existed and there were good models from which to choose. During that process, I was able to identify other ethical issues that had not previously come to mind, such as:

- How could I verify that students in the program were doing their own work?
- How could I monitor for dispositions of students in order to make sure we were not sending any potentially harmful therapists out into the world?

With regard to the second question, we developed a protocol that included having students self-monitor and having faculty monitor, via discussion questions and student writing assignments. We also implemented weekly live, online meetings for all art education classes; talking and interacting with students enabled us to get to know them well. We worked with the technology office to develop lockdown methods for administering quizzes; employed built-in plagiarism checker tools for the work turned in; and created a process for conducting proctored exams. I also had students create art as part of the program and had them present their work live to the rest of the classes, in order to determine how art making shared online worked, what its qualities were, and what the nature of student interaction surrounding the art making would be.

I used the development of the online art education master's program as a sort of pilot program in which I could test and solve ethical issues as they arose. Since students in the Master's in Art Education program were already licensed art educators, I knew that they were qualified to work in their field and would do no harm. Thus, I could experiment a little with the curriculum and with the process of online education itself, and use both as learning experiences, without the risk of graduating poorly educated or inappropriate professionals. I was able to research best practices in online education by taking courses and by getting qualified as an online instructor, as well as by training with a standard bearer for online education called Quality Matters.

The online Master's in Art Education program commenced in 2010. I decided to work with that program for at least two years, in order to gather sufficient data and resolve any issues that arose, before I would start working on the online Master's in Art Therapy program. The whole process sounds extensive, and it was, but I felt that building a solid, ethically sound, easily accessible graduate program in art therapy was critical, since, as the first online art therapy Master's program, it would come under close scrutiny.

Waiting for Technology to Catch Up

An element that was not present in the online Master's in Art Education program, but was one that I needed to explore, was the ability to do online supervision of internship students. Thus, I studied doing distance supervision with undergraduate art education teachers (Orr, 2010), exploring current research on distance supervision, the efficacy of distance supervision using Skype, and the ethical issues that arose. This allowed me to discern and address issues regarding client confidentiality, to observe and provide feedback to interns, and to facilitate case-study presentations over the Internet. At the time, there were no HIPAA-compliant emails, online platforms, or video services, so I had to develop protocols for sharing client information without using identifying information. I still felt that this did not go far enough to protect art therapy clients, but I was unsure how to complete this aspect of the online art therapy program. I decided to start building the educational side of the online program and hope that technology would catch up with me to provide those necessary platforms in the future.

Creating an Online Master's Degree Program in Art Therapy

I started working on the online Master's in Art Therapy program in 2011, using the AATA educational guidelines and those of the Council for Accreditation of Counseling and Related Educational Programs (CACREP) for program quality. I began talking with the art therapy community about online education, to elicit concerns and feedback. The reaction was immediate and very negative. I had expected the comments to focus upon ethics or quality of education, but most conveyed a conviction that the online environment was "unsuitable or inappropriate" for teaching therapy or art. Since I had already researched many of the concerns they mentioned and had found that successful online programs had been created in the field of counseling, I felt reassured that I had addressed the issues necessary to start to develop my program.

Fortunately, by the time I had finished building the educational side of the online program in 2012, technology had indeed caught up with me. There was now HIPAA-compliant document sharing (Soukasa), email (Virtru), and HIPAA-compliant online meeting and video conferencing (Zoom). My ethical concerns surrounding confidentiality had been addressed by advancing technology.

The Edinboro University (PA) Master's in Art Therapy online program accepted its first students in the Fall of 2013; was accredited by the National Association of Schools of Art and Design (NASAD) and the Middle States Commission on Higher Education; and is applying for accreditation by the Accreditation Council for Art Therapy Education (ACATE) as this book goes to press. The program will continue to evolve as new regulations and standards emerge, as new technologies are developed, and as new ethical issues arise. To date my goal of creating a program that would increase access for students is already showing success. We have been successful at attaining diversity in race, gender, age, sexual orientation, and disabilities and have provided access to persons in India, South Africa, Lebanon, and Thailand, as well as in the USA and Canada, who would not otherwise have had access to getting a degree in art therapy.

Recent Ethical Issues

Admitting Inappropriate Students into the Online Art Therapy Program

There have been a few instances in which a student looked good on paper, had decent letters of recommendation, and did fine in the interview with me over SKYPE and, thus, was admitted to the program, only for me to discover later that the student was not appropriate, due to personality characteristics or disposition. This situation occurs in Master's in Art Therapy programs at ground-based universities, also, but my concern is that it might be harder to determine and document these qualities in the distance environment. *How could I improve my ability to screen candidates for appropriateness during the online application process? How could I monitor and address inappropriateness once it arises in a student who has been admitted to the program?*

First, I researched best practices that had been established and tailored them to meet the specific needs of my program. I reviewed our dispositions policy and compared it with other universities' policies, to make sure it was legal and sufficient. I ensured that the policy was in the orientation booklet, in the online orientation module, and in the internship/practicum manuals. I added a section on dispositions to the Professional Practices course and moved that course to the first year, so that students would understand, from the outset, what was expected of them as professionals. I created a policy that called for a review of the appropriateness of students' interactions during built-in checkpoints (such as at the completion of the first 12 credits); if needed, remediation plans would then be instituted. A form was sent out with the acceptance letter, describing these policies, and students were required to indicate their acceptance of them by signing and returning the form.

To help reduce the incidence of admitting inappropriate students, in the Fall of 2016, my colleague and I started conducting group admission interviews via SKYPE, so that we could see students' interactions with each other, as well as with us, in order to better understand how each student functions within a professional and social milieu before admission to the program is granted. I also require that all students participate in counseling where they live, in order to ensure that they have support when issues arise.

Supervision Observation and HIPAA Compliance

How do we provide supervision of student interns when we are not physically present at their sites? (One of our students, for example, is in Thailand.) If we have students videotape sessions to share with their supervisors, as is required by CACREP, how can we do that in a HIPAA-compliant manner? How should students take, store, and transmit videos to ensure confidentiality?

I began by researching what CACREP and ACATE require in terms of supervision. CACREP requires all interns, even those in on-the-ground programs, to submit 3–5 videotapes to their supervising professors with a self-assessment of how they did in the session. ACATE requires that each intern/practicum student have 1.5 group supervision hours for every 10 client contact hours, and an onsite supervisor with graduate-level mental-health credentials. Providing online supervision via HIPAA-compliant Zoom video meetings allows students to show, via the camera, actual client art, and to talk about clients in a HIPAA-compliant manner.

Although the videotape requirement enables the supervisor to see the student in practice, it can be very difficult to manage and keep confidential. Some sites in the USA won't allow videotaping at all, let alone sharing that tape with an offsite supervisor. The system we developed isn't perfect and will continue to be something I struggle to improve, but it works for now. I advise students that, if they are allowed to videotape at their sites, they obtain proper release forms and they use their phones or cameras to videotape directly onto a memory stick/card. This way, the video is never on the phone. They can then transmit the video from the stick directly to our secure online HIPAA-compliant, Sookasa-secured drop box, which ensures that the video is never on their own computer. They must then break the memory stick and shred it, to ensure confidentiality of transmission and storage. If an individual site won't allow video but will allow audio recording, we handle it the same way. If the site won't allow either, I ask the site supervisor to observe sessions, using a guide that focuses upon the student's manner and actions, rather than the clients', and then to meet with the student following the observation, to review the session. The site supervisor's review form and the student's reflections are then uploaded to the drop box.

MY ETHICAL DILEMMA

Can one, ethically, teach art-making interaction online?

When all the students live at different locations and are physically in different rooms, how can rapport-building, group skills, and artistic interaction skills be taught and learned?

How would you respond?

For the writer's response, see Appendix B, page 424.

Lessons Learned

It is critical that we train future art therapists to be ethical, competent, creative, and knowledgeable. When this training takes place in an online environment, unique ethical challenges can arise. The following is a list of "tried and true" recommendations for anyone considering teaching online or developing an online art therapy program:

1. Become very familiar with the ATCB *Code of Ethics, Conduct, and Disciplinary Procedures* (2018), the AATA *Ethical Principles for Art Therapists* (2013), and the ACATE program standards.
2. Take a Quality Matters training course and become certified in online teaching before teaching online, as it is not the same as teaching in person.
3. Take an online course so that you know what it is like for a student and can identify what other online teachers are doing well or poorly.
4. Build community with your online student cohorts through scheduling weekly live online seminars, forming a Facebook group, doing group art (such as mail art and artist trading cards), and encouraging students to meet at state and national conferences. It is through community building that you get to know your students and they get to practice those soft skills that are so needed by art therapists.
5. Build, monitor, and enforce good disposition policies.
6. Design log-ins with multiple levels to ensure student identity and use tools such as "lock down browser" and "turn it in" to reduce instances of cheating and plagiarism.
7. Use HIPAA-compliant software whenever possible and constantly review changing technologies that could help your program.
8. Have students make art as part of every class and have students share their work and their thoughts about their work and the work of others. Art making can be recorded through photography and video.

The most important thing to realize is that, whether teaching in higher education or in an online art therapy program, there is no perfect solution to any problem, but we do our best, keep ourselves informed, and keep evolving in our knowledge and ethical understanding.

REFLECTIVE ART EXPERIENCES & DISCUSSION QUESTIONS

1. Have a discussion with a friend online through texting or Facebook about a relationship. Then, after you have had a discussion with the same friend in person, create an art image that explores the similarities and differences between those two interactions.
2. Do a zoom, Skype, or other form of video chat with a friend. Discuss your relationship or a mutual friend/family member. Create an art piece about that discussion. Explore what worked about this discussion and what did not work, because of the technology used. Were there advantages/disadvantages? Compare with the text discussion in the previous activity.
3. Current trends in the counseling field are embracing online counseling. If you were never able to meet your client in person, but, rather, through Skype or Zoom or other conferencing platforms, what ethical issues would you need to consider? Looking at your answer to this question, which issues are aligned with ethical issues identified by the AATA and ATCB and which issues speak only to your personal values? Are personal values/ethics the same as professional values/ethics?
4. Online education in art therapy was designed to provide access to underserved populations due to location, disability, and time constraints. Online counseling is often justified for the same reasons. Is it ethical to deny access to education or art therapy counseling because of lack of funds, lack of transportation, distance to services, or disability? Do these types of barriers to service and education effect certain populations more than others? How do we address these issues in an ethical manner?

References

Art Therapy Credentials Board (2011). *Code of professional practice.* Greensboro, NC: Author.

Art Therapy Credentials Board (2018). *Code of ethics, conduct, and disciplinary procedures.* Greensboro, NC: Author.

Elkins, D., & Deaver, S. (2015). American Art Therapy Association, Inc.: 2013 Membership survey report. *Art Therapy*, 32(2), 60–69.

Orr, P. (2010). Distance supervision: Research, findings, and considerations. *Arts in Psychotherapy*, 37(2), 106–111.

40

WIDENING THE LENS OF ETHICAL PRACTICE IN ART THERAPY

Visual Free Speech and the Inclusive Studio Environment

Michael A. Franklin

When leaving the Monet exhibit of *Water Lilies*, also known as *Nymphéas*, at the Musée de l'Orangerie in Paris, there is a sign that reads, "Thank you for visiting peacefully." I have made two visits to this unusually large gallery and observed the same phenomenon both times; as if to respect the rights of the entire random group assembled, public voices drop to a low whisper as visitors pensively observe these monumental gutsy, yet serene paintings. The communal silence seems to mirror the quiet majesty of the work, respecting the visitor's entitlement to commune with the art.

Visiting Peacefully

Similar to the self-initiated behavior observed in the Monet gallery, studio spaces invite opportunities for independent self-reflection grounded in the democratic practice of expressive equality. Hierarchy flattens as expertise is shared judiciously in unfolding artist-to-artist relationships. Designing studios that support these values requires that several factors be addressed; carefully crafted mission statements, readily understandable attendance/release forms, and ethically agreeable rules (including excusal/dismissal policies) are just a few. However, the profession of art therapy has not yet articulated ethical guidelines for this burgeoning field within our field. Our work at the Naropa Community Art Studio (NCAS), which has functioned reliably since September 2001, serves as the research laboratory for the ethical questions related to visual free speech proposed throughout this chapter (Franklin, 2010; Franklin, Rothaus, & Schpock, 2005).

Studio Approaches to Art Therapy: Looking for Guidance

The Preamble to the American Art Therapy Association's (AATA's) *Ethical Principles for Art Therapists* (2013) states that "art therapists are guided in their decision-making by core values that affirm basic human rights." The majority language imbedded throughout the document, however, privileges the consumer of art therapy services as client, not artist, highlighting the extent to which the field has aligned itself with psychotherapy. Little has been written on the ethical issues confronting community-based art therapy studios as a place to uphold and sustain fundamental human rights. This chapter describes questions and concerns faced by our students and lead art mentors who work as artists in the NCAS. Within this workspace, the environment is therapeutic, but certainly not clinical.

By therapeutic, I mean restorative, remedial, even reparative outcomes tied directly to the use of art materials and processes in community rather than to psychotherapeutic interventions delivered by an art psychotherapist. Since this approach intentionally avoids privileged, Western medical model tenets such as diagnosis, assessment, and treatment planning, the consideration of ethical guidelines from a non-clinical, community perspective is sorely needed. In fact, the first ethical points to be named in this chapter are the need to confront privileged biases including our assumptions about the practice of art therapy, our competence for cultural attunement, and when and how to offer the appropriate theoretical application.

Visual Free Speech

Free speech is a protected first amendment right that guarantees general liberties to publicly communicate and express personal views without consequences. Freedom of expression, a related phrase, infers the right to engage in artistic efforts that have a similar purpose. These privileges, often contingent upon jurisdictional regulations, are linked to considerations such as respect for basic human rights, rules set by a hosting body, and implicit communal norms. Art therapy services, whether in the studio or a psychotherapy setting, are determined by where one is working, with whom one is working, and the use of the theoretical orientation best able to support that particular client within that specific setting.

In a clinical setting, clients are encouraged to speak freely and show artwork that conveys any subject to their art therapist. They are told from the very beginning that verbal and visual speech is privileged communication, protected by confidentiality. In fact, the therapeutic relationship is surrounded by an airtight seal of privacy unless a person is of danger to them/him/herself or others.

To what degree then is visual or verbal speech in the studio free? Since therapy is not the goal of the studio approach advocated in this chapter, confidentiality is of little concern. These communal spaces do not pretend to safeguard privileged communication. Even though a broad range of liberal visual free speech is encouraged in the studio, there are limits. For example, if artwork is hatefully assaultive to another participant, the artist cannot easily claim the right to freely express these views. If this is the claim, it will be addressed by the studio community, which helps to define and impose the parameters of what is acceptable in the studio. Member tolerance for uninhibited expression is exceedingly generous; only on rare occasions is someone dismissed.

Ethical Dilemmas in the Studio: Three Vignettes

NCAS provides local marginalized populations, from teens to older adults, with access to a thriving studio environment and free art materials. We do not seek out information about diagnosis or medical history unless it is a matter of safety. We do request just enough information to enable us to make informed decisions should an emergency occur. For example, since food is often served, we want to know about serious allergies that could result in a 911 call. When working with people who have some form of mental illness, we ask for clearance from their caseworker. This authorization, intentionally thin on private details yet appropriate for the requirements of the setting, conveys whether the caseworker deems the participant appropriate for our studio, which is situated within a university setting.

NCAS Policies and Procedures include a consent form which asks participants to agree to the following:

- I will practice respect for myself and others, the artwork, art materials, the studio space, and Naropa University campus facilities.
- I acknowledge that coming to the studio means coming sober and to make art. I will refrain from illegal drug use and alcohol use while at the studio.
- I understand that the *NCAS is not a psychotherapy group* and studio personnel are there to serve as art mentors rather than as psychotherapists or counselors.
- If I am disruptive to the studio process, I agree to leave if asked.
- I will keep my time commitment. If I miss two meetings, I may lose my spot at the studio.
- Confidentially, I will comply with the prescribed medical advice and treatments suggested by my doctors.
- I will give a copy of this form to my caseworker (if applicable).
- In case of a medical emergency, I understand that the NCAS mentors will call 911.

When is Enough (Really) Enough?

Beatrice joined us with a thirst to toil on her artwork. She had a strong art background and was highly motivated to experiment with materials and processes. She usually worked independently from the other studio members, insisting upon her privacy. She would separate herself from the group, quietly blending into the background. Her artwork was thoughtful and technically sophisticated.

Beatrice took pride in her sculptures, insisting upon their safety when stored between studio meetings. Her requests to protect her work were always taken seriously. On several occasions, I helped her cover her sculptures in foam, bubble wrap, and other protective material. Upon returning the following week, she would unwrap the figures and carefully inspect her projects. Eventually, vituperative comments began to fly as she insisted that someone had tampered with her work between meetings. At first, these accusations were directed at our student mentors for not doing their job. The allegations quickly turned into punitive insults. The students and the studio members became increasingly uncomfortable with Beatrice's unreasonable, suspicious behavior.

Soon everyone was to blame, including me. As lead mentor for this group, it was incumbent upon me to privately and, when necessary, publicly, intervene to address inflammatory situations. Try as I might to calm Beatrice, her suspicions outweighed any attempt to console her. Eventually, her behavior no longer seemed to be appropriate for the studio.

The student mentors and I agonized over this assessment, believing that we could keep flexing and bending to accommodate Beatrice's errant comments and actions. The more we tried to accommodate her, the more we became part of the problem. Our policies and procedures helped us to define our concerns, confront our blind spots, and recognize that safety was increasingly being compromised. Participants were saying that they felt threatened and unsafe, and would not return, and student mentors agreed that they, too, felt insecure. The aligning responses confirmed the nature of the problem and supported our decision to ask Beatrice to leave the studio.

Initially, Beatrice did not agree to the dismissal, contending that others were at fault. She argued her points with administrative university personnel, who listened to her but kept returning to the NCAS policies and procedures, including the clearly stated rules presented on the consent form, which Beatrice had signed and, thus, accepted. It was this form and our attendance requirements that supported our decision to dismiss her.

How Far is Too Far?

Harriet, reportedly, was making romantic gestures towards another member participant that were eventually experienced as harassment. When asked to stop, she found other ways to continue her adoring intentions. The other person became increasingly uncomfortable, made phone calls to university administrators, and eventually chose not to attend the studio any longer, due to extreme personal discomfort.

Our lead mentor gently challenged Harriet, asking her to manage her impulses, a request that could not be fulfilled. Several phone calls were made to Harriet's therapist to gain additional perspective. Since Harriet wanted to continue coming to the NCAS, she and her therapist were asked to craft a letter acknowledging her actions and her awareness of their effects upon the other member and promising to maintain restraint. Unfortunately, she could not keep her promise, even denying that anything was wrong. Additional consultation with her therapist revealed that Harriet was not grasping the seriousness of the situation. Like Beatrice, Harriet had reported events to administrators from her idiosyncratic point of view. The lead mentor briefly discussed offering Harriet a place in another NCAS group, but decided against it due to her unwavering perspective and lack of insight. We try hard to accommodate marginalized community members (for example, by providing simple rules that everyone agrees to uphold) and, as with Beatrice, we struggled to balance compassion for NCAS participants with the safety of the NCAS environment. Deliberative exchanges with administrative representatives holding legal expertise clarified what had to be done. For only the second time since the NCAS began, we dismissed Harriet from the studio.

Teens, Rage, and Material Culture

Leadership is required to help support ethical acculturation to the studio setting. Since material culture abounds in the studio, at times there can be healthy tension between unrestricted creative license and unfitting imagery related to invasive behavior. Material culture, suggests Bolin and Blandy (2003), covers the entire range of purposeful, "human-mediated sights, sounds, smells, tastes, objects, forms, and expressions" (p. 250). Therefore, anything touched and manifested by human activity becomes part of material culture. At what point might someone's art, which is legitimately an extension of material culture, become a form of screaming "Fire!" in the theater of the studio environment? When suicidal messages are communicated in artwork or conversation, we have a civic obligation to protect the participant and call the right medical or law enforcement services to intervene. While norms of tolerance are customary, safety is key. Although assessing when behavior or imagery in the studio goes too far is one of my roles, as lead mentor, the goal is to share as much power as possible with studio members so they can become their own self-governing resource, especially when conflict arises.

MY ETHICAL DILEMMA

How should I respond to visual free speech in the studio?

While working with a teen new to our community studio, I told him that he could create just about anything he could think of. "Anything?" he asked. "Yes," I responded. He then took a large sheet of butcher paper and wrote "FUCK YOU" in large block letters.

How would you respond?

For the writer's response, see Appendix B, page 407.

Conclusion

Because we believe in visual free speech as a human right, we art therapists are willing to work in settings with people who live on the social-safety-net edges where poverty exists and mental illness and oppression can be the norm. In my estimation, being an artist is not enough. Kramer's "three-legged stool" advice to the art therapist—to simultaneously hold artist, therapist and teacher identities—insists that we understand psychological processes, skillfully teach the use of art materials, and intelligently grasp the complexity of human behavior (Franklin, 2018; Kramer, 1994). All three are in play within the studio model as we strive to respond thoughtfully to behavioral anomalies while curbing our clinical impulses. My identity as therapist is always in my back pocket, serving me during those rare moments when serious conflict arises. My artist identity and humanistic orientation towards others is in my front pocket, guiding my NCAS artist-to-artist relationships. Lastly, aspirational and virtue ethics help me to pre- and post-reflectively identify my values as I strive to address my relational blind spots (Corey, et al., 2015; DeSouza, 2013).

Unlike the psychotherapeutic relationship, boundaries in the studio are flexible. Together, our community has attended funerals, births, and welcomed survivors of fires and floods of biblical proportions. Yes, there are limits to outside relational contact, but the reasons vary and do not easily fit the traditional definition of dual relationships. We simply make ourselves available to each other in order to experience our collective capacity for altruism while believing that inclusion leads to self-other community wholeness.

Many members of our nine-month long groups have attended for as long as a decade. They gladly return each year, knowing that they will not be perceived as a patient, diagnosis, or case study. As at the Monet gallery, we strive to make their visits peaceful. When challenges occur, the cultivation of aspirational and virtue ethics, combined with thoughtful policies and procedures, helps us to balance the scales of fairness related to visual free speech within the studio setting.

REFLECTIVE ART EXPERIENCES & DISCUSSION QUESTIONS

1. Using various art materials, recreate a challenging therapeutic relationship by illustrating three aspects of it: (a) the inside and outside of the art therapist, (b) the inside and outside of the client, and (c) the contextual physical space of the therapeutic relationship (Franklin, 1999). As a result of this process, what did you learn about yourself, your client, and your therapeutic relationship?
2. Think of a difficult situation related to either community art studios or clinical practice.
3. Roll out three feet of butcher paper. List, and then define, the different aspects of this challenging situation. Draw a road map that takes you through the temporal steps needed for conscientious decision making.
4. Fantasize setting up your own community art studio based upon the needs of the individuals in your setting. How would you alter the structure and guidelines of the Naropa model to be responsive to the needs of those in your specific setting?
5. What would it take for you to excuse (i.e., dismiss) a participant from your community art studio? Imagine two or three scenarios and contemplate not only the ethical considerations that would guide your decision-making process, but also how you would speak to this person as conflictual circumstances dominated the interaction.

References

American Art Therapy Association (2013). *Ethical principles for art therapists*. Alexandria, VA: Author.

Bolin, P., & Blandy, D. (2003). Beyond visual culture: Seven statements of support for material culture studies in art education. *Studies in Art Education*, 44(3), 246–263.

Corey, G., Corey, M., Corey, C., & Callanan, P. (2015). Issues and ethics in the helping professions (9th ed.). Stamford, CT: Cengage Learning.

DeSouza, N. (2013). Pre-reflective ethical know-how. Ethical Theory and Moral Practice, 16(2), 279–295.

Franklin, M. (1999). Becoming a student of oneself: Activating the witness in meditation and super-vision. *American Journal of Art Therapy*, 38(1), 2–13.

Franklin, M., Rothaus, M., & Schpock, K. (2005). Unity in diversity: Communal pluralism in the art studio and the classroom. In F. Kaplan (Ed.), *Art therapy and social action: Treating the world's wounds* (pp. 215–232). London and Philadelphia: Jessica Kingsley.

Franklin, M. (2010). Global recovery and the culturally/socially engaged artist. In D. Peoples (Ed.), *Buddhism and ethics* (pp. 309–320). Ayuthaya, Thailand: Mahachulalongkornrajavidyalaya University.

Franklin, M (2018). Understanding lineage, difference, and the contemplative dimensions of Edith Kramer's art as therapy model. In L.A. Gerity & S. Anand (Eds.), *The legacy of Edith Kramer: A multifaceted view* (pp. 205–213). New York: Routledge.

Kramer, E. (1994). *A portrait of artist/art therapist Edith Kramer*. Sacramento, CA: Chuck Conners Productions.

Transference and Counter-transference

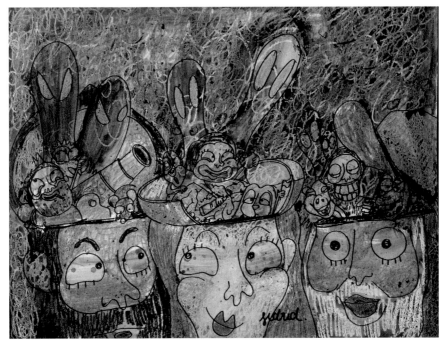

Jid Shwanpach Ratanapinyopong *(see color insert)*

41

AN OPEN BOOK

How Does a Bereaved Art Therapist Maintain Boundaries with Bereaved Clients?

Sharon Strouse

The bell rang and I moved toward the front door, just as I had a thousand times. A heightened state of anticipation marked the moment. I opened the door and entered unfamiliar territory with April, my new client.

My book, *Artful Grief: A Diary of Healing,* had just been published. April had read it and contacted me. She knew that, on October 11, 2001, I received a phone call from the New York City Police Department telling me that my 17-year-old daughter Kristin had fallen from the roof of her college dormitory. April knew that, finding no "comfort in traditional therapy and no solace in spoken and written words … I had created one collage after another in response to Kristin's suicide" (Strouse, 2013, back cover). I wondered about the impact of my book's publication; for my life, loss, and healing were graphically shared and now in the public domain. In light of that, I wondered how I would maintain professional boundaries with my bereaved clients.

I spoke with April on the phone, a few days before. I made sure that our initial conversation was extensive, as I wanted to get a sense of April and her needs. I wanted to explain how I worked and determine if we were a good fit before agreeing to set up an appointment, before meeting her face to face in the foyer of my home. Thirty years ago I never would have entertained a thought like that. I worked as an art therapist on the inpatient and outpatient units of a private psychiatric hospital. I was a professional in a professional space, within an institution that provided safety and structure. There were rules and regulations as well as codes of ethics. Boundaries were maintained, personal information was kept private. From a psychoanalytic point of view, good therapy was anchored in the notion that a "therapist was a non-specific human presence or 'blank slate' onto which the client's feelings could be projected" (Kosminsky & Jordan, 2016, p. 112). I embraced this way of thinking, especially during the early years of my art therapy training and practice. Over time, I gravitated toward more contemporary models of psychodynamic treatment which focused upon therapy as a relational process, the effectiveness of which hinged upon the therapeutic bond.

Home Studio

There were changes, within the profession and for me personally. The 15 years since Kristin's suicide had reshaped and redefined me. Through the creative process of collage, I made sense of my fragmented and torn parts. I discovered that I was more than a mother with the word suicide tattooed on her forehead. I was an artist and author, as well as a teacher and clinician, enriched by my studies in the field of grief and bereavement. I found purpose and meaning again, becoming a board certified and licensed art therapist, focused upon traumatic loss. Since I was blessed with the luxury of having an art studio in the basement of my home, I decided to offer my services in a space that was both personal and professional. Maintaining personal and professional lives that were separate, yet under one roof, brought with it a certain set of challenges, beginning with those related to safety. There was no panic button to push, alerting staff to a crisis. I relied upon my lengthy phone interview and my "gut feeling" for reassurance. I decided to see clients during the day instead of evenings so that we wouldn't have to contend with the sound of my husband moving around upstairs or inadvertently overhearing conversations. In another effort to ensure privacy, I considered having clients enter the studio through the back door, but the walk down a grassy hill presented another safety concern. Because my "office" was in my home, I was sensitive to the potential for blurred boundaries, and made every effort to delineate those spaces, which looked and felt very different.

Personal Questions

April crossed the threshold into my home and we made our way down a set of steps into the art studio. I closed the door behind us. She looked as I had expected: faun-like, skittish, her eyes glazed over with grief. Her hair was in disarray, tucked back with clips. No makeup. In the heat of summer, she pulled her heavy dark sweater around her. Her teenage son had shot himself in his bedroom just weeks before. She was the one who found him and called 911. She sat in the middle of the sofa and I sat in the rocking chair across from her. "I am reading your book for a second time," she said. "It's comforting to know I am not losing my mind. I have a lot of hope just looking at you; I know what you have been through and can see you've made it."

Although April told me on the phone what had happened to her son Justin, she began again, filling in details. At one point, she stopped and asked if I still thought of Kristin falling and of the condition of her body in the aftermath. "I can't get the image of Justin's body out of my head," she said. "I can't go into his room. There was a lot of blood." April then went on to ask if she should allow friends to come in and clean out her son's room or if she should wait and take care of this in her own time. She asked about Kristin's room and her personal things. Any concern I had about answering her direct and personal questions, which rested on the foundation of my book's content, dissolved during our time together. My personal experience and willingness to share was crucial to our exchange. I had the feeling that my "empathetic spirit," perhaps sensed by April in the pages of *Artful Grief*, would serve as "the foundation of the clinical process of facilitating [her] mourning" (Kauffman, 2012, p. 12). My own self-knowledge, the "work done by a therapist to develop insight about their own sources of emotional pain and injury" (Kosminsky & Jordan, 2016, p. 127), had created a "safe place wherein [April] was able to be with her grief, turn toward the loss and allow the loss to find expression" (Cacciatore, 2012, p. 16).

I knew that "The sudden and violent death of a loved one—whether to accident, natural disaster, homicide, or suicide—carried with it an even greater risk of a complicated bereavement trajectory" (Jordan & McIntosh, 2011, p. 34). It was especially difficult for April, who had discovered Justin's body. We would revisit this moment repeatedly, especially as we moved into the creative process of collage. The collage images that I described in my book as a visual diary of my journey were noted by April during our initial session; she could see healing in my artwork and that gave her courage (see Figures 41.1 and 41.2). After she shared, I noticed that April took a deep breath. "I am relieved to be able to talk with someone who understands," she

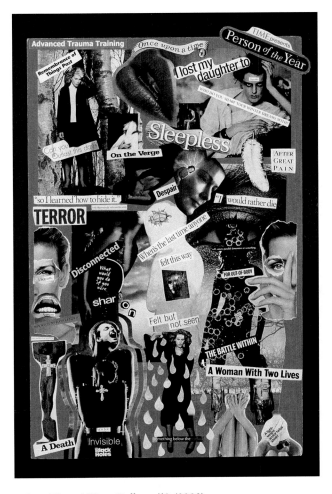

FIGURE 41.1 *Once Upon A Time*, Collage #3 (2003).

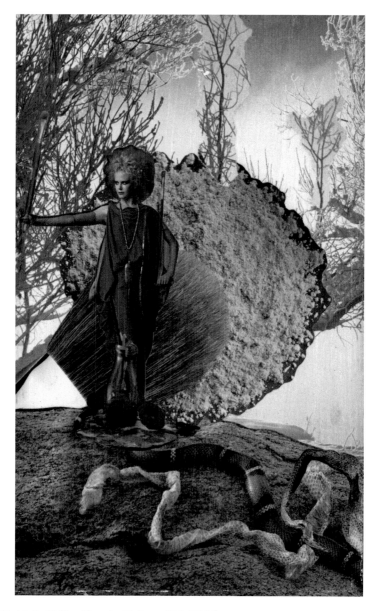

FIGURE 41.2 *Golden Creatrix*, Collage #23 (2006).

said. "There is a natural give-and-take between us, something I did not find with the therapist I saw prior to finding you."

Our initial session lasted for an hour and a half. At times, she would pause and I would hold the space for April to feel her feelings; by the end of our time together, she appeared to have relaxed into her body. Another appointment was made and I walked April upstairs. Before she left, she reached for me. I sensed, in the gesture, both an offering and an expression of need. I noticed my mind commenting on the appropriateness of being touched by, or touching, a client. I also recognized the "reciprocity of gratitude in honoring the other—in being privileged to receive the opening up of the griever and in the privilege of having one's opening up implicitly received as an honor" (Kauffman, 2012, p. 14). We hugged.

On Call

That initial session with April became a weekly 50-minute appointment that stretched over a two-year period. I recall the phone ringing one Sunday afternoon, a month or more into treatment, and hearing April say, "I am so sorry to have to call you but I'm not doing well. Could I come over right now?" I could tell by the breathless quality of her voice that something was wrong. During that morning's church service, one of the parishioners had offered her condolences, saying, "I am so sorry that Justin lost his way and turned away from God by committing suicide. I will pray for his soul, wherever he may be." I knew, firsthand, that the "suicide bereaved must not only attempt to cope with the death of someone close to them, but must do so in a likely context of shame, stigma, guilt, blame and confusion" (Jordan & McIntosh, 2011, p. xxvii). I was glad that April had reached out for help. I reflected upon the early months after Kristin's suicide, when I turned for help at inopportune times. My therapist's presence in the face of my own emotional storm was greatly appreciated. Wallin describes "the flexibility and freedom of the secure therapist—the capacity to change, adjust, and even stretch themselves beyond their usual professional comfort zone to meet the client where they need to be met" (Wallin quoted in Kosminsky & Jordan, 2016, p. 126). April arrived an hour later.

Over the next five months there were a few more calls during off hours, with requests to be seen after a cousin's wedding and on the eve of Thanksgiving. These special requests were not out of line with the needs of the newly bereaved and I was glad that I had the flexibility and freedom to see her. It was also one of the perks of a home office.

A Christmas Gift

During a session just before Christmas, April shyly removed a small gift from her tote bag; thanking me profusely, she said, "You have saved my life." I paused before accepting it, nodding as April acknowledged the possible inappropriateness of a gift. The holidays are unforgiving, especially for a parent who has lost a child. I found no need to add to her suffering. I thanked her and said, "Even though I am not supposed to accept personal gifts, I will accept your gift as a gift to the studio. Everyone will enjoy this lovely string of dragonfly lights."

Current Status

The year, filled with so many firsts, continued through the cold winter and into spring. As May and Mother's Day approached, April turned her attention to her young daughter. April was curious about my two surviving children, who were mentioned in my book. She wanted to know about their current status, although 2011 marked the end point to my *Artful Grief*. I felt comfortable sharing from the book's perspective, especially when it was in the service of April's healing process. I was very cautious about questions regarding my children, however, and answered generally, telling her that my children were fine; that my daughter went on to get her Master's in Fine Arts and that my son graduated from medical school and went on to a residency in psychiatry. Detailed information was not necessary. What April really wanted to know was, "had there been healing and were they happy." I could attest to the fact that life went on and that each had found meaning in the paths they had chosen.

MY ETHICAL DILEMMA

To attend or not to attend?

I noticed that the one-year anniversary of Justin's suicide coincided with an annual fund raising event sponsored by The Kristin Rita Strouse Foundation for Mental Health Awareness, Education, and Suicide Prevention. This was the 15th anniversary of our Yellow Dress Golf Classic and we had added a speaker event to mark the occasion. The latter was widely promoted on social media and had been advertised at many local mental health agencies, including local suicide survivors groups. April had picked up information about our event and bought a ticket to hear the speaker. At our next session, with her KRSF ticket proudly in hand, April invited me to Justin's one-year anniversary memorial service, followed by a reception at her home. As I paused and considered how to answer her, I caught a glimpse of the sun streaming through the studio window, casting light across the sofa. Healing had occurred during our year together. April was stronger and less anxious. She was casually dressed, hair and make-up in accordance with the colorful summer dress she wore that day.

How would you respond?

For the writer's response, see Appendix B, page 437.

Concluding Thoughts

After the publication of my book, *Artful Grief*, which traced my personal healing journey after my daughter Kristin's suicide, I felt like an open book. As a book, already opened, I remained open, yet respectful of my ongoing personal process. April's appearance, as the first client who had read my book, ushered in opportunities to feel along the edges of multiple boundaries, particularly in an effort to determine what was appropriate to share and what was off-limits. Issues that were tender and actively being attended to would be closely guarded, as was my current collage work, which found form in altered book techniques. I was aware that my healing journey had continued beyond what I shared in *Artful Grief*. My healing experiences are ongoing and, I believe, of benefit to the bereaved clients with whom I work. Gandhi said, "You must be the change you wish to see in the world." As a clinician, wife and mother, friend, and fellow human being, it is essential that I do my own personal grief work.

> For in order for the grief therapist to be of assistance to a client who is buffeted by the disruption of loss, they must be aware of, have reflected on, and to a reasonable degree, have come to terms with their own experiences of loss, separation and psychological trauma.
>
> *Kosminsky & Jordan, 2016, p. 125*

REFLECTIVE ART EXPERIENCES & DISCUSSION QUESTIONS

1. Do boundary issues change when the experience shared by therapist and client is mental illness (e.g., a diagnosis of depression), rather than traumatic loss? Explore that territory through the process of collaging a shoe box. The form's structure will illustrate what stays inside the box and what is revealed to the outside world.
2. Consider a moment with a client when your personal sharing could have made a difference but, instead, you held back, fearful of opening that door. Explore your feelings in a collage: give form to your fear. What actually did happen and what could have happened, both positively and negatively? Have a conversation with your image and write it down.

References

American Art Therapy Association (2013). *Ethical principles for art therapists*. Alexandria, VA: AATA.

Cacciatore, J. (2012). Selah: A mindfulness guide through grief. In R.A. Neimeyer (Ed.), *Techniques in grief therapy: Creative practices for counseling the bereaved* (pp. 16–19). New York: Routledge.

Jordan, J.R., & McIntosh, J.L. (2011). *Grief after suicide: Understanding the consequences and caring for the survivors*. New York: Routledge.

Kauffman, J. (2012). The empathetic spirit in grief therapy. In R.A. Neimeyer (Ed.), *Techniques in grief therapy: Creative practices for counseling the bereaved* (pp. 12–15). New York: Routledge.

Kosminsky, P.S., & Jordan, J.R. (2016). *Attachment informed grief therapy: The clinician's guide to foundations and applications*. New York: Routledge.

Strouse, S.T. (2013). *Artful grief: A diary of healing*. Indianapolis, IN: Balboa Press.

42

BOYS WILL BE BOYS

Men, Ethics, and Art Therapy

Michael Pretzer

The year that I applied to a graduate art therapy program was also the year I enrolled in Medicare. Being accepted into Medicare was a no-brainer, but I worried about grad school. What university would want to invest in someone whose career promised to be so brief? Wouldn't a 22-year-old yield a bigger return?

Age, however, was not as important as gender. Male and female art therapists alike assured me that I would be accepted. "Relax," they said, "You're male." I am male—apparently a valuable commodity in a profession where women outnumber men by about fourteen to one (Elkins & Deaver, 2015), which was the ratio of my graduating class, incidentally. Thinking of myself as a member of a minority group is nearly impossible. For seven decades I have been white and male. When I'm pulled to the side of the road, I really have been speeding. Yet, even in a minority, I was still getting the breaks. Where was the justice?

My foray into the art therapy profession prompted some soul-searching. I considered the ethics of benefitting from an aberration of affirmative action. I felt guilt and shame about my advantage; but I was also elated. In retrospect, I do not think gender was a factor; my previous experiences and education made me a strong candidate. But I continue to ponder my position and my behavior as a male in a profession that consists, predominately, of women.

The words *man* or *male*, *woman* or *female*, appear in neither the American Art Therapy Association's *Ethical Principles for Art Therapists* (2013) nor the Art Therapy Credentials Board's *Code of Ethics, Conduct, and Disciplinary Procedures* (2018). There are no gender-specific rules in either document. The overarching attitude is what is good for the goose is good for the gander.

Look at Principle 1.4 of the AATA code: "Art therapists recognize their influential position with respect to clients, and they do not exploit the trust and dependency of clients." There is no implication of male or female; in fact, the rule's language is neutral, with the possible exception of the word *exploit*, which has a slight bite to it. Go back

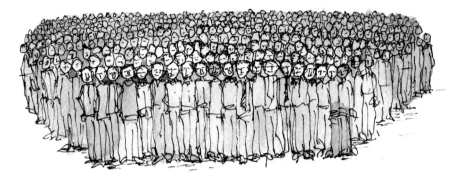

FIGURE 42.1 Author's portrait of all the male art therapists in the United States.

and read it again. This time imagine a scene in which an art therapist exploits a client's trust and dependency. In your scene, assign a gender to the exploited client, then assign a gender to the art therapist.

Bad Boys

It would not be surprising if you designated the exploiter as male. The public is offered a constant supply of examples to support the idea that men can and do act badly, that they abuse from their positions of privilege and power. An assistant college football coach gets too friendly with young boys in the shower. A former US Congressman tries to conceal his past sexual initiatives with teenagers. A Catholic priest lives out his sexual fantasies with the altar boys in his charge.

The transgressions of psychiatrists, psychologists, social workers, and expressive arts therapists seldom, if ever, reach the national stage. The public is more likely to develop its opinion of therapists from movies and TV shows, which, one might note, are fiction. With some exceptions—such as Berger in the 1981 movie, *Ordinary People*—the portrayal is not flattering (Fass, 2014). In HBO's *In Treatment*, psychologist Paul Weston breaches several ethical boundaries including a romantic entanglement with a client (Bader, 2011). But Weston is a saint compared to Carter Nix, a child psychologist whose ethical violations in the movie *Raising Cain* involve kidnap and murder (Horsley, 1992).

Male Therapists

C.G. Jung was one of the earliest real-life therapists to have sex with a patient—at least according to the 2011 movie *A Dangerous Method*. Even if their interaction was not sexual in nature, Jung's multiple relationships with Sabina Spielrein—his patient, student, and, later, colleague (Van Nuys, 2012)—would raise an ethical eyebrow if he were practicing today.

A half-dozen surveys found that between 0.9% and 12% of male therapists and 0.2% to 3.6% of female therapists have had sex with a client (Gabbard, 1991), while about 14% of men and 8% of women admitted to having sex with a former client (Pope, 2001).

Model Men

Not every male-related ethical challenge is sexual, of course. For 10 years I was a stay-at-home dad for two daughters and a son. They brought out compassion and caring that, as a male, I did not know I possessed. Had my children not enlightened me—they are young adults now—I would never have had the courage and the confidence to become an art therapist.

Female adolescents, especially, can elicit my paternal instinct. I felt overly protective of one teenage client, for example, only to realize that she reminded me of girls on my daughter's soccer team. Oftentimes, I want to embrace a troubled teenager as I would one of my own children. Yet for therapeutic—and ethical—reasons, I know I dare not offer a fatherly hug or kiss.

Several times I have been asked to work with a male adolescent, usually a boy whose father has been absent or in some way abusive. I am to be a male role model, a kind and caring man the boy would otherwise be unlikely to experience. The idea seems sound. Young boys appreciate the rare opportunity "to talk openly about masculinity with other males," and art therapy gives boys "permission to cultivate a sense of self" without negating their experience of maleness (Choi, 2013, p. 30).

When I met Robert, he was 13 years old, a skilled basketball player and a stylish dresser. He never knew his father, his biological mother offered him up for adoption, his first adoptive mother died, and his second adoptive mother proved not to be a good match. He never looked anyone in the eye. The week before I began to work with Robert, I overheard him boasting about his new basketball shoes. After he entered the studio for our first session, I closed the door, effectively blocking the view to the outside. As we sat side-by-side, I suggested that each of us take off a shoe and put it on the table to sketch. In subsequent sessions, I tried to catch his gaze, a signal that we might be connecting. I believe girls and women need good male role models, too, but if Robert had been a girl, my approach as a male would have been more considered. I would not have isolated the studio by closing the door. I would not have sat beside her. I would not have asked her to remove an article of clothing.

MY ETHICAL DILEMMA

As a male art therapist, how should I respond to the apparent boundary crossing of a female client?

Early in my career, my experience with one 16-year-old client proved instructive in many ways—including how my perceptions and reactions differ from those of female colleagues. Sylvie, whose mother had died when she was 10, had good reason to hate men. She felt emotionally abandoned by her father, and a male whom she trusted had sexually assaulted her. When Sylvie came to art therapy, she asked that the door remain partially open. During a particularly crowded and boisterous group session, I tapped her gently on the arm to get her attention. "Don't touch me," she reprimanded, and I promptly apologized. I knew that I had committed an ethical misdemeanor.

Once, Sylvie was having a hard time deciding what to paint. She was perched on a stool along one side of the work peninsula, while I stood at the end of it, my hands resting, palms down, on the counter. Abruptly, she began to paint on the back of my left hand, moving it to get a better angle. "You have soft hands," she said, then immediately recanted by exclaiming, "That's a weird thing to say." I felt apprehensive, a bit panicky. I thought about Sylvie's emotional rejection, her sexual assault, her aversion to touch. As a male therapist with a female client, I believed that a boundary had been breached. But should I halt Sylvie's art making or let it play out?

How would you respond?

For the writer's response, see Appendix B, page 429.

I have told Sylvie's story to at least a dozen art therapists, with varied reactions. Several male art therapists focused upon my behavior, suggesting ways to fix the situation: things I could have said or done to stop Sylvie, hopefully without her feeling rejected. One opined that, given Sylvie's trauma history, it had been unwise for me to see Sylvie in the first place. Female art therapists unanimously focused upon Sylvie, and they were not especially troubled. They saw a client trying to build a positive relationship with her art therapist. In their eyes, Sylvie had drawn her boundary and, when she realized she had gone too far, she appropriately backtracked with, "That's a weird thing to say." Slowly, I have come to see what my female colleagues see: Sylvie was reaching out in her way, on her terms. The client's behavior trumps my male-driven paranoia.

I ask clients of either gender questions such as: *Would you prefer the door ajar or closed? Would you like me to sit here or there? Would you like to talk or work quietly? May I make art with you? May I stand beside you so we can look at your art together? May I touch your art?* Sometimes a student shoots back, "Michael, what's with all the questions?" If I think too much about being a role model, I become confused. As a man and an art therapist, when am I not a male role model? I never say to myself before a session, "Okay. Step it up. This is one of your male-role-model clients." The paint for all my clients is squeezed from the same tube.

The Makings of a Man

Human behavior begins with our most bewitching organ: the brain. The structure of the male brain is different than the female brain, though the impact of the difference continues to be debated (Nature Neuroscience, 2005). For example, the male brain has 6.5 times more gray matter, which is thought to facilitate focused tasks, while the female brain has about 10 times more white matter, useful in assimilating and integrating information (University of California, Irvine, 2005). The amygdala, which

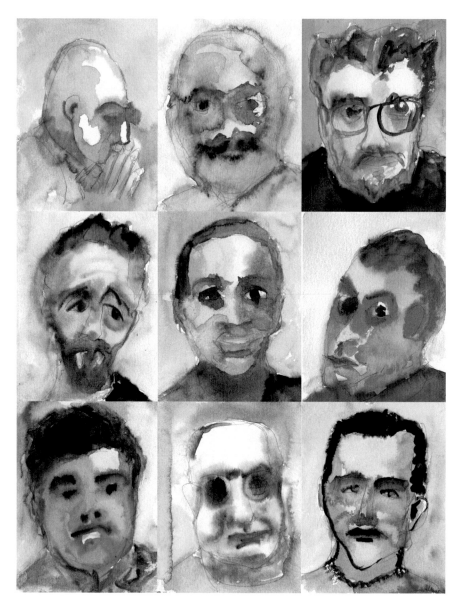

FIGURE 42.2 Male art therapists ask themselves: "Are we agreeable enough? Are we open enough? Are we nurturing enough?" *(See color insert).*

processes fear and can trigger protective aggression, is more active in the male brain, as is the hypothalamus, which stimulates sexual responses (Brizendine, 2010). The brain in males 20–30 years of age generates a sexual thought about once a minute, the female brain about once a day (Brizendine, 2006). The male and the female brain are awash in a hormonal soup. Testosterone and vasopressin, which promote competitiveness and aggression, dominate the male brain, although the estrogen and oxytocin that are plentiful in the female brain are also present. Late in a man's life, testosterone and vasopressin decrease, and estrogen and oxytocin increase (Brizendine, 2010).

Some researchers suggest that brain structure and chemistry are given too much credit for men's aggression and lack of empathy and that behavior, itself, may shape the brain to help one conform to social expectations. Although very young boys and girls seem to have an equal capacity to empathize, the *boy code* has long been credited—and blamed—for stereotypic male behavior; boys should be stoic, self-reliant, assertive, daring, aggressive, and powerful (Pollack, 1998). The adult version of the code, the *man box*, has similar marching orders: be tough and show no emotion—with the exception of anger (Porter, 2016).

Recent studies indicate that some of the brain's features may correlate as closely with gender identity as with biological sex (Eliot, 2009). Culturally, the increasing acceptance of persons of all sexual identities and orientations suggests that binary male-female differentiation is being jettisoned in favor of this masculine-feminine continuum. However, on the Bem Sex-Role Inventory—used to rate personality as masculine, feminine, androgynous, or undifferentiated—while women's scores for descriptors such as *self-reliant* and *assertive* are increasing, men have barely moved the needle on items such as *gentle* and *tender* (Rosin, 2012).

Men in Art Therapy

Although we work in a profession founded by women and more than 90% of our colleagues are female, we seem relatively secure in what we do. In a survey of male art therapists, few said they think of themselves as doing what is derogatorily termed "women's work" (Tavani, 2007). Using the Five-Factor Model descriptor for imagination, creativity, curiosity and insight (McCrae & John, 1992), female art therapists most often cite openness/intellect and agreeableness (altruism, empathy, and nurturing) as the predominant characteristics of male art therapists—the same characteristics that the women see in themselves (Pretzer, 2014). Some male art therapists have become—or are becoming—what Franklin (2007) calls middlemen, men who refuse "to identify with the disengaged, distorted bravado men are frequently taught to display. Instead there is a willingness to cultivate an identity as a nurturer" (p. 5).

Concluding Thoughts

Ethically speaking, how are the 350–400 male art therapists in the United States doing? In some ways, we are doing well. Although there is no available data from the ATCB about the ethical violations of art therapists in general (let alone categorized by gender), those familiar with the review process say that nearly all of its cases are minor and easily mediated.

With regard to the ethics of (mostly white) male privilege, we are works-in-progress. In a 2007 survey, 21% of male art therapists believed that they advanced in the art therapy profession because of their gender and 17% expected to move up in the future for the same reason (Tavani, 2007). Female art therapists recognize signs of aggression, emotional illiteracy, and hunger for power in their male counterparts. After seeing too many instances of male arrogance, one female art therapist said, "I do not want to imagine what they are like in art therapy sessions." Another said that she felt that men use their minority status to "get away with more crap" (Pretzer, 2014, pp. 35–36).

A few years ago, I heard a male art therapist complain about what he considered to be an indignity. To accommodate the many female art therapists at an AATA conference, some of the men's bathrooms had been reassigned to women. The male was miffed because he had to go to another floor to take care of his business. I am not sure if lack of generosity is an ethical issue—or just bad manners. But surely our use of male privilege is an indication that our feminine side is still evolving.

REFLECTIVE ART EXPERIENCES & DISCUSSION QUESTIONS

1. If you identify as female, create an image that viewers are likely to think was created by a male. If you identify as male, create an image that might be perceived as having been made by a female.
2. Make an image that portrays what you think of as your most feminine characteristic. Make a second image that depicts what you believe is your most masculine characteristic.
3. Describe an instance when you think you got ahead or were held back because of your gender rather than your individual effort.
4. Now turn the tables. Discuss an instance in which you may have exhibited implicit gender bias toward someone else.

References

American Art Therapy Association (2013). *Ethical principles for art therapists.* Retrieved from www.americanarttherapyassociation.org/upload/ethicalprinciples.pdf

Art Therapy Credentials Board (2018). *Code of ethics, conduct, and disciplinary procedures.* Retrieved from www.atcb.org/resource/pdf/2016-ATCB-Code-of-Ethics-Conduct-DisciplinaryProcedures.pdf

Bader, M. (2011). The biggest myth about therapy that HBO's In Treatment promotes. *Huffpost Entertainment.* Retrieved from www.huffingtonpost.com/michael-bader-dmh/the-biggest-myth-about-th_b_802668.html

Brizendine, L. (2006). *The female brain.* New York: Morgan Road Books.

Brizendine, L. (2010). *The male brain.* New York: Broadway Books.

Choi, D. (2013). From boys to men: The experience of maleness in 4 boys aged 6–12 who utilized art therapy with a male art therapist. *Canadian Art Therapy Association Journal,* 26(2), 8–32.

Eliot, L. (2009, September 8). Girl brain, boy brain? *Scientific American.* Retrieved from www.scientificamerican.com/article/girl-brain-boy-brain/

Elkins, D.E., & Deaver, S.P. (2015). American Art Therapy Association, Inc.: 2013 membership survey report. *Art Therapy: Journal of the American Art Therapy Association,* 32(2), 60–69.

Fass, T. (2014). Therapists on the big and small screens versus real life. *Huffpost Entertainment.* Retrieved from www.huffingtonpost.com/tara-fass/therapists-on-the-big-and_b_4263798. html

Franklin, M. (2007). Contemplations of the middle man: Anima rising. *Art Therapy: Journal of the American Art Therapy Association,* 24 (1), 4–9. doi: 10.1177/0022487104273761

Gabbard, G.O. & Menninger, W.W. (1991). An overview of sexual boundary violations in psychiatry. *Psychiatric Annals,* 24 (11), 649–650. doi: 10.3928/0048-5713-19911101-05

Horsley, R. (1992). *Raising Cain.* Retrieved from www.imdb.com/title/tt0105217/

McCrae, R.R., & John, O.P. (1992). An introduction to the five factor model and its applications. *Journal of Personality,* 60(2), 175–215.

Nature Neuroscience (2005). Separating science from stereotype [Editorial]. *Nature Neuroscience,* 8, 253.

Pollack, W. (1998). *Real boys.* New York: Henry Holt.

Pope, K. (2001). Sex between therapists and clients. In J. Worell (Ed.), *Encyclopedia of women and gender: Sex similarities and differences and the impact of society on gender* (pp. 955–962). Cambridge, MA: Academic Press.

Porter, T. (2016). Thinking outside the "man box." Omega Institute. Retrieved from www.eomega.org/article/thinking-outside-the-man-box

Pretzer, M. (2014). *Female perspectives of men in art therapy.* Unpublished master's thesis. The George Washington University, Washington, DC.

Rosin, H. (2012). *The end of men and the rise of women.* New York: Riverhead Books.

Tavani, R. (2007). Male mail: A survey of men in the field of art therapy. *Art Therapy: Journal of the American Art Therapy Association,* 24(1), 22–28.

University of California, Irvine. (2005, January 22). Intelligence in men and women is a gray and white matter. *Science Daily.* Retrieved from www.sciencedaily.com/releases/2005/01/050121100142.htm

Van Nuys, D. (2012). A dangerous film? Puts bad light on Jungian analysis and therapy in general. *Psychology Today.* Retrieved from www.psychologytoday.com/blog/the-happiness-dispatch/201202/dangerous-film

43

COLORING INSIDE THE ROOMS

Art Therapy in Residential Substance and Gambling Addiction Treatment

Todd C. Stonnell

I am an art therapist in a 28-day residential treatment facility that serves adults who are seeking help for addiction to substances, gambling, and video game or internet addiction. During their stay, patients who have diverse backgrounds, beliefs, and histories mingle together in a treatment potpourri (e.g., men and women seeking alcohol treatment attending group sessions with those trying to overcome the siren call of gambling) before ultimately stepping into "the rooms" (a term coined for recovery meetings such as Alcoholics Anonymous). In the process, a host of ethical issues may arise.

Reframing Creativity

Stop me if you've heard this one: "I'm not creative." How about: "I can barely draw stick figures." Art therapy is a part of each person's care at my facility, which means that much of my work is with patients who are highly resistant to making art. Whether this resistance is rooted in a belief that they lack artistic talent or that creating art is "pointless," I usually respond by pointing out a unique aspect of addiction—that, in large part, it is fueled by creativity. One only has to listen to patients sharing anecdotes about their lives in active addiction (e.g., the methods they used to maintain their substance use; the elaborate plans they concocted to make up for lost money) to marvel at their creativity. I am sometimes left speechless by the *Mission Impossible* nature of these stories. My goal is to help patients harness the creativity that has been hijacked by impulsivity or desperation, in the service of manipulation or deception, and to redirect it in ways that will enable them to meet their current goals.

There is a component of risk-taking, or rule breaking, in the creative process. A certain "screw the norm" feeling accompanies us as we approach our struggles through the vehicle of art-making, be it drawing, writing, dance, or music. In the process, patients face several specific challenges: the first is knowing that their voice can be used for more than addiction has led to them to believe; the second is believing that they can trust this voice; and the third is being able to acknowledge that others are willing to hear it. Through the use of certain materials and interventions, patients begin to loosen control, safely expressing feelings instead of being stagnated by them or believing that they should feel some other way. As they explore the role and the pull of their substance use, they encounter the paradox of discovering the power that they actually possess when they are not under the control of a substance.

Ethical Issues That Arise in Residential Treatment for Addiction

Boundaries between Peers

The coed and residential nature of the facility means that patients sometimes form unique, even romantic, bonds with one another. As patients get to know each other, timid comments may give way to the inappropriate sharing of "war stories" or to the spicing up of conversation with sexual innuendoes. Patients might speak to each other in a way that feeds into or challenges their addictions. What happens when patients begin to gamble among themselves, creating competitions out of otherwise straight-forward activities (such as tossing a wad of paper into a wastepaper basket), or when a game that was meant as a way to get to know one another suddenly becomes a battle between who can throw the hardest? Although patients are encouraged not only to be mindful of the rights of their peers, but also to set boundaries when they, themselves, are feeling uncomfortable, these situations emphasize the thin line between addictions.

Just as the omnipresent nature of food can pose an on-going challenge for individuals overcoming eating disorders, those with an addiction to some form of technology must deal with the constant presence of this "drug." Instituting harm reduction for those seeking treatment for internet or gaming addiction—rather than the abstinence-focused approach usually employed to treat addiction to substances—can, ironically, result in patients feeling that differences in the approaches to their treatment are unfair. We are tasked with explaining the individualized nature of patient treatment, pointing out that each person's journey will look different.

Physical Touch

Whether it is offered to—or initiated by—a patient or a coworker, the topic of touch can be polarizing because of the emotions attached to it; physical touch can stir up many responses and memories, not only in our patients, but also in ourselves. Individuals who have experienced sexual or violent trauma often struggle with their personal boundaries and may not know what they are truly able to handle, as a result becoming too close to others or separating from them completely. The rigid rule follower in me tends to argue with the softy who also lives there, particularly when the latter shouts "*Help her!*" whenever a patient begins to cry during session and I feel like giving her a hug. This conundrum is exacerbated when it is the patient who asks for a hug. I catch myself staggering for a moment, considering the consequences of my prospective response. The intimacy of the setting must be taken into account, as well as the fact that I might be setting a precedent. *What happens when another patient asks for a hug? What if this same patient saw me give a hug to my coworker earlier in the day? How would a hug affect the development of the therapeutic relationship?* Ultimately, the decision depends upon the specific case. The key lies in communicating clearly *about* boundaries, remaining consistent (so important within a residential setting), and remembering that once a boundary is either set or crossed, it may remain that way until further processed.

Self-Disclosure

The residential setting can be a very intimate location; patients get small, unexpected glimpses into our lives. As we pull into parking spaces in the morning, they can see what cars we drive (and how dirty my car is); see us walk into the building and pour our cup of coffee or tea; notice what food we eat, and so forth. This is not to say that patients are watching from their windows, binoculars in place, or that they even really care what we are doing when we step onto the grounds, but it is important to be aware that our daily routines and choices can be observed. I find it important to be mindful of the way in which I carry myself when I arrive to work, by brushing off a difficult evening or a slow-chugging morning before stepping into the facility. On my treks between sessions, I have overheard patients say that some therapists "only seem to be here for a paycheck" or "always look miserable." While I encourage the patients to maintain the same open mind that they hope to find in us and to consider that there may be challenging things going on in others' lives, I can't help but wonder: *Are they talking about me? Did they catch that heavy sigh I made before opening the door?* Although peppered with irrational paranoia, these thoughts do reflect a need to be extremely aware of the impact of my behavior.

Additionally, patients often ask staff if we have ever experienced their specific addictions or addiction-related struggles. Initially, I wondered whether sharing details related to substance use would in some way devalue or invalidate their own experiences in seeking treatment. Then I wondered if patients might perceive my lack of personal experience with addiction to mean that I could not provide the understanding necessary to accompany them on their journeys. Since the times that I have answered their question frankly have not appeared to deter patients from finding a connection with me, this has become less of an issue. There are times when I have encouraged some patients to talk, also, with our peer counselors, who have years of recovery under their belts, but I always let them know that I have a huge desire to join them on this leg of their journey and to offer what I can at this time, fueled by my care for them.

Burnout: Practicing Outside of One's (Functional) Competence

Burnout is an insidious force. Defined as a condition of chronic stress, it can lead to: physical and emotional exhaustion; cynicism and detachment, as well as feelings of ineffectiveness and lack of accomplishment (Carter, 2013). The progression of burnout can also be marked by stress-related illness, along with mental health issues including anxiety, depression and decreased self-esteem. Interestingly, Elman and Dowd (1997) found that counselors who work in the field of substance abuse are at particular risk for burnout, referencing the emotional investment in the patients, while also handling the brunt of possible relapse following treatment.

Burnout can be caused by any number of things both within and outside of the work environment. Within an organization, itself, the workload can become very heavy, with very little downtime between patients. Add to this a high staff turnover rate, patients' coverage cut off by insurance, and frequent changes to scheduling and/or structure, and it can be hard to maintain a sense of stability and security in the workplace. At what point does the uncomfortable safety of accepting "the way things are" shift to a need to advocate not only for the patients, but also for the team and oneself? Essentially, burnout can boil down to a belief that "I have no control here."

We have only 28 days with most patients, sometimes fewer, depending upon their insurance; the feeling that we have some control over their recovery generally ends when they are discharged. Despite our best efforts, provided within the constraints that we have, many obstacles—either environmental or personal—can cause patients to relapse. When this occurs, staff morale can take a beating. I remember sitting at a meeting table, sharing details from check-ins with former patients, and learning that several relapses had occurred. I recall a stirring feeling of frustration and defeat. "Does anyone have any success stories??" I asked. When working in the field of addiction—given the sheer number of people who are in need of help and the relatively small number of resources available to provide it—it is a hard but necessary practice to recognize that the time spent in residential treatment constitutes only a small part of these individuals' journeys toward recovery.

I recall the vigor and excitement I felt following graduation from my art therapy program; I felt a pull to jump into a job that offered the most opportunity to prove myself and use the skills I had gained. Like many graduates, this energy led me to take on challenging cases and accrue as many hours as I could and to absorb as much experience as possible, without recognizing my limits. When burnout sets in, it is as if the deficit in self-care that we have accrued throughout the years suddenly catches up with us. Often, it is accompanied by "compassion fatigue," which is identified by feelings of helplessness or even emotional numbness in response to patients' illnesses and trauma (Burnett & Wahl, 2015). Connecting with patients can become more difficult and feel less authentic. When the effects of burnout spill out onto vulnerable patients, we run the risk of doing more harm than good.

When I'm beginning to sense the effects of burnout, I can almost hear the laugh track of a comedy sitcom running through my mind as I give tips to patients about self-care and the importance of achieving a sense of balance. It can feel hypocritical to tell someone else to make time for him- or herself when I am faltering at that very task. At these times, it's as if my "burnout-brain" wants to shift the blame for my imbalance onto the patients: "Can't they tell that I am burned out and just take it easy on me today?"

MY ETHICAL DILEMMA

Disclosing burnout to patients—to tell or not to tell?

The thing is, our patients really do seem to notice how we are feeling on a day-to-day basis; there is a sense of attunement that allows them to recognize when our energy meter is nearly empty, and many do not shy away from bringing attention to it within the session. At these moments, I feel as though my stubbornly held "strong and confident therapeutic mask" has slipped or been shattered, revealing my vulnerability. The fact that it is noticed means that I am not doing what I should be doing in order to be the best presence and ally to this patient that I possibly can. At a time like this, is it all right for therapists to share that they are struggling to find balance between their work and their lives outside of work?

How would you respond?

For the writer's response, see Appendix B, page 436.

Closing Thoughts

Working within a residential treatment setting has granted me an opportunity to craft what I believe to be a more ethically sound therapeutic practice. As noted earlier, the setting serves an incredibly diverse population, which means that a diverse array of challenges needs to be addressed. As a "rookie" therapist, I found myself viewing—and I continue to view—the process of professional growth much as I would approach the task of learning to use a new art material; it requires patience, experimentation, quite a bit of failure, but ultimately can lead to something amazing. As this piece of art continues to go through the sculpting process, certain parts will require additional attention, while others will become even more solid and strong. I am a work in progress and I am excited to see what the process holds.

REFLECTIVE ART EXPERIENCES & DISCUSSION QUESTIONS

1. Picture a time when you felt truly effective in your role as a therapist. Using materials of your choice, illustrate the feelings associated with this. Now envision a time when you felt that you were not as effective. Again, use materials to illustrate this feeling. Make a third piece of art that represents a resource that can be utilized during a time of ineffectiveness.
2. What are your personal warning signs that you are becoming burned out at work? What do you do about this?

3. Imagine your own personal resilience, either as a figure in nature or as an abstract energy. Create artwork that represents this and reflect upon how you can tap into this resilience when you need it.
4. What do you feel that you need from your professional peers when you are struggling with burnout/personal issues at work?

References

Burnett, H.J. & Wahl, K. (2015). The compassion fatigue and resilience connection: A survey of resilience and compassion fatigue, burnout, and compassion satisfaction among trauma responders. *International Journal of Emergency Mental Health and Human Resilience*, 17(1), 318–326.

Carter, S.B. (2013, November 26). The tell tale signs of burnout…do you have them? *Psychology Today*. www.psychologytoday.com/blog/high-octane-women/201311/the-tell-tale-signs-burnout-do-you-have-them

Elman, B.D. & Dowd, E.T. (1997). Correlates in inpatient substance abuse treatment therapists. *Journal of Addictions and Offender Counseling*, 17(2), 56–65.

Oser, C.B., Biebel, E.P., Pullen, E., & Harp, K.L.H. (2013). Causes, consequences, and prevention of burnout among substance abuse treatment counselors: A rural versus urban comparison. *Journal of Psychoactive Drugs*, 45(1), 17–27.

44

GAZA WAS DIFFERENT

Ethical Issues That Arose on an Art Therapy Journey in the Middle East

Shirin Yaish

My art therapy journey began when, having completed my graduate training in Art Psychotherapy in the UK, I returned home to Jordan. I have always known that my true passion lies in working with refugees, orphans, and others who are in need of psychological support. This led me to found the Kaynouna Arab Art Therapy Center in Amman in 2012, the first art psychotherapy center in the Arab world (Freij, 2016). Perhaps the first ethical issue I encountered was envisioning the Center as a place where Syrian and Palestinian refugees could seek treatment for trauma; I soon realized that I needed to go to them, not expect them to come to me. I found myself spending less time at the Center and more time traveling to refugee camps and orphanages throughout Jordan, Lebanon, and Palestine. When witnessing the trauma of our children and women, I had to keep my own therapy and supervision on track, to ensure that I was able to process, contain, and deal with what I saw and heard—while continuing to provide support. Gaza was different, though.

Art Therapy with Members of Psychosocial Teams in Gaza

I had been invited to train, and to provide art therapy groups for, the members of a psychosocial team of mental health professionals whose mission was to work with children and families to deal with the traumas of war. Since the three weeks allotted to my visit were not nearly enough to explore the trauma with which the team members were dealing, I decided to focus upon the *here and now*, with the aim of helping them to build their resilience, self-empowerment, and self-soothing skills. I remember the excitement I felt to be able, finally, to enter the coastal enclave. I thought that four years of working with Syrian and Palestinian refugees and training psychosocial teams in the Arab world had prepared me for Gaza. I was wrong.

"A Foreigner?"

The art therapy group began late the first day, due to participants drifting in, one or two at a time, throughout the morning. When I asked group members to show up on time for the duration of our sessions together over the next three weeks, one person replied that starting late was a cultural norm and told me that I was acting like a foreigner. Sensing myself becoming defensive, I wondered if, in fact, my art therapy training in the West *had* blinded me to the norms of those with whom I was preparing to work (in effect, *my own* cultural norms). Given what they were going through, would it matter so much if the group didn't start on time? On the other hand, I knew that consistency can be therapeutic for people who have been through conflict and do not have control over many of the situations that surround them. Being Palestinian myself gave me the confidence to explain the reason for adopting this particular *Western* expectation, or therapeutic boundary, and to ask for a commitment to it.

Casement (1991) believes that therapists should never have expectations from a patient or group, as it restricts their growth and limits their ability to experience something new. An expectation that I had which proved to be utterly without merit was that the group might resist the art-making process and the discussion that was to follow. I was surprised by how willing the group members were to make art and by how open they were in discussing their fears, inhibitions, and experiences as psycho-social workers in a city like Gaza (see Figure 44.1).

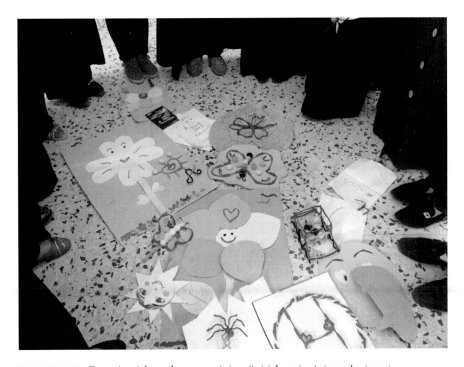

FIGURE 44.1 Experiential art therapy training (initial session) *(see color insert)*.

In the End, Only Cockroaches

Having drawn a picture that she said reflected the ugliness and hopelessness she felt (Figure 44.2), Layla, a woman in her twenties, explained that the siege had finally eliminated any signs of hope, love, or belief in a better life or a better world. This resonated with other group members, who shared stories of pain and loss, some speaking of the smell of flesh and blood during the worst of times.

It was as if the trauma and constriction of the siege had been internalized.

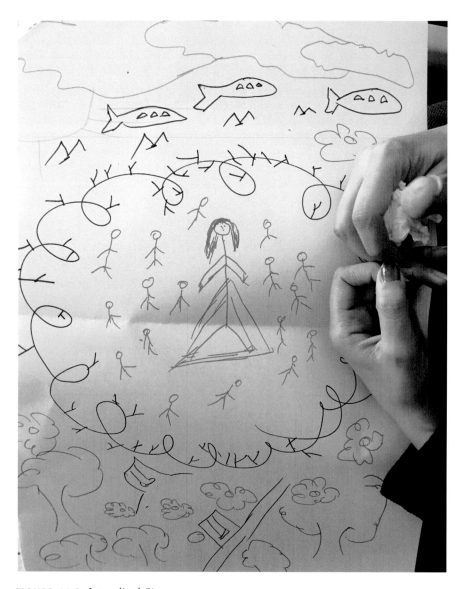

FIGURE 44.2 *Internalized Siege.*

Drawing a picture of a cockroach, Dima explained that cockroaches survived wars; people didn't (see Figure 44.3). If the siege killed their humanity and their dreams, someone asked, "Would the shells of cockroaches be all that remained?" Another person wondered whether the ongoing siege had killed humanity in the outside world so that all that was left there were cockroaches, watching in silence as Gaza suffered.

"Superhuman"

Group members discussed the pressure of being a psychologist or therapist in Gaza, where it seemed as though they were "on-call" 24 hours a day. The people of Gaza were suffering from severe anxiety, fear, and loss, and, as a result, neighbors, relatives, even people they didn't know would continually seek their advice on subjects such as how to deal with their children's panic attacks, bedwetting, pain, and depression.

Ali, a male therapist and father of two, created a card that presented a happy appearance on the outside, but a dark inner world (see Figure 44.4). "If *we* cannot

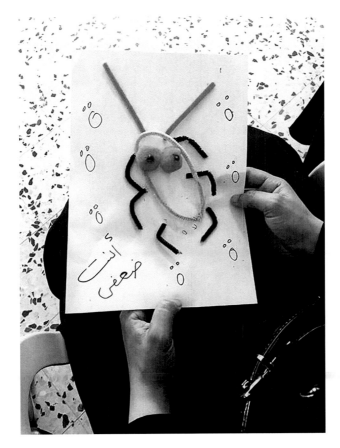

FIGURE 44.3 *Cockroach Within.*

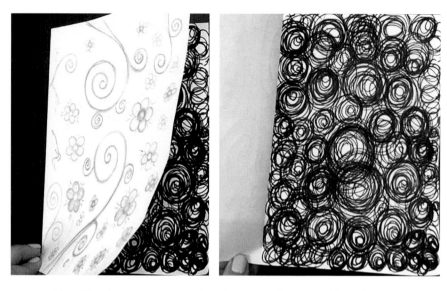

FIGURE 44.4 "People see a rosy me—they do not see the war inside me."

survive the trauma, then how will regular people survive it?" he asked. "We have to pretend that we are not suffering, in order to empower others," he explained.

Lama reflected upon an image she had made of a strong, patriotic Palestinian woman, yet spoke of how fragile and stuck she really felt. The bird, she explained, was being pulled down by the weight of others' expectations of her and by the trauma she had witnessed and felt in her soul (see Figure 44.5).

While group members shared the burden of their jobs and the cultural expectation of appearing "superhuman" before other Gaza residents, they agreed that Ahmad, a social worker and father of three, summed up the worst part of it all when he said that, "Everybody around us is acting like the lives we lead are normal, as if the siege is a way of life. There is nothing *normal* about this *normal.*"

I understood the group's confusion over what was normal and what wasn't. About this time, we were invited for a heartwarming meal by a lovely older couple who lived in the neighborhood. Their daughter had recently given birth to a child who had a heart condition. The young mother explained that her baby was in a hospital in Jerusalem, but that she had not been granted a permit that would allow to be with her child. I choked on my food. I wanted to put my spoon down and cry for her, her daughter, and her parents. It was not normal for a mother to be away from her baby while the child needed to be in a hospital, but in Gaza it was common.

Armour

Not being able to say "no" to family members and neighbors or to set boundaries for themselves was a recurring theme in the art. Yasmin, a therapist and an artist, explained that people expected them to be therapists all the time, yet she was overwhelmed by

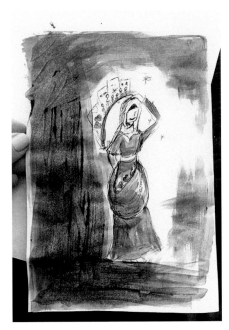 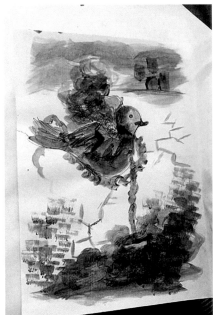

FIGURE 44.5 *A Strong Woman on the Outside, a Caged Bird Inside.*

her own pain and that of others. When the group was asked to visualize imaginary armor that would protect the self from outside and inside pain, Yasmin drew a forest. Expressing a need to be alone, she said that the darkness and the trees would keep others away during her time of seclusion (see Figure 44.6).

Von Franz (1991) explains that sinking into a forest has to do with the psycho-somatic realm of the psyche, which is associated with the bodily unconscious. I felt that there was a fine line between hiding in the body and sinking into depression and, having found that most of the amour that was created reflected depression and a sense of helplessness, I expressed this concern during the group discussion.

Drums of War

The night before one of our art therapy groups met, an air strike resulted in loud explosions. The next day, the group made art that symbolized their own ongoing panic attacks, the continuous drums of war, and the lingering smell of burnt bodies. Drawing a horn speaker, Jamal explained that it felt as if there were people screaming in his ears every night, reminding him that his trauma was permanent and had become a way of life.

"Selfies"

I was deeply moved by the group's candor and reflected (aloud) upon how difficult it must be to connect to one's self when there are continual reminders of aggression and

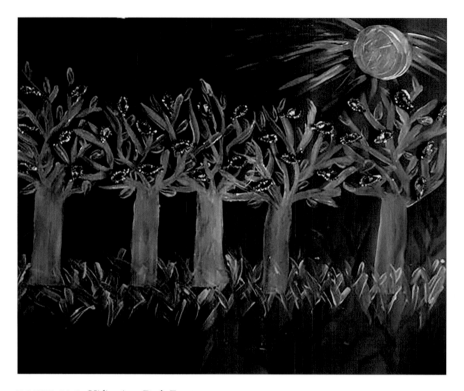

FIGURE 44.6 *Hiding in a Dark Forest.*

trauma, as well as the need to be available and giving. The psychosocial workers did not have time to be alone or the opportunity to process and reflect upon their feelings. We reviewed the concepts of ugliness, internalized siege, and armor, and I asked group members to create a "selfie" of their "higher self"—a self that was healthy, present, dealt with its trauma, and was able to set boundaries to protect itself not only from aggression, but also from unrealistic expectations from without and within. My aim was to remind, and assist, them to connect to a part of them that seemed unavailable and under siege from all sides.

The "selfies" they created reflected hope and desperation at the same time; they conveyed a continuous struggle to stay human within an inhumane environment. The youngest of the group members, an artist called Farah, pictured her "self" as a tree that was still able to love and to give hope in the form of flowers. The siege was pictured as a wall that physically and mentally forced her to stay where she was, yet the wall was penetrated by her love and humanity. When I asked about the sun in her picture, she said that the tree would eventually burn down (see Figure 44.7). I left the session, went home, and had my first panic attack ever.

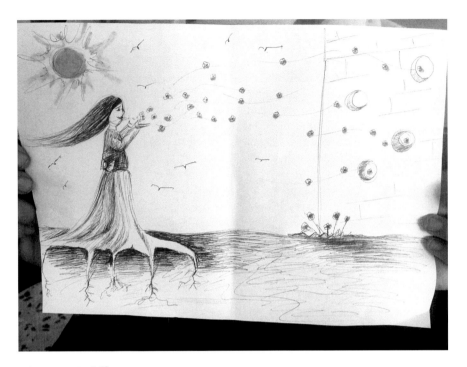

FIGURE 44.7 *Selfie.*

MY ETHICAL DILEMMA

What do we do when the experiences shared by others feel so overwhelming that we question whether our supports are sufficient to the task?

Much like Lama's portrayal of the strong Palestinian woman who felt like a fragile bird inside, I, too, was experiencing an overpowering desire to be there for everyone, and guilt that I was giving the team members just "a taste" of art therapy, only to leave them. I was also feeling overwhelmed by the force of the emotions that had been stirred up in me by the graphic and verbal images that had been shared so passionately and so eloquently by this group of individuals who were, themselves, helpers. How could I help these helpers, when I felt in need of help, myself? Supervision and therapy seemed a long way off.

How would you respond?

For the writer's response, see Appendix B, page 441.

Mandala Making

The following day, I introduced the groups to the concept of the *mandala*, its history and its capacity to help one reflect, find the "self," and meditate when one needed time alone. For the first time since we began our experiential art therapy training, the group made art for two hours in complete silence. Completely immersed in the art-making process, it was as though what they needed most was time to themselves, time to reach within, time to remember that their "selves" were, indeed, alive and kicking underneath the rubble of all the trauma that they had experienced. Upon completing their *mandalas*, they said that they had experienced a sense of relief that they hadn't thought possible.

Although a three-week experience of art therapy was not enough to deal with the trauma the members of this psychosocial team had experienced—and would continue to experience—it seemed to bring to light the power of art to help when they needed to express themselves, to process or contain their pain, or to connecting with their "selves." We discussed ways in which art making might continue to be of use to them as part of the process of self-care that they so desperately needed (see Figure 44.8).

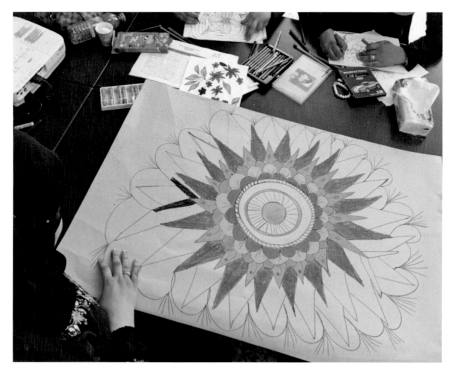

FIGURE 44.8 "I don't remember the last time I enjoyed silence as I did today" (final session) *(see color insert)*.

Concluding Thoughts

Gaza is the site of an ongoing collective trauma that will undoubtedly be carried for generations. I left the besieged territory feeling both humbled and moved beyond words by my time there and hoping that the team would continue to make art. As I continue my journey as an art therapist—having worked with thousands of refugees and underprivileged children, youth, and women, at the time of this writing—I can see how my experiences have come to shape both my vision of art therapy and the art therapist I have become. I expect them to continue to so do. This is not a comfortable process, nor should it be. How much easier it would be simply to apply the lessons learned in our training, with the assumption that, if done properly, they will "work." But the people with whom we work are complex and ever-changing—as are the art therapists with whom *they* work—and defy categorization. The very least we can do is to rid ourselves of expectations and, instead, attend to the unique human being who sits in front of us—as well as to the individual who has chosen to pursue this profession called art therapy. This should prepare us for the next leg of the exhilarating, demanding, never-ending journey of discovery we have signed up to take.

REFLECTIVE ART EXPERIENCES & DISCUSSION QUESTIONS

1. Using basic art materials, create a "selfie" that depicts how you believe people see you (i.e., what you show to others). Then, using basic art materials, create a "selfie" that depicts how you really feel on the inside (e.g., your worries, fears, inhibitions).
2. Share an instance when you felt so overwhelmed by the material being presented by a client that you were not sure what to do. Discuss how you felt, what helped you at the time, and what has helped you to deal with similar situations since that time.
3. Reflect upon a time when you had expectations of what a session with a client would be like, only to discover that your expectations had been wrong. How did that make you feel? Have you been in similar situations since then? Discuss ways in which your expectations can not only alter sessions, but also affect clients.

References

Casement, P. (1991). *On learning from the patient.* New York: Guilford Press.

Freij, M. (2016, November 13). Orphans turn to art as a form of therapy. *Jordan Times.* Retrieved from www.jordantimes.com/news/local/orphans-turn-art-form-therapy

Von Franz, M. L. (1991). *The cat: A tale of feminine redemption.* Toronto: Inner City Books.

45

IS ALL ART MAKING ETHICAL?

Dilemmas Posed in the Making of Response Art by Australian Art Therapy Trainees

Patricia Fenner and Libby Byrne

Therapist art making, both in-session or related to clinical work such as in supervision, has become known as *response art* (Fish, 2008, 2012; Havsteen-Franklin, 2014; Marshall-Tierney, 2014). Discussion of therapist art making directly with clients has shifted from being viewed as clinically unhelpful (Case & Dalley, 1992) to being considered positively. Research exploring the impact of in-session therapist art making from the perspective of the client is absent from the discourse, however. Art making within art therapy supervision has become accepted as an integral component of good practice (Brown, Meyerowitz-katz, & Ryde, 2003). In this chapter we review the functions of *response art* and show how—amid its positive contributions—ethically problematic practices can emerge within the context of the therapeutic relationship or in supervision, focusing upon its impact on the training and formation of new therapists.

What is Response Art?

Response art has been defined as art made by the therapist in- or post-session as a response to material arising in therapy. Some limit the use of the term to art made by the therapist to influence relational dynamics in-session, usually while the client makes art (Havsteen-Franklin, 2014; Marshall-Tierney, 2014). Others refer to post-session supervision about client work (Elkis-Abuhoff et al., 2010) or to art as a self-care strategy (Fish, 2008). Marshall-Tierney's experience of making *response art* in the clinical setting when the client is not present (2014) adds a further dimension to this practice. The numerous applications of *response art* serve multiple functions, such as offering containment for therapists' emotions (Fish, 2008); a self-soothing strategy and tool for depth exploration of counter-transferential responses; and a way to invoke interplay with the unconscious in supervision. The *art response* is understood to enhance the empathic grasp of client's experience through processes such as replicating the client's imagery, art making style, or preferred materials (Fish, 2012; Havsteen-Altamirano,

2014). It can support the development of the therapeutic alliance by modelling and be effective as a form of active listening (Fish, 2008).

As with many therapist skills, proficiency is dependent upon experience. In his provisional guidelines for the clinical use of *response art*, Havsteen-Franklin (2014) invokes the therapist to maintain a constant or alternating focus upon both the emotional content contained in his or her image and the interpersonal dynamics and imagery of the client(s). We support his assertion that guidelines will benefit clinical practice and, for our purposes, be of use to the emerging art therapist. As University lecturers, charged with ethical responsibilities in how we educate our students, we have decided to place these art-based practices under scrutiny.

Bragge and Fenner (Fenner is first author of this chapter) published an article (2009) illuminating the benefits of therapist art making with autistic children within an intersubjective practice framework, proposing the notion of the Interactive Square as an alternative conceptualization to Schaverien's triangle (Schaverien, 2000). The Square represents the various communication patterns which occur when the therapist makes art in therapy in response to the images of the autistic child, creating a dialogic art-based interaction. The results of the study were evidence of how social engagement and enhanced meaningful verbal capacity were possible for these children when therapy incorporated therapist art making.

We revisited the under-examined concerns of Case and Dalley (1992), who considered the prospect of being fully present to clients while, simultaneously, making art to be an unachievable goal, voicing concerns that "honest" art making by the therapist in session placed "holding the client in mind" at risk (p. 209). The experience of Bragge and Fenner (2009) demonstrated that, when therapist art making is firmly centered in deep listening to the images and narratives of the client—in much the same manner as an attuned therapeutic conversation—this concern is unfounded. We are sympathetic, however, to the potential vulnerabilities of the entry-level, student experience, in the early days of therapist learning. It is on this period that we focus, when the role and function of the student's art making is required to shift in order to address the needs of the other; to make art in the service of the client.

As published researchers using art-based methods, located in art-based epistemologies, we affirm that knowledge is produced by means other than words alone. We do not question the positive value of *response art* per se. We do wish to examine questions such as the following:

- Is it always clear whose needs are being met in the practice of response art?
- Do art materials and creative expression provide a safe haven for the student when the content of therapy is overwhelming?
- What is the impact upon the student therapist when no images are being made in therapy?
- Does the use of materials and art making sometimes represent acts of avoidance or resistance when client content is disquieting?

We will pursue this discussion by way of scenarios which exemplify how such issues can arise within the context of therapist education.

The Art Therapy Student

The decision to study art therapy requires the investment of considerable personal resources and inevitably results in highly motivated students. These students bring passion that is often borne of having experienced the power of art making. Indeed, the desire to learn about art therapy, and to qualify as an art therapist, may have begun many years prior to actual commencement. During the course of study, the personal commitment to engage with others through art becomes channeled into an identity as a practitioner. If, as Gadamer claimed, work is desire restrained (1975)—or, perhaps, re-trained—the transformation of the function of art making, from being essentially a private expressive event to being a process used in the service of another, will also be under challenge. The formation of a therapist identity can be painful for students as they experience the push and pull of transition. We concur with Hendriksen (2009) that art making fuels and satisfies our desires of self-expression as it connects us to the world, giving shape and form to internal impulses. If art has the capacity to awaken us to our desires and work restrains those desires, the friction between these two forces could be palpable, at least for some of us.

Though maintaining an art practice enriches a therapist's clinical capacity on many levels, many art therapy students are challenged by a reduction in the time available to make art in the manner to which they have been accustomed. If, as Moon (2002) stated, our artist identities are "the constellating force that informs practice" (p. 22), students and therapists alike will seek out the opportunity to express themselves inside and outside clinical practice. Thus, a tension can exist within our profession between the desire to maintain an art practice and to fulfil the other responsibilities we have as students and therapists.

High levels of anxiety and fluctuating self-confidence are present during the transition to becoming a therapist, especially as client contact progresses. One key element in therapist development has been identified as the building of a reservoir of internalised experience. In the initial absence of such, a high level of reliance upon the supervisor and peers is present in clinical supervision to assist in skill development (Folkes-Skinner, Elliott, & Wheeler, 2010; Skovholt & Ronnestad, 1992). Just as the image plays a dynamic role in art therapy's therapeutic triangle or interactive square (Schaverien, 2000; Bragge & Fenner, 2009), so can the image create a potent force in art therapy supervision.

Ethical Challenges Posed by Some Response Art Making

The following fictitious scenarios of trainee-client communication on placement demonstrate the kinds of challenges we have experienced within the university group supervision context. In each case, the making of *response art* might have had a productive intention and might have reaped some positive outcomes for the client. However, ethical dilemmas lie embedded within each, in that the attraction to making art can serve as self-protection against the often overwhelming emotion that arises when one is in relationship with people who are suffering deeply. Each of these scenarios poses opportunities to discuss what is taking place for the student and to examine the role *response art* making has played. We wish to emphasize that it is through such experiences that students learn and that all therapists make errors of judgement from time to time.

Sandy's Drawing of Her Client's Brain

Working in a hospital rehabilitation ward, Sandy became overwhelmed by compassion for a female client who had Multiple Sclerosis (MS), and was challenged to form words clearly. The sound of her newly slurred speech was distressing not only for the woman herself, but also for Sandy, who responded by drawing an image of how she understood her client's brain to have been changed by the progression of MS. Sandy hoped that this visual representation might help her client to understand this alarming experience within a newly informed context.

What function did the art making fulfil in Sandy's response and for whom?

In this situation, Sandy employed *response art* in the face of overwhelming feelings such as the inability to remedy or relieve her client of her difficulties. Sandy assumed that her client lacked insight into what was happening to her. Adopting a rational framework, Sandy assumed that a level of cognitive awareness would shift her client's emotionality. In doing this, Sandy failed to bear her client's emotional experience of isolation, grief, pain, confusion, and loss. Sandy made art, herself, as a way of taking control and placing limits upon the overpowering nature of what she and her client were experiencing. The problems in this act were many, not the least of which was that, in drawing her imaginary representation of her client's brain, Sandy went beyond her area of expertise and level of authority. Instead of becoming aware of and examining her own counter-transferential response, she made this part of her client's world. She crossed a boundary not only with her client, but also with other members of the multidisciplinary team, all of whom held particular areas of responsibility in relation to this client. By making art, Sandy felt that she was taking up the role of art therapist. By making art in this way, her client was no longer required to inquire into her own experience and was reduced to a passive role. At this moment, art making of any kind may not have been a useful response. Instead, simply listening or responding with words may have been both compassionate and therapeutic. Art making was employed as a form of rescue when it was not called for.

Ray's Portraits of His Clients

Ray was on placement in a palliative care ward of a major public hospital where, during this time of transition, patients were often restricted by their limited physical capacities and powerful emotional responses. One of Ray's patients had lost an eye to cancer and became despairing of whom she now saw in the mirror, as though cancer had taken her identity. In response, Ray asked permission to draw her portrait, as a means of supporting her in seeing this new appearance in a different, perhaps helpful, way. His patient enjoyed spending time with Ray and so agreed to this. When the portrait was finished, the patient was pleased with the outcome and Ray felt rewarded by the process and by this new way of creating positive relationship. Over time, Ray regularly sought and received permission to create portraits of his patients on the ward, who found spending time with Ray this way satisfying. The images were such a success with others on the ward that, after several months, hospital management held a public exhibition of the portraits.

What function did the art making fulfil in Ray's portrait making and for whom?

Under a clear contract, such as a legacy project, this art response might facilitate productive outcomes for patients and their families. Ray's portraiture evolved spontaneously and provided a way to be present with patients with whom he otherwise struggled to identify a therapeutically productive response. The images also became gifts which could endure after the patients had died. What commenced as a strategy for embracing physical change and altered identity created by the cancer was transformed into a legacy program. As the intervention gained steam, more patients sat for, and received, portraits. As families and staff celebrated the moving portraits, Ray was affirmed that his artist skills were productive for the benefit of others.

What Ray, patients, and family members risked losing sight of was that—in turning patients into passive sitters and receivers of portrait gifts—Ray not only risked engaging the agency of the sitters to participate in making art for themselves, but also closed off the explorations that art therapy can facilitate at times of existential crisis, such as that of making meaning through loss.

Ray avoided the more difficult struggle to find an active way for his clients to engage in art therapy. The portrait became a container of emotion and issues prior to death, a resolution created by the art therapist rather than by the client. In supervision, Ray resisted seeing the activity as other than positive for the hospital community. The celebrations and accolades made it difficult for Ray to consider that the intervention might be meeting his owns needs and assuaging feelings of discomfort on placement.

The needs of highly dependent patients with little in the balance of relational power must always come first. This circumstance risked disavowing patients, close to death, of the right of refusal, to express needs which were counter to the positive celebration on the ward. Inadvertently, the images risked becoming agents of unintended coercion.

OUR ETHICAL DILEMMA

What function did the art making fulfil?

Tanya's placement was with adolescents hospitalized in an acute mental health ward. Over time, she recognized that many of these young people were discharged from hospital well before they were fully recovered. Back in the supervision group at university, Tanya struggled to find a way to speak about her work on the ward and decided to make a visual representation. After being fully absorbed in her drawing, she choked back tears, stating that she didn't want to speak about the image. She stated that the drawing told the whole story; that words are not important in the work she does.

What function did the art making fulfil for Tanya and how might her supervisor address Tanya's insistence that her drawing "tells the whole story" and that "words are not important in art therapy"?

How would you respond?

For the writer's response, see Appendix B, page 406.

Conclusion

From an ethical perspective, making *response art* in situations such as those raised here can risk becoming a refuge for overwhelming feelings, thus functioning as a deceptive coping strategy, and leading, paradoxically, to a reduced awareness of self and other. As art therapists, making art may seem to be the legitimate response; it can answer the question of competence, coping, and being seen to manage well, especially as trainee therapists. While art is particular to our form of therapy, in some circumstances making *response art* may be equivalent to a psychotherapist over talking. And, yet, our art can seduce us into misjudging resolutions through the power of the successful image. Although critiquing the primary tools of our trade can feel perilous, whenever we reach for our art materials in sessions, we would do well to ask ourselves: *Why am I doing this (now)? What might I be avoiding? What feelings might be threatening to overwhelm me? Making art with my client might be helpful for me, but is it what my client needs right now?*

Art made as a response in therapy requires the same ethical parameters as do all other practices in our work.

REFLECTIVE ART EXPERIENCES & DISCUSSION QUESTIONS

a. Create an image to explore a particular experience of making art with a client.
b. Create an image to explore a particular aspect of your own art-making process.

1. What stands out to you in each of these images?
2. Explore the resonances and dissonances in the emerging similarities and differences.
3. What are the ethical implications that emerge from the above?

References

Bragge, A., & Fenner, P. (2009). The emergence of the "interactive square" as an approach to art therapy with children on the autistic spectrum. *International Journal of Art Therapy*, 14(1), 17–28.

Brown, C., Meyerowitz-katz, J., & Ryde, J. (2003). Thinking with image making in supervision. *International Journal of Art Therapy*, 8(2), 71–78.

Case, C., & Dalley, T. (1992). *The handbook of art therapy*. New York: Routledge.

Elkis-Abuhoff, D., Gaydos, M., Rose, S., & Goldblatt, R. (2010). The impact of education and exposure on art therapist identity and perception. *Art Therapy: Journal of the American Art Therapy Association*, 27(3), 119–126.

Fish, B. (2008). Formative evaluation research of art-based supervision in art therapy training. *Art Therapy: Journal of the American Art Therapy Association*, 25(2), 70–77.

Fish, B. (2012). Response art: The art of the art therapist. *Art Therapy: Journal of the American Art Therapy Association*, 29(3), 138–143.

Folkes-Skinner, J., Elliott, R., & Wheeler, S. (2010). "A baptism of fire": A qualitative investigation of a trainee counsellor's experience at the start of training. *Counselling and Psychotherapy*, 10(2), 83–92.

Gadamer, H. (1975). *Truth and method*. London: Sheed & Ward.

Havsteen-Franklin, D. (2014). Consensus for using an art-based response in art therapy. *International Journal of Art Therapy*, 19(3), 107–113.

Hendriksen, J.O. (2009). *Desire, gift, and recognition: Christology and postmodern philosophy*. Grand Rapids, MI: William B. Eerdmans.

Marshall-Tierney, A. (2014). Making art with and without patients in acute settings. *International Journal of Art Therapy*, 19(3), 96–106.

Miller, A. (2012). Inspired by *el duende*: One-canvas process painting in art therapy supervision. *Art Therapy: Journal of the American Art Therapy Association*, 29(4), 166–173.

Moon, C.H. (2002). *Studio art therapy: Cultivating the artist identity in the art therapist*. London: Jessica Kingsley.

Schaverien, J. (2000). The triangular relationship and the aesthetic counter-transference in analytical art psychotherapy. In A. Gilroy & G. McNeilly (Eds.), *The changing shape of art therapy* (pp. 55–83). London: Jessica Kingsley.

Skovolt, T.M., & Ronnestad, M.H. (1992). Themes in therapist and counsellor development. *Journal of Counselling and Development*, 70, 505–515.

46

MULTIPLE ROLES IN ART THERAPY SUPERVISION

Using *El Duende* One-Canvas Process Painting

Abbe Miller

O body swayed to music, O brightening glance,
How can we know the dancer from the dance?
William Butler Yeats, "Among School Children" (in Yeats, 2010)

I dance the roles of clinician, professor, supervisor, faculty advisor, thesis advisor, and director at a Graduate Art Therapy Program in New England. Who I am, my fuller self, is really more the *dancer*, weaving a rich choreography over my 60 years as an artist/art psychotherapist, wife, mother, daughter, friend, sister, journeyer, visionary, athlete, scholar, and more. This is not atypical for art therapy instructors, who are—at minimum—both instructor and clinician.

The use of expressive arts in supervision raises ethical concerns such as boundary issues, dual relationships, and the use of supervisory power; concerns that are potentiated by the intimate processing that occurs with arts modalities (Purswell & Stulmaker, 2015). These ethical challenges can also be learning opportunities, made visible via engagement in the depth-oriented *el duende* one-canvas process painting (EDPP) supervision seminar (Miller, 2012; Miller & Robb, 2017). EDPP is an art-based approach inspired by the artistic struggle of *el duende*, a Spanish term used in the arts to mean a mysterious power of emotional vibrancy that can be felt but not always seen or explained (Maurer, 1955/1998). The method combines clinical insight with archetypal awareness arising from painting on a single canvas throughout the internship semester. EDPP supervision is composed of three main components: (a) spontaneous painting, (b) complex reflective processing, and (c) aesthetically focused attention to imagery.

The relationship between supervisee and the single canvas becomes the primary container for transformation, while the sequential layering stimulates tension, curiosity, expression and integration of authentic professional and personal voice (Miller, 2012).

This chapter explores ethical issues that arise from the multiple relationships that exist between instructor and student during art-based supervision. Boundaries and containers play an important role in supervision; depth-oriented models are of particular interest for art therapists because complexity in relationship to the therapeutic art process and product is central to learning. Goren (2013) points out that it is not so much the complex ethical conflicts about roles but the subsequent secrecy about these conflicts that can stimulate difficulties. EDPP offers unique ways to reveal, in an ethical manner, material that might otherwise remain concealed.

Part I. Diving Deep

> Turning and turning in the widening gyre
> The falcon cannot hear the falconer;
> Things fall apart; the centre cannot hold;
> Mere anarchy is loosed upon the world.
> > *William Butler Yeats, "The Second Coming" (in Yeats, 2010)*

Why dive deep? Because that's where transformation occurs; where a deep and abiding trust in the creative process as a healing agent becomes illuminated. It's where the animated, passionate juiciness of art therapy resides. Learning how and when to dive deep guides discovery of *who* the dancer is—the authentic self of the art therapist.

In this realm, things must fall apart. It can get messy, even chaotic, mirroring the therapeutic relationship. Miller (2012), Moon (2015) and McNiff (1998) encourage depth-oriented art-based learning, and Robbins (1999) connects the power of chaos with supervisory responsibility to create strong enough containers to hold charged material. Art therapists know that the creative process, itself, can be container, while students learn it through experience and reflection. For their *center* to hold it must be felt, witnessed, and processed in relational space. The supervisor's role is not to be the center, but to guide students to develop their own ways of centering, while attending to the container of supervision, itself.

Containers and Boundaries

Students need boundaries and containers to help them center when anxious, listen deeply to explore power dynamics, and learn agency by reflecting upon ethical concerns as they arise.

Supervision is an experiential modeling container. How tensions are welcomed and worked with, both among peers and with a supervisor, directly affects the building of trust. The essential quality for nurturing trust is the release of judgment, yet, as a professor, I am always judging the students' performance and capabilities while witnessing their painting journey with a non-judgmental stance. As supervisor, teacher, and clinician, I bring complexity to the container; as faculty advisor, I weave my observations into professional performance reviews; as program director, I am generally aware of "back stories" between students and faculty. A conceptual container that can hold complexity is parallel process work (Doehrman, 1976); combined with depth artwork, as in EDPP, it deepens the supervisory alliance while creating opportunities to increase a sense of professional autonomy (Mills & Chasler, 2012) and a space to explore ethical issues.

The EDPP seminar is both a literal and a metaphorical container with boundaries that are not too tight, not too loose (Gilligan, 1997). Its fluid five-step model (archetypal invocation; warm-up identification of tension; one large canvas painting with photographing progression; active imagination journaling and witnessing; and final project) provides the container for the transformation of activated supervision material. The large (24" × 36") canvas is the boundary/container within which students layer spontaneous imagery, offering a direct experience with complex reflective process, aesthetically focused attention, and opportunity to explore multiple relationships. This often activates deep layers of professional and personal identity material and sets the stage for metamorphosis of thoughts, beliefs, and awareness. The canvas becomes a metaphor and reflection of the student's evolving self (Miller, 2012; Moon, 2009).

The canvas size acknowledges the "bigness" of the work. EDPP uses the prominence of the canvas as primary tangible container to respond to the somewhat blurry boundary between supervision and psychotherapy (Mills & Chasler, 2012). Ethical concerns arise in the subtle differences and similarities between supervisory and therapeutic trust development. In EDPP, the canvas takes on the therapist role, welcoming the "problem" into an artistic container. Trust grows within the inter-subjective relational layer of knowing (Van Lith, 2014). Imagery shifts from "it" to the beloved "thou" (Buber, 1958), grounding ethical exploration in compassion.

Amy expressed feeling insecure and was unsure that this was acceptable. I directed her to paint the "insecurity" (it) into her canvas as a means of exploring acceptance. An embryonic figure emerged (other). A vulnerable part was made visible and her peer group and I were able to offer compassionate witnessing. Amy also embraced the embryonic form with self-compassion (thou); "she" grew while her canvas "therapist" served as a safe, expansive container.

Power Dynamics

Goren (2013) identifies the intrinsic issues of power and authority that are part of the supervisor/trainee/patient triad. EDPP uses spontaneous, directed, or responsive imagery in addressing concerns in supervision. Historically, the grayer areas of ethics emerge as personal material arises or when students face particularly charged counter-transference issues in regard to patients and supervisors. Authority figures are always ripe targets for projection. The complexity of guiding students through these projections is heightened within the hierarchical power systems of academia, particularly around issues of grading. Having two supervisors (site and seminar) can blur boundaries. What happens when I disagree with a site supervisor's feedback about student performance? Ethically, I do not want to feed into splitting, yet, as program director, I often feel protective of my students. I defer to the canvas as a space for students to process, guiding them to bring their supervisor(s) into the painting and then process insights gleaned via art making.

Fish (2008) notes the importance of building trust among peer group members in supervision, typically an area where unconscious sibling power dynamics play out. EDPP peer reflection aims to do this, as well as to address dilemmas with interpersonal reflection. When coupled with dual roles, being the central authority figure can generate additional ethical dilemmas, so I oscillate between central and side witnessing during time structured for verbal interaction, personal journaling, and peer feedback. This facilitates a shift from a hierarchical ("power over") structure towards an interactive ("power with others") dynamic among the group.

Depth-oriented art-based models of supervision (Miller, 2012; Robbins, 1999; Moon, 2009) value spontaneous potent imagery as part of the voice of the developing professional. When it emerges, which *"dance"* will be activated between supervisor/ supervisee—one of anxiety or of curiosity?

Anxiety

Edwards (2010) has found that the flow of the creative process can be inhibited by the oscillation of anxiety levels that occurs among peers, supervisor, and the art making.

EDPP's boundaries and containers conceal and reveal both professional and personal anxieties. I try to address ethical concerns that might arise from my having multiple roles with all the students in my program by explaining how my various roles do, and do not, influence one another.

Purswell and Stulmaker (2015) note the importance of helping supervisees to develop a tolerance for ambiguity before seeking a solution in response to this anxiety. Students' verbal and non-verbal expressions of discomfort with vulnerability and self-disclosure (AATA, 2013, 8.5) can also signal the emergence of an ethical dilemma. While the supervisor's responsibility is to help students grow at the edges of tension, when parallel material is overtly personal, navigating these edges can feel like therapy, even though it is not. I use a body awareness ethics orientation (Taylor, 1995) to help categorize non-verbal tension (e.g., power struggles are often located in the solar plexus; grounding issues, in the sacral spine). Somatic expressions are then invited into the art making, integrating a body-up (Dennison, 2014) orientation with artistic awareness. If a student cannot physically settle, it informs me that the student cannot emotionally settle as well.

Curiosity

Purswell and Stulmaker (2015) suggest considering the developmental stage of the supervisee when making decisions about which expressive techniques to use, while Lett (1995) stresses that students should have expressive agency, enabling them to guide their mode of artistic curiosity intuitively, leading to authentic moments of discovery. Ethical concerns regarding materials agency can appear early in the EDPP process because the directed use of acrylic paints on a single canvas can feel limiting. As the semester continues, students see that creative curiosity is welcomed with varied media. Three intentions, ethically grounded, guide awareness about choice of materials in supervision, providing simultaneous learning about how their use can affect the supervisory and therapeutic container:

1. Respect student agency and capabilities while respecting the EDPP process.
2. Recognize that learning about various media comes from comfort and discomfort.
3. Encourage curiosity about the unknown.

When Gina asked for a ruler and pencil to use on her blank canvas, I felt conflicted, since the process always begins with acrylic painting. I spoke with her about anxiety and curiosity to support her tuning into her emotional process. She responded by first using pencil, then watercolors, and finally acrylics. Had she been a client, I might have directed material choice more overtly but I watched and encouraged each effort to push the edges of her comfort zone; by the end of class, everyone noticed that she was more playful. El duende's chaotic imagery was emerging into the canvas container.

Part II. A Journey to Hope

> Through creativity we are saying that in putting fragments and pieces together, hope is possible.
>
> *Robbins, 1999, p. 124*

During art therapy supervision, I try to foster an environment in which supervisees may explore many levels of vulnerability via artistic expression. My work with Ciara illustrates some of my own vulnerabilities when navigating ethical dilemmas that arise, in part, from the many hats I wear in the graduate program. Ciara entered the EDPP seminar in her second year, during her second internship rotation, at a graduate art therapy program approved by the American Art Therapy Association (AATA). As an art psychotherapist for 35+ years with a private practice specializing in treatment of trauma, I always approach the seminar with passion. We began her process painting journey—a journey that was to span the 15-week semester—with the concepts of inter-subjective relationship and parallel process.

In the first class, students create small, warm-up canvases (3" × 3") of their personal and professional selves; this thrusts them into an expressive world that explores opposites, while I assert a certain level of power by inviting tension (*duende*) into the

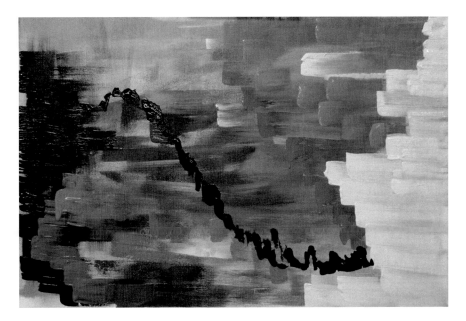

FIGURE 46.1 First painting.

container. Ciara created two visually distinct images, signaling a desire for separation of emotional and cognitive processes.

Next, students are directed to surrender to the struggle of opposite energies, painting on the large canvas without focusing upon the product. Ciara began with an abstract display of color, expressing feelings about her internship experience at an alternative high school setting, while verbally expressing discomfort (Figure 46.1). I trusted that the painting itself would reveal imagery that would challenge her to deepen her personal and professional growth.

Ciara became frustrated by what she perceived as a lack of beauty in her image, while I noticed body discomfort as she applied layers of color. A sense of chaos and

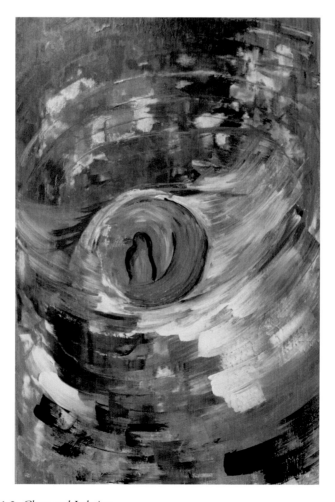

FIGURE 46.2 *Chaos and Isolation.*

isolation (note the lone figure in the center of Figure 46.2) seemed to vie with an attempt to create a grid-like order. I sensed, via body language and art imagery, an oscillating pull towards and away from her canvas. As she began to outline the shape of Italy, Ciara expressed aesthetic discomfort, but was unsure how to address this tension. I suggested that she explore the concept of boundaries and she layered colored tissue paper in a circle around Italy, perhaps an unconscious effort to contain the emergent chaos (Figure 46.3). The red area at the bottom of the "boot" was compelling and I asked if she wanted to explore that more deeply. Immediately, her subtle energy shifted into a freeze-like trauma response, coupled with an upwelling of tears and an apparent sense of shame.

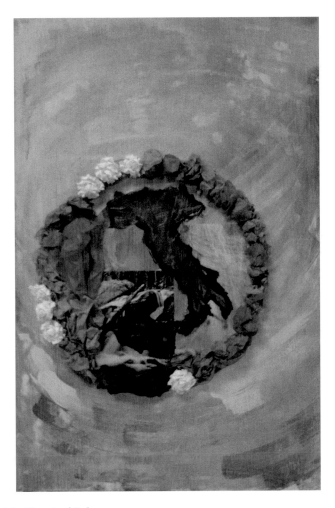

FIGURE 46.3 *Contained Italy.*

MY ETHICAL DILEMMA

How should I proceed when the boundary between supervision and therapy starts to slip?

I was aware of the potential for blurring boundaries as potent material was emerging. The concept that vulnerabilities (tears) are also strengths is initially quite foreign to most students, so I was aware that my role as program director and professor might be heightening her discomfort. With parallel awareness, I sensed a trauma connection and guided her to grounding and centering techniques. Overwhelmed by tears, Clara left the classroom. She did not yet trust the seminar or me as containers to hold the tides of emotional discharge that were spilling. While I felt deep compassion towards Ciara and might have wanted to respond as I would as a therapist, as mentor/supervisor I needed to effect a strength-based approach and the concept of the *"wounded healer"* came to mind. I hoped that, by sharing this, Ciara might begin to believe that her personal wounds, when made conscious and attended to, would aid her in guiding her own patients towards balance and hope. Listening to my *wise mind*, heart and gut—three very important guides in all matters ethical—I went out into the hallway to encourage Ciara to rejoin the class. Spontaneously, she disclosed a history of childhood sexual abuse that was activated by her map of Italy in the painting and by her work with adolescent girls.

How would you respond?

For the writer's response, see Appendix B, page 420.

Ciara approached the next class with trepidation, not unusual after a layer of challenging depth material arises. I focused her upon the strong container of her canvas, noting that the process painting had led her to an important awareness and that, if more emotional energy were felt, it could also be painted/collaged and that this process would ultimately help her to develop an appreciation of the skills needed to guide patients through art. She courageously proceeded to express pain and anger, both hers and her patients', by layering with black and red tissue. When, during peer processing, the image of a gagged face was noticed (Figure 46.4) and she received support. By trusting her use of the canvas as primary container I was able to settle into focused orientation as supervisor, attentive to nuances of integration of parallel process, and some of my ethical concerns were allayed. During the following class, Ciara's incorporation in her art of plaster gauze—material that, literally, is used to mend broken bones—seemed to signal a shift in her psyche from descent to ascent, towards light (Figure 46.5).

At major shifts, changing the orientation of the painting encourages awareness of multiple meanings. When Ciara turned her canvas and intuitively covered everything

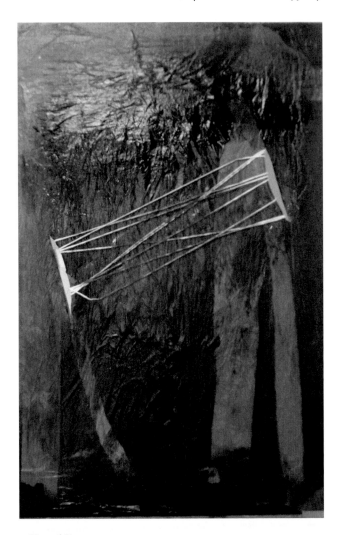

FIGURE 46.4 *Gagged Face.*

in a layer of white, the image of a young girl's head and upper torso emerged. Painstakingly, with open compassion for the wounding, Ciara fleshed out the girl's portrait until the word "HOPE" appeared (Figure 46.6).

During the final class, sparkling silver glitter (reminiscent of the glitter that she had first used, with the color blue, to soothe) and a fragmented but complete heart—all surrounded by confetti-like iridescent glass pieces—graced her canvas. Ciara named her progression, *Journey to Hope* (Figure 46.7).

> Hope and Memory have one daughter and her name is Art.
>
> *William Butler Yeats, "The Celtic Twilight" (in Yeats, 2010)*

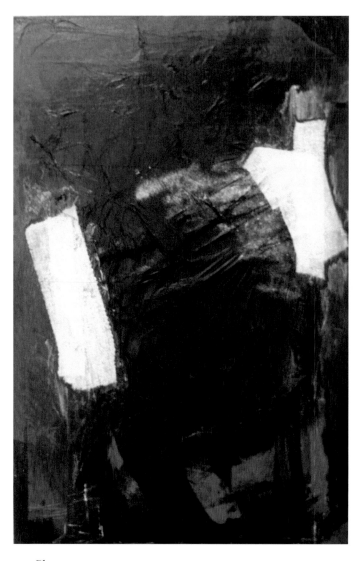

FIGURE 46.5 Plaster gauze.

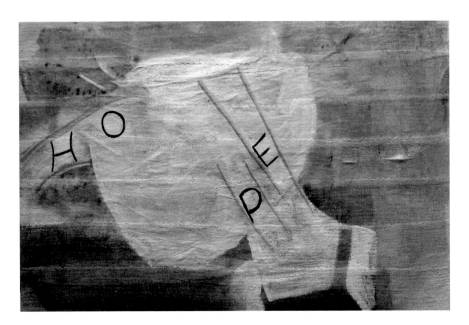

FIGURE 46.6 *Hope Appears.*

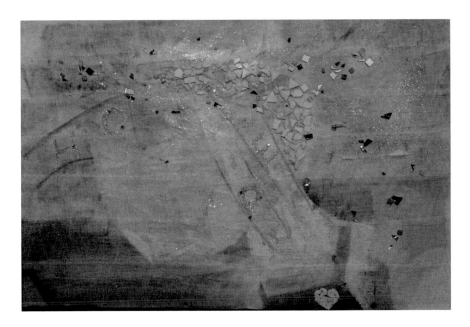

FIGURE 46.7 *Journey to Hope.*

REFLECTIVE ART EXPERIENCES & DISCUSSION QUESTIONS

1. Create an image/artistic reflection of the multiple roles that you carry as clinician, supervisor, faculty member, etc.
2. By reflecting upon your artwork, what tensions do you notice between roles? Where do they seem to enhance one another? What kind of aesthetic resolution arises as you sit with the image?
3. Choose a challenging moment as supervisor and create a piece of art that reflects the specific challenge. Photograph the piece. Continue to follow the energy of the image by creating a layered response work of art. Witness and reflect upon the transformation.
4. What does the impulse to layer tell you about that challenging moment? What is concealed, revealed, and/or transformed during the layering process and how does this shift the meaning of the challenging moment?

References

American Art Therapy Association (2013). *Ethical principles for art therapists.* Retrieved from www.arttherapy.org/upload/ethicalprinciples.pdf

Buber, M. (1958). *I and thou* (2nd ed.). New York: Charles Scribner's Sons.

Dennison, B. (2014). Speaking & teaching. Retrieved from www.clearingtrauma.com/Speaker.html

Doehrman, M.J. (1976). Parallel processes in supervision and psychotherapy. *Bulletin of the Meninger Clinic,* 40, 1–104.

Edwards, D. (2010). Play and metaphor in clinical supervision: Keeping creativity alive. *The Arts in Psychotherapy,* 37, 248–254.

Fish, B. (2008). Formative evaluation research of art-based supervision in art therapy training. *Art Therapy: Journal of the American Art Therapy Association,* 25(2), 70–77.

Gilligan, S. (1997). *The courage to love.* New York: W.W. Norton.

Goren, E. (2013). Ethics, boundaries, and supervision: Commentary on trauma triangles and parallel processes: Geometry and the supervisor/trainee/patient triad. *Psychoanalytic Dialogues,* 23, 737–743.

Lett, W. (1995). Experiential supervision through simultaneous drawing and talking. *The Arts in Psychotherapy,* 22(4), 31–328.

Maurer, C. (Ed.) (1955/1998). *Federico Garcia Lorca: In search of duende.* New York: New Directions.

McNiff, S. (1998). *Trust the process: An artist's guide to letting go.* Boston, MA: Shambhala Publications.

Miller, A. (2012). Inspired by el duende: One-canvas process painting in art therapy supervision. *Art Therapy: Journal of the American Art Therapy Association,* 29(4), 166–173.

Miller, A., & Robb, M. (2017). Transformative phases in *el duende* process painting art-based supervision. *The Arts in Psychotherapy,* 54, 15–27.

Mills, J., & Chasler, J. (2012). Establishing priorities in the supervision hour. *Training and Education in Professional Psychology,* 6(3), 160–166.

Moon, B.L. (2009). *Existential art therapy: The canvas mirror.* Springfield, IL: Charles C. Thomas.

Moon, B.L. (2015). *Ethical issues in art therapy* (3rd ed.). Springfield, IL: Charles C. Thomas.

Purswell, K., & Stulmaker, H. (2015). Expressive arts in supervision: Choosing developmentally appropriate interventions. *International Journal of Play Therapy*, 24(2), 103–117.

Robbins, A. (1999). Chaos and form. *Art Therapy: Journal of the American Art Therapy Association*, 16(3), 121–125. doi: 10.1080/07421656.1999.10129652.

Taylor, K. (1995). *The ethics of caring: Honoring the web of life in our professional healing relationships.* Santa Cruz, CA: Hanford Mead.

Van Lith, T. (2014). A meeting with 'I–Thou': Exploring the intersection between mental health recovery and art making through a co-operative inquiry. *Action Research*, 12(3), 254–272.

Yeats, W.B. (2010). *The collected works of W.B. Yeats, volume I: The poems* (R.J. Finneran, Ed.). New York: Simon & Schuster.

47

TRAUMA AND DISPLACED AGGRESSION

An Art Therapist Works with Refugees in Sweden

Catherine Rogers Jonsson

The Beginning …

I fell in love with a Swede, we married, and I moved from Fairbanks, Alaska to Sweden 20 years ago. My husband Jan and I live in a century-old, typically Swedish, red and white house, surrounded by fields of wheat, oats, barley, and canola. Ancient northern forests stand on the edges of the grain fields in every direction. Our land still holds remnants of the ancient Viking culture that dwelt here more than 1000 years ago. Several rock outcroppings reveal rune markings and carved, cup-like shapes used to hold food offerings to the Viking gods and goddesses. Archeologists have told us that on a nearby hill there is a burial mound for a Viking chieftain.

A Personal Perspective on the Refugee Experience in One Small Village

In a tiny agricultural village of a few hundred Swedish citizens, there is a kiosk, a café with a gas pump, a primary school, and a church that is nearly a thousand years old. A few years ago, refugees and asylum seekers began moving to the village to await the Swedish Migration Agency's decision on their resettlement and residency status. At one point, about 50 refugees and asylum seekers lived in temporary accommodations in several four-flat apartment buildings and a block of row houses. The refugees were assigned to housing without apparent consideration of their country of origin, language, or religious affiliation, in that one could find four women or four men of very different backgrounds living in the same studio apartment in four single beds or two bunk beds. While visiting a group of refugees to invite them to art therapy sessions, I noticed that one of the lower bunk beds was entirely closed off from the others, completely draped with curtains, towels, and bed sheets. This makeshift tent afforded its occupant a bit of privacy and, perhaps, a sense of safety. The sound of jet airplanes taking off and landing day and night at a Swedish Air Force base is retraumatizing to refugees from war-torn countries such as Syria and Afghanistan, who instinctively flinch and cower, fearful that the planes are coming to bomb them.

A few retired primary school teachers offered the refugees an informal introductory class in the Swedish language and culture. The teachers had had no prior experience with refugees or asylum seekers and had never taught Swedish to adults or as a second language. Still, they wanted to help. Their initial strategy was to teach the adult refugees as if they, too, were young children, handing out work sheets designed for first-graders and teaching them simple songs.

A few years ago, two dozen refugees were attending the informal Swedish school in the congregation building two mornings per week. The other refugees and asylum seekers stayed in their apartments. Depression runs high in refugee communities, as does trauma. For weeks, and sometimes even months, even a simple walk around the block can be a frightening task. Most of the refugees ventured outside only to shop in the village or bravely take the county bus into a nearby town for *halāl* grocery shopping. Even in the absence of trauma, Swedish is a difficult language that takes years for most people to master. Victims of trauma find it even more difficult to focus upon learning. I've worked with refugees who have PhDs and MDs and those who are illiterate. Illiteracy in one's own language is a huge barrier to learning to read, write, and speak another language.

Almost all refugees and asylum seekers apply for Swedish residence by petitioning the Swedish Migration Agency for asylum. The Agency assesses whether the person seeking protection has the right to a residence permit in accordance with the Swedish Aliens Act. The refugees who attended the informal Swedish school did so with a belief that it would help their candidacy for permanent residency in Sweden. After some months, they realized that it had no bearing upon the decision-making process. Whether they had attended school or not, some of the refugees began to be deported to their EU country of entrance and some were repatriated to their home countries. School attendance dropped off dramatically.

Introducing Art Therapy to the Refugees

As an *Auktoriserad Bildterapeut* (an authorized art therapist), I, too, wanted to help. My first step was to find a way to explain what art therapy is and what the refugees and asylum seekers might gain from it. I contacted a local Iraqi poet who is a long-time Swedish citizen to assist me in translating a basic introduction of myself, along with a brief explanation of the principles and practice of art therapy. I turned this into a PowerPoint program that utilized photos of art materials and art-making processes.

I began working with the refugees by donating an hour, one day a week, during their school time. After showing the PowerPoint to the refugees and the school teachers, I passed out large drawing paper, chalk pastels, oil pastels, tempera paints, brushes, and paper plates as palettes. Everyone participated, including the teachers!

Immediately, an ethical issue arose. The teachers, who had had no social service experience and seemed to be unaware of therapeutic protocol or psychodynamic group process, stayed throughout the art therapy session, trying to assist the clients as though they were children and making comments and suggestions such as "How pretty!" "That's so nice!" or "You need more blue there." During that first session, I realized that the PowerPoint material I had presented was insufficient to address the topic of appropriate adult support during art therapy sessions, which wasn't the role of the teachers anyway. I was also well aware of the fact that I was conducting my art therapy sessions during their "school time." I came to the conclusion that I had to separate my art therapy group from the school if it were to be of therapeutic benefit to the refugees.

About that same time, the pastoral deacon of the area asked me to present a program about art therapy to the Church leaders in the district. I created an introduction to art therapy PowerPoint lecture describing who I am and what I do. As a result, I was offered contractual work as an art therapist through the Church of Sweden and have been employed by them ever since. I was then able to separate my art therapy group from the Swedish school by holding my sessions on different days.

I knew that I would face many challenges in creating a multinational, multicultural, and multi-faith art therapy group, but, as the sessions continued, week after week, the challenges multiplied and deepened. The refugees brought every kind of situation with them to the art therapy groups: infected teeth, eyes, and ears; a crushed and badly set elbow; psychological issues such as depression, phobias, extreme startle responses, tactile defensiveness, grief, insomnia, and nightmares due to PTSD; and a host of social service issues. The stories they shared were heart-wrenching. One of my adult clients had (literally) lost her child while they were staying in a German refugee camp. Another client, forced to drink bacteria-ridden water while she was in a Libyan refugee camp, had gone into liver failure. Fortunately, she had received a liver transplant while she was in an Italian refugee camp. She arrived in Sweden a year after the operation and continues to need constant medical monitoring for infection and other signs of organ rejection. Several female clients hinted at the daily and nightly terrors they had experienced in camps in Libya, Turkey, Germany, and Italy. Both male and female refugees had been terrified by groups of men that roved the camps at night. I suspect that some of them had been raped. Looting was common. Due to language and cultural barriers, the details of these events were sketchy at best.

My Eritrean clients reported that human traffickers in Libya had demanded extra money to let them onto the refugee boats that were bound for Italy. Handing the refugees a cell phone, the traffickers had instructed them to call their families in Eritrea and tell them to deposit sums of money into the traffickers' bank accounts. If the money wasn't forthcoming, the refugees were given a choice: they could return to Eritrea by foot or give the traffickers one of their kidneys. I was told that a make-shift surgical tent was located in the camp for the sole purpose of removing kidneys; although none of my clients reported having lost a kidney, all had been deeply disturbed by the horror of being confronted by those who sold human body parts on the black market.

Clinical and Ethical Issues in the Art Therapy Group

How was I going to administer and interpret viable art therapy assessments to this mixed group of refugees from Syria, Eritrea, Somalia, Sudan, Iran, Iraq, and Afghanistan? How could I offer art therapeutic interventions to non-Swedish speaking, non-English speaking, and limited-English speaking refugees and asylum seekers? How was I to structure a session? How would I clinically interview, interact with, and assess new members, as well as departing members?

I conducted one-and-a-half hour art therapy groups twice a week. Attendance was sporadic at best. A core group of three clients came regularly; seven to ten clients came on an irregular basis. Women constituted the majority of clients, with African women coming to group more consistently than Middle Eastern women and single women attending more readily than married women. Most clients came 15 minutes late; others appeared any time after that. At the close of group, every client spontaneously and actively participated in pick-up and clean-up without any prompting from me: thoroughly cleaning tables, chairs, and other work surfaces; sweeping floors, cleaning brushes, and wiping down the sink; then bagging the garbage, replacing the plastic liner, and carrying the bag to the garbage can outside the building. In this way, they seemed to express their appreciation, as well as their collective ownership, of the art therapy space.

Selecting Appropriate Art Therapy Assessments and Interventions

Art therapists have an ethical responsibility to provide interventions with care. Some assessments and approaches didn't help the refugees; others could be detrimental. Someone who has lived all his life in a desert environment would find it difficult—if not impossible—to respond to a request to "Draw a person in the rain." Likewise, an invitation to "Draw a person picking an apple from a tree" doesn't work with people from Eritrea, Somalia, or Sudan, where apple trees don't grow; I substituted Beles cactus fruit, instead. For similar reasons, a number of refugees found it difficult to respond to the "bird's nest" assessment. The prospect of body tracing can be extremely confronting, depending upon one's religious beliefs, cultural traditions, and personal history of sexual assault and genital mutilation. Some of the women (remaining seated) chose, instead, to place their arms, heads, and chests on a sheet of mural paper that had been affixed to the table and then to have their fellow female group members trace around those areas.

By contrast, most of the refugees actively invested themselves in the creation of "a safe place." A Syrian man sculpted a dead woman lying on the ground in front of the soldier who had killed her; the artist's safe place was behind that wall. He then created a clay tank to protect and hide himself, his wife, and their six children from the soldiers. An Eritrean woman in her forties created a buoy—the only safe place she could see from the terribly over-crowded refugee boat; alligators encircle it. A Somali woman in her 30s sculpted a mother, a child, and a grandmother walking; snakes lie on their path.

Supporting the client's freedom of choice in the selection and use of art materials was crucial.

MY ETHICAL DILEMMA

How should I respond to projection and displaced aggression?

Due to the popularity of my work with the refugees in the village, the Church of Sweden in a larger town offered to sponsor my art therapy work with refugees in their congregation hall, too. I provided participants with an hour-and-a-half open art therapy workshop one day a week. One afternoon, a man from Afghanistan, his wife, and two children came to my open workshop art therapy group. Although his speech seemed a bit strained when I greeted him, he spoke English very well. His wife and children sat down at a table and began to paint with tempera. When I demonstrated how we could make monoprints with the paint, they gladly joined in the process.

The man engaged me in conversation at the art supply table where I was filling plastic cups with paint. When I asked if he wanted to paint or draw, mentioning that we had clay as well, he looked at me as though he were clearly upset about something.

Suddenly, he blurted out, "Did you know that Hillary Clinton started ISIS in Afghanistan?"

I replied that I didn't.

"Well, she did!" he said emphatically. "Before her, we had no ISIS in Afghanistan!"

I said that I wasn't aware of that and became very calm, focusing exclusively upon him, to show him I was respectfully listening to him.

In a louder voice, he continued. "Hillary Clinton sent more troops into Afghanistan—then there was more ISIS coming!"

Now he was really angry and he shouted at me, "We *never* had ISIS like that before!"

I responded, "Please tell me more about it. It's the first I've heard about this."

The man's eyes bulged and his face turned red. He clenched his fists against his sides. It was clear that he wasn't just speaking to me anymore. He was speaking to Hillary Clinton. It was as if I were responsible for the ISIS insurgents in Afghanistan.

The man's wife and children remained at the table but were clearly upset. The children's eyes darted back and forth between their artwork on the table and their father's face. The other refugee clients in the room were Eritreans who had very little understanding of English. The man's outburst appeared to have made them apprehensive and frightened and they watched him closely. The therapeutic milieu of this art therapy group was now threatened. The sense of safety in the space had vanished. A hush came over the room and tension filled the air.

How would you respond?

For the writer's response, see Appendix B, page 415.

Concluding Thoughts

In 2016, Sweden, a country of fewer than 10 million people, granted protection to nearly 70,000 people who were seeking asylum.

My experience with the refugees and asylum seekers in one small village showed me that art therapy can be a powerful resource for those who are struggling with displacement and trauma, but it is a drop in the bucket. I plan to turn to the Svenska Riksförbundet för Bildterapeuter (SRBt), the Swedish National Association for Art Therapists, to see whether any of its 205 other members (25 supporting members, 19 authorized members—a credential similar to that of the ATR in the US—and 161 regular members) are engaged in working with this population. Besides providing each other with a supportive forum within which to discuss and explore best practices in working with the refugees and asylum seekers in our country, perhaps we will be able ignite interest in working with a population whose needs are all too often misunderstood.

REFLECTIVE ART EXPERIENCES & DISCUSSION QUESTIONS

1. As a way in which to empathize with clients who have been traumatized and/or displaced, select an egg from a carton, paint it if desired, and create a safe place for it from natural materials, such as moss, leaves, flowers, branches, dirt, sand, clay, and bark, in addition to construction paper, twine, yarn, tape, or hot glue. Tell a story about your egg; if the egg breaks, note how you respond to the event (e.g., saving the shell, mending the pieces; getting a new egg and trying again).
2. Create artwork about the place that you call home. Then, imagine it taken away from you. Create a second piece that reflects what you have left and what you might be able to do with that.
3. Have you ever felt displaced, out of your "element," and unable to communicate how you felt and what you needed? What helped you most in that moment—or what do you believe might have been most helpful to you at that time?
4. Have you ever spent time with refugees or asylum seekers? If not, why not?

The Abuse of Power

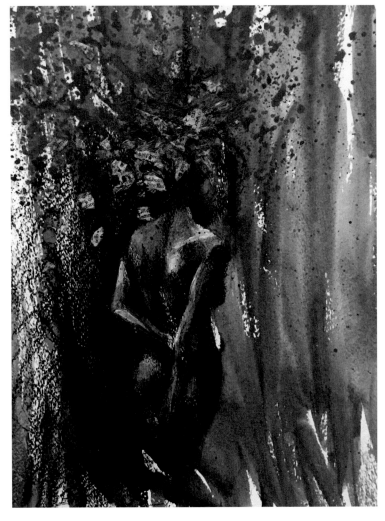

Kristina Nowak *(see color insert)*

48

IF YOU DON'T STAND FOR SOMETHING, YOU'LL FALL FOR ANYTHING

Finding Courage When Asked to Do Wrong

Leslie Milofsky

Have you ever been asked by a supervisor or administrator to do something unethical or illegal? Have you ever been treated in an unethical manner by your "superiors"? The members of regional art therapy associations throughout the United States were asked these questions and, assured of anonymity, were invited to share their answers by email, phone, or post (with no contact information requested or provided). They were asked to include how they had reacted to those requests or situations and if, in looking back, they wished that they had responded differently, to describe how they wish they had reacted and what they believe had prevented them from responding in that way. Many art therapists felt that they had betrayed their own convictions due to fear of retribution, job loss, or isolation if they didn't "go along." They expressed regret for not having had the moral courage to stand up to those in positions of power. I hope to convey that self-compassion and forgiveness can replace regret and shame for choices made due to youth, inexperience, or fear.

The selected narratives that follow are presented in a de-identified format, categorized by topic. I wondered whether the relatively small pool of respondents could be attributed, in part, to apprehension about resurrecting feelings associated with experiences that linger in the form of discomfiting, long-buried memories; to fear of reprisal should the de-identified anecdote somehow be linked to a particular site or supervisor-subordinate relationship; to reluctance to admit to feeling helpless. When we lose trust in the boss who picked us from a stable of applicants, who believed in our strengths and bore the promise of literally and figuratively supporting us, how different is it from losing trust in a parental figure?

Why Are Ethical Dilemmas Involving Supervisors and Supervisees So Difficult?

Most of us carry vestiges of our child-like desire to trust "the big person" in our relational dyads into adulthood, our university studies, and our workplaces. Many articles have been written about the power disparity between employer and employee, supervisor and supervisee. That dynamic is terribly strained when trust becomes tenuous. According to the Deloitte Consulting's 2010 Ethics and Workplace Survey, of the 34% of employed Americans who planned to look for a new job, 48% cited loss of trust in their employer and 46% cited lack of transparent communication from their companies' leadership as the primary reasons for pursuing new employment (Harris, 2012, p. 1).

Guest notes that, in three studies involving 30,000 employees, Mayer found that about 20% of the participants said that they had witnessed unethical behavior. People chose not to report their observations because of "a feeling of futility [or] a fear of retaliation" (Guest, 2013, p. 1). Gerhardt (2011) noted that "research indicates that as many as 50% of all supervisors do not adhere to ethical behavior guidelines ... Too often, supervisors adhere to unethical practices, such as sexual overtures, discrimination between the employees, lack of transparency" (p. 1). This results in mistrust, decreased work efficiency, absenteeism, and increased employee anxiety, "a condition where the supervisee is in a constant state of apprehension, stress, uneasiness and fear whenever [he or she] has to interact with the supervisor" (p. 1).

In his article, "Help! My Supervisor is Unethical," Reamer (2013) addresses the clinicians' inherent sense that he or she must "blow the whistle on ethical misconduct if more moderate efforts fail" (p. 1), but notes that "agency-based politics and organizational dynamics are such that management of these ethical dilemmas requires considerable skill and nuance" (p. 1). Although the Art Therapy Credentials Board (2018) expects credentialed art therapists to "file a complaint with the ATCB when they have reason to believe that another art therapist is or has been engaged in conduct that violates the law or the Standards of Ethics and Conduct contained in this Code" (Standard 1.2.10), most art therapists are supervised not by art therapists but by other mental health professionals.

As clinicians, we want to believe that our supervisors have the best interest of our clients, ourselves, and the organization in mind. As you will discover in reading the following vignettes, this is not always the case.

The Ethical Dilemmas

Because the following vignettes are self-contained accounts of ethical dilemmas experienced and responded to by the art therapists who submitted them, they do not directly ask the reader, "How would you respond?"—nor are they accompanied by pages in Appendix B that describe the resolution to their dilemmas.

Nevertheless, while reading these vignettes, readers are invited (indeed, encouraged) to ponder how they might have responded, had they encountered the ethical challenges presented.

Don't I Have a Duty to Report?

When I was an art therapist at a school for children and adolescents with emotional disturbance and learning disabilities, I worked individually with a quiet adolescent who suddenly began revealing aggressive impulses towards others in her artwork. Her teacher brought me sketches and writing that suggested that the teenager was hearing voices that the latter attributed to Charles Manson; the student had recently watched the movie, *Helter Skelter*. The student told me that "Charlie" was telling her whom to kill and she mentioned the names of two students.

I reported this information to the staff psychologist, who agreed that the student should be sent for a psychiatric evaluation as soon as possible, but the director of the school did not take the situation seriously. In our following session, the student told me that she wanted to kill three staff members, drew pictures of gravestones bearing their names, and said that she planned to bring a kitchen knife with her on the bus the next day. I reported this immediately and the people in charge finally took notice. The three staff members were warned, the teenager was watched carefully, and that afternoon she was hospitalized and subsequently diagnosed with schizophrenia. In retrospect, I believe that the two students who were also intended victims should have been protected and their families warned. I wish I had been more adamant about what I regarded as a potentially dangerous situation instead of acquiescing to those with more power than I.

Years ago, as I stood outside a bathroom at the school for emotionally disturbed, latency-aged children where I worked, I repeatedly heard the "thwap" of leather striking skin, followed by a child's screams. A parent (who had been called in by the teacher) was whipping his young child with a belt. I ran to the main office where the principal and the clinical coordinator demanded that I not intervene and not call Child Protective Services (CPS). They stated that the child needed his bottom beaten. I was too "green" and too frightened of retaliation to stand up to them.

Recently, noticing that—with staff support—parents had taken their child to a wing of the school where an isolation room was used for students who were deemed violent, I demanded that the father step aside from the door of the room he was guarding while his wife berated and repeatedly struck their cowering disabled child. I reported the incident to an unsupportive administration and then called CPS. The fact that I now have the courage and experience to act with integrity in such moments doesn't erase my earlier memory of not having protected the small child for whom even school had become an unsafe place.

I once worked as an art therapist in a large hospice with dedicated units for patients who had end-stage AIDs. It was common knowledge among staff that the calmer, more compliant residents actually were ingesting drugs (heroin or crack cocaine) that were furnished by friends and family. Despite the ethical and legal implications, nursing staff looked the other way and I did not report what I observed. I still feel that it was the right decision; the practice seemed to be an act of compassion.

As I was leaving the girls' unit in a private residential facility one day, I spotted, in the seclusion room, a patient I knew to be HIV positive. Although her clothing had been replaced by a hospital gown, she had been permitted to keep her flannel shirt which she was using to self-harm by creating friction burns on her arms. I reported this at the nursing station, assuming that they would take the shirt away. The next day I saw the girl sitting in the day room having dressings changed on the multiple burns she had been able to inflict because the shirt had not been removed from her. Meanwhile, her contaminated gauze bandages sat on public surfaces, exposing others to her bodily fluids.

Another day, I heard a resident yell from the bathroom near the nurses' station that she needed toilet paper. She was told to use her hand and then wash it in the sink. I reported these troubling incidents to my supervisor but saw no changes. Another incident on the unit involved two girls who had bored a hole through the wall separating their respective rooms so that they could fondle each other; despite this being reported, it was weeks before the hole was fixed. Shortly thereafter, one of the social workers assigned to the unit phoned me at home to share that she was reporting the daily violations of patients' rights to an outside governing agency. Although I was relieved that she was taking action, I felt an obligation to let my employer know that an investigation would be forthcoming. When I shared what I knew with my supervisor, I was promptly swept to the CEO's office where I was questioned, told not to engage socially with my colleague (whom they deemed unstable), and asked to phone her surreptitiously to obtain details about her plans to report malfeasance. I refused. I wish that I had had the strength to do what my social work colleague did; I've carried the memory of her courage in my heart for decades as a reminder of what can be done to defend patients' rights.

A large storage room across from the classroom where I provided art therapy services in a public school was being worked on by an outside plumbing contractor who asked if he could dump buckets of water into my sink. While doing so, he said that he was chopping away large quantities of asbestos insulation from the pipes. When I asked, he said he was not using protective measures because he'd been doing the work for so long that his health was already compromised. I reported my concern about the storage space not being properly sealed off from the students/staff and was curtly dismissed by my supervisor. I then contacted the facilities office, which assessed the situation and found that, indeed, asbestos was being disturbed without proper procedures being followed. Corrective measures were instituted immediately.

During the first week of my very first art therapy job, in a psycho-educational facility, the sound of a child yelling and crying made me open my office door and go to investigate. Turning a corner in the hallway, I spotted the principal kneeling on the back of child, apparently in an effort to subdue him. "What's going on?" I blurted out. The principal looked up at me, furious, and shouted, "I won't ever tell you how to do your art therapy and don't you ever tell me how to run my school!" Stunned and speechless, I backed away, returned to my room, and closed the door, feeling as if I were closing my door on a child in trouble, intimidated by a bully who could have me fired. I'm ashamed to say that I also felt a little relieved to know that he would "never tell me how to do my art therapy." At the time, I was young, worried and defensive about my ability to do my job, and uncomfortable with conflict, so tended to go to great lengths to avoid it. No call to CPS was made. Later, as a result of staff members sharing their collective observations of the principal's inappropriate behavior, a report was made and the principal was dismissed.

While working as the director of an end-stage residential treatment facility for patients with AIDS, I coordinated pastoral services, volunteer programming, and special events, in addition to providing art therapy services. One evening I walked into a patient's room to find two nurses pinning the patient to the bed while pressing a four-inch crucifix against his forehead, imploring Jesus to "renounce [his] sins, release the demons that dwelt within, and save [his] soul." I told the nurses to release the patient, advised them that they couldn't define what should happen to him based upon their own beliefs, and said that the patient was too compromised to be a willing participant or to express his own spiritual needs. Although I disrupted the exorcism, I did not report the nurses to their supervisor. They appeared to be acting out of desperation and seemed to want to do right by him. I still believe that my decision was appropriate.

Isn't This Fraud?

At an agency where I worked, the clients were asked to sign in as soon as they arrived for group sessions. Since many of the clients were very low functioning and unable to tolerate group work, they did not stay very long; nevertheless, the company billed for the group even if the client stayed for only five minutes. I made it a practice to ask clients in my art therapy groups to sign in at the end of their sessions and worked with others to send a complaint to Medicare. As a result, the facility was investigated and subsequently disciplined, then later shut down.

Just as I was leaving work one day in a large public school system, I was asked by the principal to sign an Individualized Education Plan for an IEP meeting that had not taken place. When I declined to sign the document, the principal told me that the other members of the team had done so. I stated that I was willing to stay late if he wanted to contact the parent via phone in order to conduct a brief meeting. He responded that there wasn't time and, as I turned to leave, remarked that the educational system would lose the money designated for that special education student. I felt proud of myself for standing up to my supervisor, ensuring that the parent and student were given the voice that was mandated to them by law. Looking back, I wish that I had also reported his request to his superiors.

I worked in an outpatient setting with clients who had a high "no show" rate. Since the therapists' time was not being "used," the facility was not receiving reimbursement for their time. As a result, we were instructed by the director of the facility to start "double booking" our clients (i.e., scheduling two clients for the same appointment time). This meant that, if one client didn't come, we therapists would be free to see the other clients. Of course, it also meant that, if both clients came, the clients would have to be squeezed into the same time slot—with one waiting while the other was seen and both clients receiving shortened sessions. Despite strong pressure to double book, I refused to comply, but took no steps to ensure that the unethical practice was discontinued.

While working as an art therapist in a hospital rehabilitation program, I was asked to do work that was typically done by an occupational therapist who, in turn, was doing work that a physical therapist usually did. By doing this, the program was saving money, as they still billed for occupational therapy and physical therapy services, respectively. I refused to do the work. It put me in bad graces with the occupational therapy supervisor, and I was let go a year later.

Racial and Religious Discrimination

As the only white (and Jewish) staff member in a public school program, I was the recipient of many bigoted remarks. Once, when I knocked on the door of a classroom, one staff member announced to another, "It's your little white friend." On numerous occasions, the principal of the school—after saying disparaging things about my race—turned to me and said, "You know I don't mean you …" These, as well as anti-Semitic remarks, underscored my "otherness." I felt vulnerable and isolated because of my skin color no matter how hard I worked to create a sense of community and was ashamed of my silence. I learned years later that a colleague had reported the same supervisor for making anti-Semitic remarks to her, and she—not the supervisor—was transferred to another school.

Sexual Harassment

My first job out of graduate school was at a residential psychiatric hospital where I provided art therapy for sex offenders, aged 13–19. During one treatment team meeting, the director of the unit—a seasoned, attractive clinician a decade or two my senior—was addressing the members of a multidisciplinary treatment team about how to respond to the residents' sexual overtures, when he turned to me and said, "For example, if I were to suddenly grab 'Jane's' breast …" I have no idea what he was trying to illustrate. I only know that I was humiliated, and that he had focused the group's attention on the fact that I had breasts.

Another time, some of the patients on the offenders' unit alleged that I was conducting group work with splayed legs and nothing on beneath my dress. The director's response was to bring me into the offenders' day room to process the allegation with all of the residents. The clients were aggressive and intimidating, and corroborated each other's outrageous story. The director provided the opportunity for them to see me in discomfort and near tears, and undermined my ability to work effectively with them. It is likely that he gave them more gratification than they had hoped to achieve with their initial allegations. They emerged empowered and I felt helpless and ashamed.

I wish that, in each situation, I had had the courage to speak to the director about his actions. Instead, I processed my feelings with my direct supervisor, which felt like a safer alternative. In doing so, I deprived the director of the sex offenders' unit of the opportunity to learn from his mishandling of both situations and deprived myself of the feelings of catharsis and empowerment that would have come from confronting him. To be honest, a complicating factor was undoubtedly the attraction I felt for him—something I was not willing, or able, to acknowledge at the time.

When I worked in a public school system, my principal would often hold me up to staff as an example of dedication and efficiency—which did not earn me any friends. On a few occasions, he put his arm around me while praising my efforts, calling me his "star" employee. This made me feel uncomfortable, but I deemed it better to be in his good graces than the alternative. I'm sure that I also felt flattered. I imagine that many young women experience this type of power imbalance and have difficulty expressing their feelings for fear of retribution.

When Supervisors Undermine One's Role

On an in-patient unit, I conducted individual art therapy sessions with a female adolescent who had a history of anxiety, depression, and trauma. In our work, the patient used an *altered book* project to process and contain intense emotions including the urge to self-harm. During a session with her psychotherapist, the patient shared the intense imagery within her altered book. Without consulting me, the talk therapist prompted the patient to cover her artwork with "positive affirmations" and then described the artwork to the patient's psychiatrist, who put in an order that the altered book be treated as contraband and taken away because the imagery could be triggering to other patients. I was given no say in the matter and had to uphold the doctor's order. The patient then started dressing differently, presenting with a mask of brightened affect, and making superficial art in our sessions. After the patient was discharged, she made a suicide attempt. Upon readmission to the hospital, she said that she had been afraid to express her feelings because she felt shamed and punished by the message that the feelings expressed in her artwork were "bad" and needed to be censored.

At the time I felt frustrated that the patient was given the message that her feelings were too intense to explore in the artwork and undermined by the other members of the treatment team, who made their decision without consulting an art therapist. I also felt guilty when the patient was readmitted, because I knew that she had been presenting in a superficial, defended manner, but had felt unable to express my dissenting opinion in rounds with her psychiatrist and therapist. I should have taken the time to address their concerns by explaining the role of an art therapist and the purpose of the book project.

I was working as an art therapy intern at a psychiatric hospital when my clinical supervisor took a leave of absence for two months. The psychiatrist who was appointed to supervise me while she was gone was someone who had previously asked me out, an invitation that I had declined. During the two months that followed, despite how much effort I put into getting him to keep our weekly supervision appointments, he was disinclined to do so. When we did meet, he exhibited what seemed like smugness or disinterest in processing what I perceived as concerns. I really had no one else to turn to and experienced feelings of helplessness and shame, in addition to anger, at how he responded to my need for supervision. When my supervisor returned, I didn't share my experience with her because I knew that she and the psychiatrist were friends. I wish I had discussed my disappointment with the psychiatrist directly; I had nothing to lose and much to gain in terms of confidence.

I vividly remember taking an art therapy course that included a workshop led by a guest speaker, a renowned art therapist. After creating artwork, we were to come to the front of the room as our names were called, where we were to stand, holding our artwork for comments by the speaker. My face reddened as the art therapist proceeded to interpret my piece. Her assessment was painfully accurate and tears ran down my face as I stood in front of the class. She made no mention of the effect of her words. She had demonstrated her skill … at the expense of a student. In the decades that have passed since that workshop, the experience has profoundly influenced not only my clinical work, but also my work as a teacher of art therapy students. I don't "make" students share their artwork with each other or with me; when they do, I don't interpret it. I respect the line between education and therapy.

After not ever being able to get a requisition order filled for art supplies, I raised the issue in a staff meeting. When I explained that I could not do my job as an art therapist without art materials, the director of the department responded, "You're an art therapist—be creative!" I was young and inexperienced but I decided that I would try to show him that I was creative. Knowing that the drawing classes I took had gotten complimentary end-of-lot rolls of paper from a local publishing company, I contacted them and arranged to pick up some free rolls of paper that would otherwise have been discarded. When I proudly showed the director the results of my effort to show incentive, he shouted that soliciting donations was against the law. I still remember how embarrassed and angry I felt. If something similar happened today, I would take the matter to the director's supervisor.

Many years ago, while working an art therapist in a psychiatric hospital, I was required to put on an annual exhibit of artwork that included something from every patient. I was opposed to doing this, as the patients were creating art for therapeutic purposes and not for display and many of the patients did not understand what was being asked of them. As a newly trained art therapist, I was not able to convince the authorities that this practice was not in the best interest of the patients. If such a demand were made today, I would include only those patients who wanted to participate and they would have to be able to give a truly informed consent.

Putting On Your Own Oxygen Mask First

It is easy to blame supervisors and administrators for their transgressions. Many of the contributors, however, indicated that they are still haunted by how they, themselves, handled some of the situations they encountered. We often judge ourselves harshly for not responding in a manner consistent with our values; it is ego-dystonic for us not to treat our clients' needs as paramount. When someone or something compromises our ability to act in accordance with our beliefs, it is important to learn from the experience by considering what we might have done differently, but it is important, also, to treat ourselves with compassion. Neff (2015) developed an eight-week program on learning self-compassion (http://self-compassion.org/about/) which I've found to be useful.

When our best efforts might not be what we'd hoped because we are tired, ill, dealing with counter-transference, or having difficulty maintaining the boundary between our professional and personal lives, it is important not only to seek supervision, consultation, and therapy, but also to practice self-care—which, for art therapists, includes doing artwork. Because most of us work in places where there is only one art therapist, we can experience feelings of isolation, particularly when we believe that our profession is not well understood by staff. Forming and participating in art therapy supervision groups with trusted peers can help to ward off those feelings as we endeavor to learn from our own experiences and those of others. Although "do-overs" don't exist outside of grade school games, it's important to remember that, with subsequent efforts, we will continue to have opportunities to "get it right."

REFLECTIVE ART EXPERIENCES & DISCUSSION QUESTIONS

1. Create an image of *shame* being "held" within a safe space.
2. Draw a continuum from birth to self-forgiveness/self-acceptance and place yourself on that continuum.
3. Imagine you are mentoring yourself when you were new to the profession of art therapy. If possible, recall an actual experience when you felt that you compromised your integrity in a work or practicum setting. How does your more experienced art therapist self respond (emotionally, as well as verbally)?
4. Think of your most positive experience when you were a subordinate or supervisee. Explore why this experience stands apart from others.

References

Art Therapy Credentials Board (2018). *Code of ethics, conduct, and disciplinary procedures*. Retrieved from www.atcb.org/resource/pdf/2016-ATCB-Code-of-Ethics-Conduct-DisciplinaryProcedures.pdf

Gerhardt, P. (2011, September). Ethical supervisor behavior: Why it is so important. Retrieved from https://leadershiplessonsblogdotcom.wordpress.com/2011/09/05/the-ethical-supervisor- behavior

Guest, G. (2013, April). Blowing the whistle on bad behavior takes more than guts. Retrieved from www.highbeam.com/doc/1G1-327987845.html

Harris, D. (2012, July). How to work with the biases you bring to every decision. Retrieved from https://diversitymbamagazine.com/leadership/trust-and-ethics-for-leaders-the-impact-of-biases-by-doug-harris

Neff, K. (2015, September). The five myths of self-compassion. Retrieved from https://greatergood.berkeley.edu/article/item/the_five_myths_of_self_compassion

Reamer, F. (2013, June). Help! My supervisor is unethical. Retrieved from www.socialworktoday.com/news/eoe_062113.shtml

PART III
Drawing to a Close

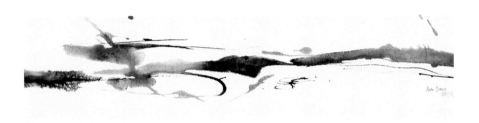

Anne Corson *(see color insert)*

49

FINISHING ART THERAPY WITHOUT THE WORK UNRAVELING

Ethical Issues in Terminating Long-term Therapy with Children

P. Gussie Klorer

It's Just a Little Fox

"I wish I could have this little fox," four-year-old Julie said as we were putting sand-tray toys away at the end of her third-to-last session (for a detailed analysis of this case, see Klorer, 2000, 2017.) Julie was in therapy because her mother had shot Julie and her brother in a murder/suicide. Unlike the others, Julie didn't die.

"Well, we want to keep that toy here for next time you come, so you can play," I said.

"Could I have this to borrow?" she hoped.

"I don't think so. I need to keep all the animals here so that when kids come, they have the animals to play with. Kids like you. You wouldn't want to come here and have an animal not here, would you?"

"I would bring it back the other day."

"Let's leave it here and you can play with it next time."

"I'm mad!" Julie shouted.

The session quickly deteriorated into tears and anguish. Julie stomped out of the room, crying that all she ever wanted was a little fox like that.

"Julie, I think I understand why you want that fox," I said. "I think maybe you want it because you want to have something that represents you and me. I think you've had a good time coming here and you want something to take with you."

"Yeah … *no!*" she shouted as she put her hands over her ears.

"What? You don't want to talk about that? I'm going to really miss you. I wish you would come over here by me so we can talk about it."

"No, I don't want to talk. I'm upset!"

Julie continued to run in and out of the room, while her father and I put away the rest of the toys. She cried that her arms were too tired and that's why she couldn't help clean up. Then she cried because she lost her shoes and, when she remembered where they were, said she was too upset to pick them up. It was a difficult and prolonged ending to another intense session.

Although I had been working with severely traumatized children for over 20 years, I was attached to Julie and my counter-transferential feelings were overwhelming. I didn't want to terminate either. It was a premature termination and she (I?) was not ready, but it was court ordered that she would move out of state to live with her father. The little plastic sand-tray figurine cost less than a dollar and wasn't particularly important in the collection of hundreds of animals. No one ever sought it out and it wasn't even one of her favorite toys. Termination was so hard and she was so sad. I had two more sessions to decide what to do, as I endeavored to terminate our four months of work successfully.

MY ETHICAL DILEMMA

Couldn't I just give her the little fox?

Consider the ethics of simply giving Julie the fox.

How would you respond?

For the writer's response, see Appendix B, page 416.

The Ethics and Challenges of Termination

The Art Therapy Credentials Board's *Code of Ethics, Conduct, and Disciplinary Procedures* (2018) states, "Art therapists shall terminate art therapy when the client has attained stated goals and objectives or fails to benefit from art therapy services" (principle 2.8.1), neither of which was true in the above case. Ethics documents of the American Art Therapy Association (2013) and the American Counseling Association (2014) note that it is the therapist's responsibility to engage the client in a termination process that provides enough time to complete a smooth transition to either another therapist, or independent functioning. But for children in the foster care system or residential treatment centers, placements can be disrupted without notice and judges seldom consider our ethics documents in issuing court orders.

The most important work of therapy often occurs at termination, when issues of loss and abandonment are fully triggered. Because it can be so difficult both for therapist and client, many ethical challenges emerge at termination. Challenges that frequently arise in work with children include a child perceiving termination as punishment rather than a reward (Hutchinson, 1990), a therapist becoming protective or possessive about a client at termination (Kranz & Lund, 1979), and a therapist's rescue fantasies intruding into his or her objectivity. Questions surrounding termination are varied and answers are never simple. For example, is it appropriate to give the client a goodbye gift? Is it appropriate to go back to visit clients in a treatment setting after one has terminated employment there? If a client brings up a bombshell issue at the end of the last session, is it okay to schedule another session so you can reach closure? It would be nice to have clear-cut rules, but frequently the answer is the dreaded "It depends." In 36 years of practice, I have broken the rules on more than one occasion, but always with the client's best interest at heart and after a thorough examination of my own counter-transference.

MY ETHICAL DILEMMA

What happens when a therapist disagrees with a decision made on behalf of a client?

I began working with Lila when she was five years old. Three years later, she had come a long way in her therapy for sexual abuse. She was no longer masturbating and showing children her private parts at school, though symptoms of post-traumatic stress disorder were still prevalent. She had persistent nightmares after visits with her mother and, when she turned 8, she refused to go on any more visits. I testified against the mother in court, whereupon the mother's attorney requested my removal from the case. I was given three weeks to terminate our three years of work together, though the therapy was far from being completed and Lila had formed a therapeutic attachment with me. Explaining to Lila why I could no longer see her was complicated, as I could not speak against the judge despite the fact that I totally disagreed with the ruling. How was I to present this to her when I was just as upset as she was?

How would you respond?

For the writer's response, see Appendix B, page 416.

MY ETHICAL DILEMMA

May a client and a therapist ever become friends?

After termination, the foster mother continued to send me updated pictures of Lila on her first day of school each year and on her ninth and tenth birthdays. The foster mother and I spoke by phone again two years after termination. She said that Lila still talked about and missed me, and we pondered whether a visit would be appropriate. She was still seeing another therapist by court order, so I clearly could not be her therapist. Could we meet in another context, such as a friendly visit? If so, where would be an appropriate place?

> ### How would you respond?
>
> *For the writer's response, see Appendix B, page 417.*

Influence of the Population, Type of Setting, and Length of Treatment

Gil and Crenshaw (2016) devote an entire book to challenging terminations, particularly with child clients, noting that even seasoned therapists are often both stymied and emotionally affected by termination. One of my most challenging terminations occurred when I was leaving a long-term residential treatment center for abused children. I had worked there for nine years and had watched many of the children grow up. Helping children experience themselves as lovable, an important goal of therapy for these children, can be completely undone if the termination is not adequately handled. As the relationships that one develops with maltreated children in this kind of setting are deeply complex, many complications can arise (Klorer, 1993; Nell, 1988). Because of the absence or inconsistent involvement of the parent, the maternal transference and the therapist's counter-transferential reactions can be acutely intense. For example, in addition to providing art therapy, I went swimming, horseback riding, and camping with the children, ate meals with them, and visited with them in their rooms—all things that one does in a family. Although this far exceeded the usual boundaries of a therapist/client relationship, it was perfectly appropriate in a residential setting.

Maintaining professional boundaries at termination was extremely important, so as not to interrupt the work the child would go on to do with a new therapist, yet I also needed to be attentive to the children's inclination to feel abandoned yet again by a parental figure, reinforcing their sense of worthlessness. I decided to meet with each child on my caseload individually—all in the same day—so that they would hear the news directly from me. I allotted four weeks to process with them the reasons for my leaving, their feelings, and their accomplishments in therapy. Although I wanted to give each child a personal gift, that desire reflected my own guilt at leaving, and it would only cause problems when they inevitably compared gifts. Instead, I worked with each child individually to plan how we would say goodbye. When we had begun our work together, I had told the children that, once I got to know them, I would draw their portrait—hoping that they would find this to be an incentive to be open in therapy. At the news of my leaving, many of the children began to ask me to draw their portrait. I honored every request, and on my last day I brought every child a flower, which in retrospect was probably for my own benefit.

What Does an Ethical, Healthful Termination Look Like?

Clients who have time to prepare for termination express feelings about it in advance, reflect upon their growth in therapy, tend to leave therapy feeling more positive than those who have abrupt, unplanned terminations (Knox, 2011). When should one start talking about termination? Leaders of time limited, solution-focused groups might begin talking about termination in the first session. Otherwise, one prepares for termination at least three or four sessions in advance, providing enough time to explore the client's feelings, reflect upon what has been accomplished, review artwork, and plan a way to say goodbye. Co-constructing a meaningful termination through art making eases the stress of termination and provides a tangible symbol of the relationship that the client may keep as a reminder (Dallin, 1986; Franklin, 1981; Gil & Crenshaw, 2016; Headley, Kautzman-East, Pusateri, & Kress, 2015). Today, my work is primarily with children and families in a private practice, so most often I use an "open door" approach to termination (Gil & Crenshaw, 2016); I assure parents and children that I am available if they need to come back, but strongly support their accomplishments and their "graduation" from therapy.

Concluding Thoughts

Termination brings up issues of attachment and loss and strong transference and counter-transferential feelings. It doesn't matter how much experience a therapist has, having someone neutral with whom to process clinical material at termination is imperative. A supervisor or a professional colleague can bring some objectivity to the situation so the therapist can make decisions based solely upon the needs of the client, rather than those of the therapist.

REFLECTIVE ART EXPERIENCES & DISCUSSION QUESTIONS

1. Envision a termination you have experienced that you would love to have an opportunity to "do over." Using art materials, illustrate both versions of this termination.
2. Termination brings up the therapist's issues of loss as well as the client's. Think about a loss in your own life and how a particular client profile might activate feelings of counter-transference.
3. What might you do to stay neutral and boundaried with this client population?
4. Create an art piece to honor the clients you will never see again.
5. Have you ever disagreed with a treatment team's decision about a client on any important issue?
6. How did you handle it then, and would you handle it differently today? Using clay, create a sculpture representing the treatment team and your role on the team.

References

American Art Therapy Association (2013). *Ethical principles for art therapists*. Retrieved from www.americanarttherapyassociation.org/upload/ethicalprinciples.pdf

American Counseling Association (2014). ACA *Code of ethics*. Retrieved from www.counseling. org/docs/ethics/2014-aca-code-of-ethics.pdf?sfvrsn=4

Art Therapy Credentials Board (2018). *Code of ethics, conduct, and disciplinary procedures*. Retrieved from www.atcb.org/resource/pdf/2016-ATCB-Code-of-Ethics-Conduct-DisciplinaryProcedures.pdf

Dallin, B. (1986). Art break: A two-day expressive therapy program using art and psychodrama to further the termination process. *The Arts in Psychotherapy*, 13(2), 137–142. doi:http://dx.doi. org/10.1016/0197-4556(86)90021–3

Franklin, M. (1981). Terminating art therapy with emotionally disturbed children. *American Journal of Art Therapy*, 20(2), 55–57.

Gil, E., & Crenshaw, D. (2016). *Termination challenges in child psychotherapy*. New York: Guilford.

Headley, J.A., Kautzman-East, M., Pusateri, C.G., & Kress, V.E. (2015). Making the intangible tangible: Using expressive art during termination to co-construct meaning. *Journal of Creativity in Mental Health*, 10(1), 89–99.

Hutchinson, R.L. (1990). Termination of counseling with children: Punishment or reward? *Journal of Mental Health Counseling*, 12(2), 228–231.

Klorer, P.G. (1993). Countertransference: A theoretical review and case study with a talented client. *Art Therapy: Journal of the American Art Therapy Association*, 10(3), 32–40.

Klorer, P.G. (2000). *Expressive therapy with troubled children*. Northvale, NJ: Jason Aronson.

Klorer, P.G. (2017). *Expressive therapy with traumatized children* (2nd ed.). New York: Rowman & Littlefield.

Knox, S., Adrians, N., Everson, E., Hess, S., Hill, C., & Crook-Lyon, R. (2011). Clients' perspectives on therapy termination. *Psychotherapy Research*, 21(2), 154–167.

Kranz, P.L., & Lund, N.L. (1979). A dilemma of play therapy termination anxiety in the therapist. *Teaching of Psychology*, 6(2), 108–110.

Nell, R. (1988). Transference and countertransference in a therapeutic commmunity. *Dynamic Psychotherapy*, 6(1), 61–66.

50

WHEN THE ART THERAPIST IS READY TO LEAVE BEFORE THE CLIENT IS

The Ethical Challenges of Closing a Clinical Practice

Deborah A. Good

I don't remember anyone ever talking about ending a clinical practice and the challenges that must be confronted in order to make the best ethical decisions for the clients involved. How do you leave a client who suddenly has a debilitating stroke, or a client whose daughter dies unexpectedly during the last week of treatment? These are some of the challenges I faced when I closed my practice a few months ago.

After working in the mental health field for 44 years and in a group practice for 26 years, after extensive thought and consideration, I made the decision to retire from the group practice. Although the agency did not have clear guidelines as to how to go about closing a long-term practice, I found guidance in the ethical codes of the associations to which I belong—the American Art Therapy Association, the Art Therapy Credentials Board, and the American Counseling Association. My main concerns were to ensure that all my clients—with whom I had worked from 2 to 20 years—were well informed about my retirement date; were given referrals to new therapists if needed; understood that their records would be kept safe by the agency where I worked (Hartsell & Bernstein, 2008); and were provided with a thorough and thoughtful ending to our therapeutic relationship. To prepare them for the inevitable end of our relationship, in January I informed them that I would retire later in the year. Even so, when I spoke with my clients during their scheduled appointments four months before my retirement date, several said that they were disheartened to learn that therapy was coming to an end. As the termination process proceeded, most clients were grateful and encouraging. Some were not.

Responses to My Impending Retirement

MY ETHICAL DILEMMA

Saying goodbye first

Six months before I set my retirement date, I had to undergo a medical procedure. I informed Caryn, a client of mine diagnosed with dissociative identity disorder (DID) and post-traumatic stress disorder (PTSD), that I would be out of the office and unavailable by phone for a few days due to the procedure. Caryn works in the medical field and is rightfully proud of her professional abilities. Even so, the thought of me having a medical issue that needed immediate attention interfered with her sense of stability in our therapeutic relationship. Her diagnosis and serious attachment issues prevented her from digesting the information she was receiving and she immediately chastised me for neglecting my self-care. To her, the affective engagement of our therapeutic or "attachment relationship" (Bowlby, 1969/1982) was threatened and, therefore, she was threatened. She verbally attacked me so viciously that several other therapeutic sessions that were being conducted near my office were interrupted. I let her vent her feelings, then informed her that I had heard her concerns but that the session had become out of control and I hoped that we could talk about this during her session the following week. To continue the discussion with her now would have been futile and would have seriously delayed my sessions with several other clients.

Returning the next week, Caryn apologized for her behavior and stated that she expected an apology from me for yelling at her. I could not agree that I had yelled at her and stated that we would need to *agree to disagree* on that point. Later that evening, Caryn left a message on my private voice mail that she was terminating therapy due to my lack of belief in her perception of the situation. I had hoped that we could use this incident to clarify her reactions to other situations in her past and to address the attachment concerns in an empathetic manner, thus helping her to gain insight into current behaviors that were being influenced by her past trauma.

How would you respond?

For the writer's response, see Appendix B, page 409.

For the writer's response, see Appendix B, page 409.

MY ETHICAL DILEMMA

Too many changes

Ralph's father had recently passed away after a short illness, leaving his mother unable to care for herself. Ralph began having to make frequent cross-country visits to settle the estate, find a healthcare facility for his mother, clear out the house (his childhood home), and prepare it for sale. Ralph had just finished building an addition to his own home so that he and his wife could retire. He had been dealing with some irritating physical problems over the past few years and had developed a facial tic that was embarrassing to him, given his profession as a performer. After undergoing several medical procedures and physical therapy to relieve the condition, he had begun to feel that he could control it by calming his body, relaxing his mind, and being patient with himself. Meditation became an important part of his daily routine.

In January, I informed Ralph that I would be closing my practice in the summer. Over the next few months, he was unable to make regular appointments, due to numerous trips to take care of his mother and her home. His siblings relinquished all responsibility for their mother's well-being to him, leaving him little time to grieve the death of his father and the changes in his mother. He became extremely stressed and overburdened, considered taking medication for anxiety, and thought about being evaluated for situational depression. I encouraged him to speak with his primary doctor.

In the six months before my practice closed, I saw Ralph four times, with long gaps in between. Although I had reminded him of the date of my last day at work and he had promised to see me several times before I retired, he was unable to do so. When I called him to schedule a session during my last week of work, he said that he had to be out of town that week. Ralph was upset. His primary care doctor had just retired, I was retiring, and Ralph felt abandoned. I made a referral to a clinician in my group practice who I thought would be a good fit for him. When I called Ralph to give him information about the referral, he made a comment about me "dumping" him. Since I had Ralph's permission to discuss his case with the clinician to whom I was referring him, I immediately spoke with the therapist to set up the earliest appointment available with Ralph and to monitor his emotional state.

How would you respond?

For the writer's response, see Appendix B, page 409.

MY ETHICAL DILEMMA

Refusal to terminate

Betsy was a middle-aged woman who had begun therapy with me 20 years before. She had been having nightmares of childhood abuse and trauma and thought that art therapy would help. She was obviously very wounded and reported numerous abusive relationships as a child and as an adult. She was sarcastic and often verbally abrasive, which irritated her coworkers and impacted her work performance.

Betsy was able to feel safe in art therapy and came weekly, often creating art between sessions to stabilize her emotions. Over two decades of therapy, she created images that expressed great pain, internal fragmentation, and extreme loneliness, complicated by haunting memories of abuse. Although Betsy was diagnosed with PTSD, her behavior reflected perceptual and interpersonal distortion indicative of a personality disorder (van der Kolk, McFarlane & Weisaeth, 2007), specifically Borderline Personality Disorder (American Psychiatric Association, 1994). Her therapy focused upon helping her to understand the way she presented herself to others and how that affected her relationships, increasing her self-regulation skills, reducing intrusive memories, and enhancing her self-care. When it became evident that Betsy experienced dissociative episodes as a means of coping with intrusive traumatic thoughts, therapy also included grounding techniques and art activities that she could do at home to remain focused on the present.

Betsy's relationships were intense, followed by feelings of rejection. Friendships never lasted and social interactions diminished. Therapy seemed to be her one consistently safe place. Over-dependence upon the therapeutic relationship colored the transference; instead of serving as a foundation from which to move to healthier relationships, it became a place from which she could not bear to move, a state that indicated a lack of proper attachment at an early age and the development of attachment insecurity (Ein-Dor, 2015).

Throughout our work, Betsy drew many pictures that depicted her intense fear that "something" would happen to me. She seemed to believe that if something dreadful happened to me, then something terrible would happen to her. Figure 50.1 reflects her intense fear of flying and shows me parachuting out of a burning airplane.

While approaching Betsy with compassion, it was continually necessary to construct and model healthful boundaries and reframe situations as they arose. Retraining behavioral responses takes hours of restructuring situations and the reactions they generate. Art therapy provided an excellent place to explore these issues, as diagramming or cartooning her interactions was extremely effective. Drawing paper became a place on which to work out appropriate and inappropriate reactions to situations by illustrating the possible consequences of each behavioral choice. Betsy seemed to be doing better and changed her appointments to every other week.

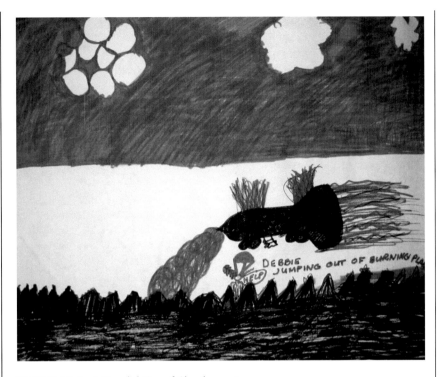

FIGURE 50.1 *A Dreaded Fear of Abandonment.*

Betsy decided that she would like to increase her social activities and find ways to use her talents. She decided to join a choir where she could sing and possibly play one of the many instruments she has mastered. When I met with her after I'd returned from vacation, she reported that her anxiety had lessened during my absence. She had employed the art and grounding techniques that we had discussed and had found a choir to join where she had met several people with whom she felt comfortable. When asked to tell me more about the choir she had joined, she said it was at a church—a church she knew to be my church.

I must admit to being stunned by Betsy's announcement. The city in which I live often seems like a small town and, at times, my life crosses those of clients and former clients. I deeply respect my clients' privacy and approach them only when invited or when they approach me. It can be awkward when asked by a friend or family member who it was that I greeted. When pressed for an answer, I respond with a comment suggested by a client, "I know them professionally." I've found this explanation to be sufficient and to cover a wide sweep of possibilities. Initially, it seemed as if Betsy respected my privacy and our out-of-session interaction was minimal. I held in highest confidence the fact that she was my client and no one in the church was aware of our professional relationship.

Betsy often spoke about retiring from her job in a year and finding something else to do to supplement her retirement income. When I told her that I would be closing my practice the summer that she planned to retire and encouraged her to use the time we had left in therapy to work out the issues around her retirement and our relationship ending, she reluctantly agreed. That was a year before I closed my practice. Six months later, Betsy started the session by telling me that she had gone to our pastor to let her know about her past sexual abuse and had mentioned that I was her therapist. She said that she told the pastor that I was changing and seemed more distant; she feared that I was about to retire and she was not prepared for that to happen. When I reminded her of our conversation six months earlier, she said that she didn't want to think about that. I reassured her that I had given her plenty of notice and that we had six more months to work on issues related to her retirement. She drew triangles, the safe drawing that she reverted to whenever she felt threatened or stressed. Triangles, heavily colored in and outlined, denote a level of emotional stress in a much-regressed state (Bender, 1938, 1946; Drachnik, 1995). Research by Rhyne (1979) and Spring (1993) states that wedge forms or triangles appear in drawings when the client feels threatened, anxious, or excited.

Betsy was stressed about the changes in her life. She was being forced to end a therapeutic relationship in which she felt unconditionally accepted and the thought of beginning therapy with an unknown person was frightening. As much as she wanted to quit her job, she didn't have another one and financial security was a major concern. Although she had plenty of time to secure supplemental employment, Betsy made no effort to apply for jobs before I closed my practice.

If I see Betsy now at church, she often wants time to talk privately. She sent a card to my home saying that she misses me and she has called my private voice mail to give me updates on her situation.

How would you respond?

For the writer's response, see Appendix B, page 410.

MY ETHICAL DILEMMA

No one saw it coming

Carina is chronically depressed, with a chemical imbalance that often throws her into the depths of despair. When her depressive episodes occur, she cries inconsolably and doesn't leave her home for days. Multiple physical ailments hinder her from consistently working. She was referred to me for art therapy 10 years ago because of her creative interests. Despite chronic pain, Carina continues to make art of various forms, which brings her great joy and satisfaction. Over the years, we have discovered that, when she loses interest in her artistic endeavors, it is a sign that her depression is getting worse; when her medication is working, her creative production is prolific. Several of her fiber and ceramic creations are shown in Figure 50.2.

Carina lives alone, with no close relatives nearby. Her parents are deceased and she has a strained relationship with her sisters, who live out of state. She continually grieves family relationships that she wishes were more nurturing and berates herself for not being more likeable, pretty, or loved. She blames herself for the death of her mother, who passed away right before we started working together, believing that there had to be something she could have done. Her mother died of complications from Alzheimer's disease. Carina worries that she may be developing symptoms similar to those of her mother and is concerned about who would care for her if something happened to her.

Carina's church is the center of most of her activities and the church community has become a surrogate family for her. The church also supports her therapy, which she attends weekly. The consistency of a nurturing, unconditional relationship seems to fill a void in Carina's life. When I told her that I was going to retire, she became very worried. Although we had arranged for her to be transferred to another therapist within the agency, that work had not begun by the time I retired.

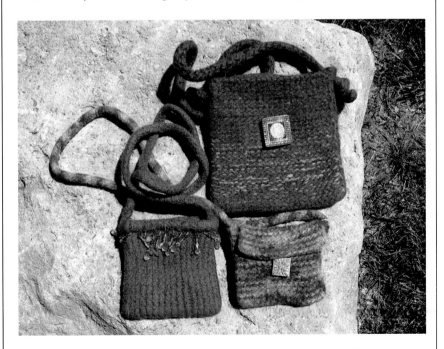

FIGURE 50.2 Boiled wool knitted purses with ceramic buttons, by Carina.

One week after I retired, Carina had a massive, debilitating stroke that left her bedridden and unable to walk or use her hands. Her depression increased with her inability to understand what had happened to her. I was called and informed that Carina had had a stroke and that she had been asking for me. She was hospitalized and her sisters were arriving in town to make permanent arrangements for her care. She would be restricted to a nursing home for the rest of her life.

How would you respond?

For the writer's response, see Appendix B, page 410.

MY ETHICAL DILEMMA

Impossible termination

Noreen was searching for answers to questions about her past that haunted her but were ill defined, other than causing a deep feeling of unrest. She had been married several times and had two children when she was a teenager. She had one friend and participated in few social activities. Several physical problems prevented her from doing many of the things that had previously brought her satisfaction. Noreen hoped that therapy could help her to deal with the changes in her life and with the feelings of angst that were associated with her past.

Since Noreen didn't want to draw, I offered her a range of collage materials and paper. Immediately, she began to tear out magazine pictures and place them on the paper, carefully moving them around until they were exactly where she wanted them. After making several collages, she turned to me and said, "Tell me about them." I began by asking her questions about the placement of images on the page, the relationship of each image to another, and why she chose the images she did. Slowly, the collages began to tell a story. One day, Noreen brought in several framed pictures of her mother and her aunt and told me stories about their relationship, their characters and personalities, and, eventually, about their lives and deaths. Through continued collage work, she remembered sounds and smells that triggered memories. About this time, Noreen's cousin came to visit her and they talked for an entire afternoon about the family and what each of them remembered. By the end of the day, they had pieced together a comprehensive memory of their family's past. Noreen was saddened by what she discovered, but relieved to know the truth about her family.

Art therapy and a rekindled relationship with her cousin helped Noreen to uncover what had been bothering her and what had been missing in her life. She started sleeping better and began to work on health issues that had remained unresolved for months. She told me that she was ready to end therapy and did not want a referral to another therapist when I retired. I felt good about her progress and agreed with her.

A week before my last day at work, Noreen's daughter died unexpectedly. She was devastated, guilt-ridden because she wasn't with her, and at a loss as to how to deal with her grief. She had to cancel our last session, because she had to leave town to take care of her daughter's remains.

How would you respond?

For the writer's response, see Appendix B, page 410.

Concluding Thoughts

It is important to maintain an emotional distance when working with people who have DID, severe PTSD, or dual diagnoses. A balance must be kept between engaging with the client to resolve the presenting dilemma and becoming emotionally entangled in the client's story and past trauma. I easily could have become angry, hurt, or offended by the way in which Caryn and Betsy treated me. Remembering that this is how the client's pathology presents itself helps to depersonalize acts of aggressive or passive-aggressive behavior. It also demonstrates how the client interacts with other people in their lives and explains their lack of ability to maintain healthy, long-term relationships.

Clients who are dealing with any level of depression are not thinking clearly and depend upon the therapist to help them to make decisions that are in their best interest. The deep relationship between client and therapist provides a safe place for self-expression that is difficult to find in other aspects of many clients' lives. Helping clients to find a new place of intimate safety can be challenging, but an important part of the process of closing a practice is empowering clients to start over with a new therapist.

In closing my clinical practice, I was not aware of the many layers and possible scenarios that could be involved in the process of ending so many therapeutic relationships at the same time. On the day that I finished cleaning out my office, my responsibilities to the clients with whom I had terminated did not end. The dilemma of how long to continue to assist clients in transitioning out of therapy with me and into a new therapeutic relationship could be answered only on a case-by-case basis.

REFLECTIVE ART EXPERIENCES & DISCUSSION QUESTIONS

1. Ending a clinical practice is an emotional, as well as a professional, experience. How would you depict the emotional feelings related to transitioning into a different persona in your life? What would it look like to make this professional shift? Create an art piece that reflects your emotional responses to making these life changes and then a piece that reflects your professional responses

to making these changes. Compare the two art creations and dialogue with them in a journal.

2. Envision what it means to have your ethical boundaries tested over and over again. Give that image shape, color, and form. Now, envision those boundaries broken. Give this image shape, color, and form. Compare them and journal your reactions to this creative experience.

3. How do you deal with the emotional stress of hearing and seeing images of your client's pain and angst? What kind of self-care do you do on a regular basis?

4. How do you know what therapist would be a good clinical referral for your client when you are not able to continue as his or her therapist? What criteria would you use to make that decision?

References

American Psychiatric Association (1994). *Diagnostic and statistical manual of mental disorders* (4th ed.). Washington, DC: Author.

Bender, L. (1938). *A visual motor Gestalt test and its clinical use.* New York: American Orthopsychiatric Association.

Bender, L. (1946). *A Bender motor gestalt test.* Washington, DC: American Orthopsychiatric Association.

Bowlby, J. (1982). *Attachment and loss. Volume 1: Attachment.* New York: Basic Books. (Original work published 1969.)

Drachnik, C. (1995). *Interpreting metaphors in children's drawings.* Burlingame, CA: Abbeygate Press.

Ein-Dor, T. (2015). Attachment dispositions and human defensive behavior. *Personality and Individual Differences*, 81, 112–116.

Hartsell, T.L. & Bernstein, B.E. (2008). *The portable ethicist for mental health professionals.* Hoboken, NJ: John Wiley & Sons.

Rhyne, J. (1979). *Drawings as personal construct: A study in visual dynamics.* Unpublished doctoral dissertation. University of California, Santa Cruz, CA.

Spring, D. (1993). *Shattered images: Phenomenological language of sexual trauma.* Chicago, IL: Magnolia Street.

van der Kolk, B., McFarlane, A., & Weisaeth, L. (Eds.) (2007). *Traumatic stress: The effects of overwhelming experience of mind, body and society.* New York: Guilford Press.

Appendix A
THE PRIVATE PRACTICE CONTRACT

Anne Mills

What appears on the following six pages is the private practice contract that Anne Mills developed in 2017. As mentioned in Chapter 2, as society, ethics codes, and laws change, clarifications must be made and new issues addressed. For that reason, she updates her contract three times a year.

Anne states that readers are welcome to use all, or to adapt any part, of her contract. However, readers should also be warned that it is their responsibility—and theirs alone—to adapt the contract in accordance with the laws, regulations, and ethics codes to which they are subject at the time that they make use of this document, and to have it reviewed and revised by a lawyer specializing in mental health law.

Anne writes as the sole proprietor of an unincorporated business in an American city. She is the only therapist in the practice. She offers art therapy and other mental health services to children and adults, as well as supervision and consultation to mental health professionals. To whatever extent this description does not match you or your practice, your policies (and thus your contract) may differ substantially. Preferences and solutions that work for Anne's business may not be appropriate for yours. Other cautions can be found throughout Chapter 2.

Anne Mills, MA, ATR-BC, LCPAT, LPC
Registered and Board Certified Art Therapist
Licensed Professional Counselor #PRC 1127

Art Therapy Services
P.O. Box 9853, Alexandria, Virginia, 22304
phone (703) 914-1078 fax (703) 663-8817
<annemills@cox.net> http://www.anne-mills.com/

Studio/Office: 3811 Porter St. NW, 2nd floor, Washington, D.C. 20016

Welcome to my practice. I am pleased to have the opportunity to serve you. Please ask questions at any time. This document contains important information about my services, business policies, and your privacy and other rights. Summary information is given about the Health Insurance Portability and Accountability Act (HIPAA), a federal law that covers the use and disclosure of your Protected Health Information (PHI).

Services Offered

I am a licensed professional counselor in the District of Columbia, where I practice, and am a registered and board certified art therapist. I am a licensed clinical professional art therapist in Maryland. I offer art therapy evaluations, art psychotherapy, counseling, consultation by Skype, Intensive Trauma Therapy, hypnotherapy, family art evaluations, sandtray, Eye Movement Desensitization and Re-processing (EMDR), and other related services. I have no specialized training in distance counseling.

The process of making art may be tremendously beneficial to some individuals while, at the same time, there are some risks. The risks may include increased awareness of feelings, facing unpleasant thoughts, or alteration of an individual's ability to deal effectively with others. I am available to discuss any possible negative side effects of our work together.

Art therapy is not like a medical doctor visit, and there are no guarantees of what you will experience. Instead, it calls for a very active effort on your part. In order to have a successful experience, you will have to work on things we talk about, during our sessions and at home.

Should you become involved in legal proceedings that require my participation, you will be expected to pay for my professional time and expenses, even if I am called to testify by another party. Court proceedings are often adversarial experiences. You may have the right to protect certain information that I may be called to testify about. I strongly encourage you to engage an attorney to advise you about your rights. My role and my fees differ for this service and I will provide you with my fees in the event that I am called to testify. I would appreciate it if you would discuss this with me in advance and I also refer you to the section below regarding confidentiality.

Because of the nature of my practice, I often require as a precondition that you have a treatment team. In this way, I can best serve the needs of the client who is dealing with especially difficult issues, is distressed, or where the use of medication or hospitalization may be required. When I am working as part of a team, I will ask that you sign a release form to allow me to discuss our work in order to collaborate as a team. When you have a treatment team, it is

46 important that you are clear about who is your 'primary therapist'—that is, the person who you
47 see most often and your main professional resource outside of sessions. My expectation is that
48 the primary therapist will be updated at regular intervals on the work you are doing with other
49 team members.
50
51 <u>Contact Information</u>
52
53 Please tell me how you wish to be contacted for routine matters: ___ personal e-mail
54 ___ work e-mail ___ mobile phone ___home phone ___ work phone ___ postal mail. Your
55 signature on this contract authorizes me to contact you by the check marked methods.
56 Due to my work schedule, I am usually not immediately available by telephone. You can
57 leave a confidential voice message for me at the number above. I check for messages once a day and
58 I use my best efforts to return calls within 24 hours or the next business day.
59 If you need to contact me between sessions, the best way is by texting. Telephoning is
60 second best, and my voicemail is a safe and confidential place to leave personal information.
61 Normal unencrypted e-mail is good for setting up appointment times. Encrypted e-mail is a good
62 way to update me with feedback or detailed information.
63 If you use e-mail to send content related to your therapy sessions, please know that it may not
64 be secure or confidential. If you choose to communicate with me by e-mail, please be aware that all
65 e-mails are retained in the logs of your and my internet service providers. While it is unlikely that
66 someone will be looking at these logs, they are available to be read by the system administrator(s) of
67 the internet service provider. You should also know that I print out and store electronically all e-
68 mails and texts that I receive from you and all e-mails and texts that I send to you, and they become
69 part of your treatment record. **If you contact me between sessions, I will understand that you are**
70 **giving me permission to respond using the same medium, which may not be secure or**
71 **confidential.** For example, if you e-mail me using normal unencrypted e-mail, I will understand that
72 you are giving me permission to respond using normal unencrypted e-mail.
73 For encrypted e-mail, I use Hushmail <arttherapyservices@hushmail.com> You can get a
74 free Hushmail account, but you have to log in once every three weeks to maintain the account.
75 Please note Hushmail has size limitations that will affect your ability to send and store large files like
76 art images. Please notify me by telephone or e-mail to <u>annemills@cox.net</u> when you have sent a
77 message to me by Hushmail; I may not see it otherwise.
78
79 <u>Safety and well-being</u>
80
81 Your safety and well being are very important to me. During sessions I ask that you not harm
82 yourself, or the office, or me. I expect you to inform me by a telephone message if you are in distress
83 between sessions and I expect you to follow your self-care plan. You are informing me so that I will
84 have the information and you will know that it is time for you to activate your own supports.
85 **If you need an immediate response, are unsafe, or are experiencing a life-**
86 **threatening emergency, go to the nearest hospital emergency room and request to**
87 **be seen by a mental health professional immediately.**
88 Should updates or requests for support between sessions become lengthy or customary, we
89 will discuss instituting a prorated fee for these services.
90

91	<u>Timely payment and late cancellation policy</u>
92	
93	Your initial fee is $\_\_\_\_$ (co-pay is $\_\_\_\_$) for a 45 minute session, and $\_\_\_\_$ for a 53
94	minute or longer session. I may make an annual adjustment to this fee and will provide you at least
95	60 days notice of any change to your fee. The charge includes art supplies, record keeping,
96	collaboration with other members of your healthcare team as needed, preparation for sessions and all
97	other related tasks. Charges may differ for family, group, or extended sessions. I charge an
98	additional prorated fee for specialized reports that you may ask me to prepare, and for customized
99	CDs or mp3s for relaxation, etc. Your signature on this contract indicates that you understand you
100	are responsible to pay me in full at the time service is provided, regardless of whether the fee is
101	covered by your insurance, such as co-pays or deductibles.
102	You must pay for the session before it begins, unless other arrangements are made.
103	A $20 late fee will be charged per month on any overdue balances of 30 days or more.
104	Consistent therapy appointments develop a rhythm that is conducive to steady progress. My
105	services are by appointment only, and I commit to a specific time just for you. If either of us is
106	unable to keep an appointment, every effort should be made to tell the other well in advance. My
107	schedule is usually very busy; thus, the cancellation or re-scheduling of an appointment without
108	sufficient notice means the loss of a therapy appointment that could have been scheduled for
109	someone else. My policy is that if you fail to arrive for your session or cancel it with less than 24
110	hours advance, a charge at the usual rate for a 45 minute session (not the copay amount) will be
111	levied. I cannot bill your insurance company for such a charge. It is your responsibility.
112	Payment can be made by cash, check, PayPal, or credit card. Please let me know if you want
113	a receipt for your insurer, a statement for tax purposes, or to leave your credit card on file with me
114	with permission to run charges as above. I do not send monthly statements. Upon request, I will
115	provide you with a receipt for your payment, or a summary of charges and payments received. Your
116	signature on this contract serves as your "signature on file", authorizing me to use electronic billing
117	as needed.
118	
119	<u>Distance counseling</u>
120	
121	You have the right to choose to work with a counselor face-to-face rather than on the phone
122	or by electronic means.
123	A benefit of phone counseling is it may lower the barriers to receiving help. A risk in phone
124	counseling is the absence of non-verbal information, which may slow communications down and/or
125	result in inaccurate or incomplete impressions. I use a cell phone, which is unsecured and therefore
126	may limit the confidentiality of our conversations.
127	Our successful work will depend on maintaining a private meeting time without
128	interruptions, and preventing potential misunderstandings arising from the lack of visual clues or
129	equipment failure. My expectation is that we will both strive to state what we observe out loud in
130	the moment. This will allow us to double check the accuracy of our perceptions.
131	Claims submitted to health insurance companies for distance counseling or teletherapy may
132	be denied.
133	When feasible, we will meet face-to-face.
134	
135	<u>Beginning and ending treatment</u>
136	

137   Your signature on this contract is your consent to treatment by me. Although the chances for
138 achieving your goals for therapy will be best met by adhering to therapeutic suggestions, you
139 understand that you have the right to discontinue or refuse treatment at any time. When you are
140 ready to leave, I will assist you with your transition and would appreciate receiving several weeks
141 advance notice. When you provide notice of terminating therapy, it will allow me to assist you as
142 your counselor. I also reserve the right to terminate counseling sessions if you fail to perform any
143 responsibilities as set forth in this contract or if you threaten or harm me in any way. If I terminate
144 my services, I will endeavor to provide you with several weeks notice, if possible. If you request a
145 referral, I will make my best efforts to provide you with a referral to another therapist. Additionally,
146 if you terminate working with any member of your treatment team, you need to notify me of that in
147 advance, as well.
148   I feel strongly about the importance of allowing adequate time and discussion for your
149 feelings about termination and other disruptions of treatment. If it is at all possible, I will make
150 arrangements so that you can do that work with me directly. However, if, due to circumstances
151 beyond my control, I am unable to continue my counseling practice or keep any further
152 appointments, I ask that you allow another therapist to assist you in that process. I have designated a
153 colleague as my professional executor, in the case of my death or disability, to have access to your
154 records to update you, to provide psychological services if needed, or to refer to another qualified
155 professional if needed. I have every confidence my professional executor will handle this transition
156 period ethically, confidently, and discreetly for us all.
157   If you stop seeing me and do not respond to my attempts to reach you, you are no longer in
158 therapy with me. Our work will be considered to have ended 10 days after my first attempt to reach
159 you.
160   Art produced in our sessions, which is your property, will remain in my safekeeping during
161 the course of our work. Your artwork is kept strictly confidential. When our relationship ends, you
162 will take your art with you and I will take photographs of your work to retain for my records.
163
164 Social media policy
165
166   It is NOT a regular part of my practice to search for clients on Google or other search
167 engines. This is out of respect for your privacy. If there are things you wish to share with me from
168 your online life, I strongly encourage you to bring them into our sessions where we can talk about
169 them together, during the therapy session.
170   I do not accept or make friend requests of current or former clients. Please be aware that I
171 will not follow you or friend you. This holds true on LinkedIn and all other social networking sites.
172 If you have questions about this, please feel free to bring it up during a session.
173   If you use Foursquare, Uber, or other location tracking services, please be aware that
174 appearing at the location of my studio/office regularly may compromise your privacy. You may
175 want to bear this in mind, or turn apps like this off when on the way to a session.
176
177 Referrals
178
179   My practice operates on referrals, and I welcome working with clients you think may benefit
180 from therapy with me.
181
182 Limits on Confidentiality

183
184   The code of ethics of the American Art Therapy Association, the Art Therapy Credentialing
185 Board, the American Counseling Association, state law, and the federal HIPAA Act all protect the
186 privacy of communications between you and me. In most cases, I can only release information
187 about your treatment to others if you sign a written authorization. You can revoke the authorization
188 at any time, unless I have taken action in reliance on it. However, there are some disclosures that do
189 not require the client's authorization, as follows:
190   -where I am subpoenaed by a court and you have not filed a timely objection;
191   - where a Court order has authorized the release of information
192   -if a government agency is requesting the information for health oversight activities
193   -if a client files a complaint against me, I may disclose relevant information in order
194 to defend myself
195   -when a client files a worker's compensation claim, upon appropriate request, I must
196 provide a copy of the record to the D.C. Office of Hearings and Adjudications, the employer, or
197 insurer
198   -if required by health insurers whose involvement the client has requested
199   -if I know or have reason to suspect that a child has been or is in immediate danger of
200 being neglected or mentally or physically abused
201   -if I have substantial cause to believe that an adult is in need of protective services
202 because of abuse, neglect, or exploitation by someone other than my client
203   -if I believe that a client presents a substantial risk of imminent and serious injury to
204 another individual, I may be required to take protective actions. These actions may   include
205 notifying the potential victim, contact the police, or seeking hospitalization for the client.
206   -in an emergency, if I believe that a client presents a substantial risk of imminent and
207 serious injury to him/herself, I may be required to take protective actions, including notifying
208 individuals who can protect the client or initiating emergency hospitalization.
209   I strongly encourage you to consult an attorney who would be able to advise you in these
210 situations. In all other situations, I will ask you for an advance authorization before disclosing any
211 information about you or showing your art.
212
213 <u>Professional Records</u>
214
215   You should be aware that, pursuant to HIPAA and as of April 2003, I keep Protected Health
216 Information about you in two sets of professional records. One set is your Record of Consultation;
217 the other is my Notes. The Record of Consultation includes information about your reason for
218 seeking my services, a description of the ways in which your problem affects your life, our goals,
219 your progress, your treatment history including records I have received from other professionals, and
220 dates on which we have met. Except in unusual circumstances that involve a substantial risk of
221 emotional impairment or serious physical danger to yourself and others, you may examine and/or
222 receive a copy of your Record of Consultation, if you request it in writing. Because these are
223 professional records, they can be misinterpreted or be upsetting to untrained readers. For this reason,
224 I recommend you initially view them in my presence, or have them forwarded to a mental health
225 professional so you can discuss the contents. If I refuse your request for access to your records, you
226 have a right of review, which I will discuss with you upon request.
227   The Notes are for my own use and are to help me provide you with the best services. The
228 Notes contain contents of our conversations, my thoughts on those conversations, and how they

229 affect your work with me. The Notes also contain sensitive information that you may reveal to me
230 which is not required to be included in your Record of Consultation. The Notes are separate from
231 the Record of Consultation, and cannot be sent to anyone without your signed authorization.
232 Insurance companies cannot require your authorization as a condition of coverage nor penalize you
233 in any way for your refusal to provide it.
234
235 Your Consent to Treatment and Your Rights
236
237 You have certain rights with regard to your Record of Consultation and disclosures of
238 protected health information. These rights include: requesting that I amend your record; requesting
239 restrictions on what information is disclosed to others; and requesting an accounting of disclosures
240 of protected health information that you did not authorize.
241 If you are concerned that I have violated your privacy rights, or you disagree with a decision
242 I made about access to your records, you may send a written complaint to the Secretary, U.S.
243 Department of Health and Human Services. I can give you the address if needed. The Art Therapy
244 Credentials Board oversees the ethical practice of art therapists and may be contacted with client
245 concerns (3 Terrace Way Greensboro, NC 27403-3660 Toll Free - (877)213-2822).
246 When you sign this agreement, you acknowledge that you have been given HIPAA-related
247 information about your personal health information, and that we agree to work together according to
248 this agreement. You may revoke this agreement in writing at any time. That revocation will be
249 binding unless I have taken action in reliance on it (for example, if you have not satisfied any
250 financial obligations you have incurred).
251 I again welcome you to our work together. It is my honor to be of service to you.
252
253
254
255 _____
256 Anne Mills, MA, ATR-BC, LCAT, LPC
257
258 I have read the above material and accept its terms.
259
260
261 _____
262 Signature and date
263 If signing as the legally authorized custodial parent, please give me a copy of the appropriate
264 papers for my records.

Appendix B
CHAPTER WRITERS' RESOLUTIONS TO THEIR ETHICAL DILEMMAS

(Alphabetized by author surname)

Maria Regina A. Alfonso

When there is a power dynamic between a psychosocial support team and the survivors of a disaster, should it be addressed? If so, how?

We decided to engage with the community despite our concern about some volunteers' perceptions of indigenous people, because of our trust in the character, professionalism, and competence of the volunteer team, and the process of art-making. To address our concern, trainers accompanied volunteers during the visits, gently reminding them of our role to facilitate the community's rediscovery of their own power and capacity for self-healing. We also led by action, approaching each community with compassion and respect for the Tagbanua culture and practicing heart-based listening, confident that the volunteers would follow suit.

After returning from the islands, we discussed the volunteers' perceptions of the community's needs, capacities, and resources, based upon the intercultural-indigenous storytelling (Macneill, 2014) in which we had engaged. One story among many stood out to illustrate the community's strength in solidarity: a mother recalled how, at the height of the storm, families from all over the island spread out in a successful attempt to find a neighbor's missing daughter. A deeper awareness and respect for the self-efficacy of the communities emerged, as did the volunteers' appreciation of the rich, intangible yet palpable treasures in each community: solidarity, hope, a love of music and dance.

Is it ethical to introduce mainstream arts-based approaches into an indigenous community that has its own cultural heritage and practices?

If one decides to engage, how does one proceed?

Learning about the "*suring*" helped us decide how to begin our next visit. The usual "*kamustahan*" was followed by the volunteers asking to learn the "*suring*"—a request that was met with incredible enthusiasm, as community elders and children jumped to their feet, eager to share. After demonstrating the "*suring*," they went on to teach the volunteers other dances, songs, and chants. This allowed the facilitators to ask if they might share some other things that might also be helpful for relaxing, which led to the introduction of the basics of breathing and tapping, and the use of local art materials to create nature sculptures. The community's eager response equaled if not surpassed their excitement to teach us their ways of coping. First honoring the practices of the Tagbanua made all of the difference to this community-centered, cross-cultural arts integration process and dissipated any (albeit unintended) power dynamic.

Would it benefit a community to take part in a post-disaster psychosocial support program that does not have a long-term plan for sustainability?

Little did we realize that part of the solution to the critical issue of sustainability would be—a boat! The reconstruction of boats, which was part of the ongoing collaborative rebuilding program for the islands, of which Cartwheel Foundation was a part, meant that the means by which the Tagbanua earned their livelihood was restored. As harvesters of seaweed, boats are essential to their survival. Upon selling their harvest in Culion, they were able to buy basic necessities, including coffee (fuel for their spirits!) and fuel for their boats! This also resolved the issue of access to health care and to continued psychosocial support from the team on the mainland. In addition, each island school's Cartwheel volunteer teachers (who are part of the support team) would be trained to integrate art-based psychosocial activities in their classrooms, to establish long-term healing spaces for students and their parents. Follow-up visits to the islands by the teams would take place over at least the next four years.

If the community has expressed a need for coffee, why bring art supplies?

While we wanted to bring coffee as a gift, since it was identified as a way of coping, we were concerned that doing so might perpetuate what we'd learned was an existing culture of dependence upon outsiders for material goods. As we thought this through, we wondered if other realities, such as the Tagbanua community's generally timid nature, due to their marginalization in society, might also be related to this issue. While the unavailability of coffee might be considered a life threatening concern by mothers (given the scarcity of food for their babies), we decided to use this information to inform our health and nutrition program focused on mothers and children, which was under way. Fortunately, we were pleased to observe that our gift of art making nourished the community in another way, awakening them to the beauty of their own indigenous art forms and providing something that was more sustaining than coffee!

Reference

Macneill, P. (Ed.). (2014). *Ethics and the arts*. New York: Springer.

Mercedes Ballbé ter Maat

To work effectively with immigrant families, must I unlearn what I've been taught about conducting art therapy and psychotherapy?

Although the art therapy that I practiced in the school system didn't look like the art therapy that I'd practiced at the psychiatric hospital, yes, it was ethical. I had bent a few rules and guidelines to incorporate cultural norms that would create a sense of community and set the stage for trust and positive therapeutic interventions. I would do it all over again.

Could I lead an effective art therapy group, given the current group's cultural norms and social psychology orientation?

My decision was neither to change nor to conform, but to compromise. I chose to stretch boundaries without crossing them, by incorporating the positive aspects of both worlds—strengths from my art therapy training and practice in the US and from what I was learning in this community setting. I picked and chose the behaviors and standards that I thought would work best from the fields of art therapy and social psychology, the gray areas of ethics, and, just as importantly, both cultural ways.

I introduced art therapy as an alternative way of communicating, connecting, and sharing thoughts and feelings. One important difference in the structure of this group was that now everyone had a chance to participate, not just two or three, as in the past. We continued to meet in the kitchen, the same casual, friendly environment where *mate* was passed around and cake and *masitas* were eaten. I kissed everyone on the way in and on the way out, and at the end of the day I caught car rides with participants to the center of town to catch the bus home. Smoking was an issue for me; I could not tolerate the amount of smoke in the room, so we compromised by cutting down the smoking to a few puffs near the opened window. I added a table so that all had a place to draw and introduced the basic tenets of art therapy, possible themes, and two-dimensional art materials. The participants were willing to try something new because I was "one of them."

The last thing to work out was the concept of time. Should I continue the tradition of members arriving for group at leisure and leaving when the conversation was exhausted? This practice had worked well due to minimal expectations regarding attendance and participation. Or should I suggest an alternative structure, one that was more in line with my adopted whiteness, training, and practice in the US; one that I knew to be effective? Imposing my values was never my intention, yet I wanted to introduce a structure that would enable everyone to draw, share, and experience the benefits of group art therapy. So, I announced that I would start the group at 17:00 hours and end it at 20:00 hours. To my surprise, almost everyone arrived on time that first group, eager to follow the suggested themes and begin to draw. With very little guidance, they took turns sharing their drawings, giving feedback to each other, and supporting the bond that they had already developed. They even agreed to stay past 20:00 hours when everyone hadn't yet had the opportunity to share. At the end of the group, participants brought up the group rules, encouraging each other to arrive at the center on time the following week, otherwise they would be late for the art therapy group.

The transformation was astonishing—for them and for me. They devoured art therapy. They seemed hungry for structure, for the opportunity to draw and to work on their issues while listening to each other in a supportive way. They appreciated my gentle yet confronting style, in contrast to that of the social psychologists, which was more "in your face." I learned to observe, to remain quiet, and to broaden an understanding of art therapy that incorporated what I knew in my head with what I felt in my heart.

Heidi Bardot

Can biases ever be right?

We made an executive decision to pull the students out of the internship for their own emotional well-being. We recognized that it would be unfeasible, and possibly damaging, for them to continue and could greatly affect their learning and experiences. Before contacting the site, we communicated the situation to our local contacts and brainstormed regarding not only how to tell the site in a culturally sensitive manner (rather than as *Westerners* coming into their organization and telling them what they were doing wrong), but also what we could do to affect the practice. Our local contact got in touch with a friend who was a human rights lawyer to determine what laws governed the treatment of disadvantaged children. She then contacted another psychiatric facility to determine what common practices were. When it was found that the second facility's approach was more humane, we suggested cooperative training and mentoring from one facility to the other by a local expert in the field who worked at the second site. This allowed the approach to be supportive and educational rather than judgmental and punitive and the intervention came from a local rather than an outsider.

A class discussion concluded that a bias could be correct when a human being is harming another human being. However, the discussion becomes complicated when the definition of harm is discussed within a cultural context: *Is corporal punishment harm? Is circumcision (male or female) harm? Is euthanasia harm?* Additionally, if the bias is now *right,* then is it actually a bias? I leave that up to your own discussions.

Hayley Berman

What is our ethical responsibility (in terms of informed consent) to children who show up for services on their own?

What is our ethical responsibility to minors? Do we turn them away as we haven't received consent? What is considered elsewhere to be the norm of informed consent, whereby parents provide written authorization for their children to receive services, does not usually occur. There is very little interaction with the majority of the parents of children who arrive at Lefika to join our open studio or holiday programs. Although some parents are invested and involved, many seem to lack a sense of agency, because they are depressed, disempowered, and/or working shifts to earn a living. Illiteracy is sometimes a factor. Another complication is that those who take care of the children are not always "legal guardians" but older siblings. So, when children take it upon themselves to seek, and become part of, a community of care that is supportive and nurturing, we welcome them.

Charlotte G. Boston

When hospital policy and the patient's needs conflict, how should I proceed?

Empathize with the patient and ask how she wants to be addressed. Talk with her individually about ways in which she can focus upon treatment despite issues she can't control. Consider seeing her individually in art therapy. Address discriminatory issues in community meetings and whenever they arise in art therapy, establishing rules as needed.

Check in with staff before group to discuss and discreetly identify patients whose preferred names are different from those on the census; request that unit staff write "preferred name" on the census next to the given name. Advocate for patients' rights by meeting with administrators (individually or with other staff) to revise existing policies, in order to provide:

(a) space for a "preferred name" on the census sheet
(b) private rooms for adolescent or adult transgender patients.

When the latter can't be arranged due to high census, roommate assignments for those who have had gender reassignment surgery should be based upon gender identity, rather than gender at birth. In the case of adolescent patients [minors], inform parents of the rationale for this policy.

Richard Carolan

How could I determine whether a community mural-making project would pose a scope of practice issue?

When I realized that no art therapists were among the participants in the proposed research project, I decided to ask the proposal authors for clarity on each of the following issues. Lack of a satisfactory response to any of the issues would result in a rejection of the IRB proposal. Just because the researchers were not art therapists did not, in itself, mean that the use of art in a protocol was unethical.

1. Are the researchers identifying themselves as art therapists or presenting the proposal and advertising material in such a way that the participants or the public would be led to believe that they are art therapists? If so, this could infringe upon a protected domain, as well as mislead the public.
2. Is the proposed research within the scope of competency of the researchers? Do they have the requisite education and experience to lead a vulnerable population in a collaborative group art process? Do they have the education and/or experience to create a mural of this type?
3. Have the researchers made provisions to adequately inform the participants of the risks of this study? Have they taken appropriate steps to both minimize the risks and identify solution-based alternatives should the risks occur?

Deirdre M. Cogan

How can I best serve both the Hospital Review Board and my clients?

Even though I found neutrality difficult to maintain, my role as a review board member superseded my clinical goals. I decided to take an objective approach, regardless of my counter-transference. Acting upon it would have been unethical and might have led other team members to view me as inept. I did, however, share my feelings with the board members.

There is difference between being empathic towards individuals and colluding with their pathology. I voted along with the Board to delay the patient's transition to day treatment until he had demonstrated control over his aggressive impulses. Since I generally feel that—when conflicted about how to resolve an ethical dilemma— respecting a patient's autonomy should prevail, this was an exception. This decision not just protected the community from potential harm; it delayed the patient's transition to day treatment to a time that would be more conducive to his success.

Donald J. Cutcher

Why is it that I seem to be doing all the work?

First, I check to see if, in fact, I *am* doing all the work. If I am, I stop!

Second, I make sure that the expectations and responsibilities of all parties were addressed and formalized at the beginning of the therapeutic process; that they were the subject of periodic review; and that they were brought up in a timely manner whenever they ceased to be observed by either party—in other words, prior to becoming an issue that was so significant that it could jeopardize the very existence of the therapeutic process.

Third, I investigate my own counter-transference toward the patient and the situation! Is this the client's therapy process or mine?

Fourth, I consider initiating a three-pronged approach with the patient:

(a) I work to enhance the therapeutic relationship by reintroducing the responsibilities of all parties and the expectations for change and the advancement of the established goals of therapy. I use various art therapy techniques (e.g., shared drawing, scribble drawings, art journals) and verbal interchanges to explore issues such as the resolution of any conflict perceived in the art therapy sessions.

(b) I set limitations on myself and my patient through contracting; the contract should contain the following elements:
   - Clear definition of the issue.
   - Goals to be met in regard to all parties.
   - A clear timeline to be followed, reviewed, and modified if necessary.
   - Defined outcomes and consequences for lack of adherence to contract.
   - Written consent by all parties to the contract.

(c) I make appropriate referrals for additional services needed, noting all such changes in my patient's treatment plan. I ensure that I am competent to provide for the specific needs of the client. If I am not, I obtain appropriate training and supervised experience or transfer the treatment of my patient to someone who has the skills needed to meet the patient's needs.

Michelle L. Dean

What should I do in this situation, considering the multiple factors that are at stake?

I never told the minister about my prior religious affiliations and, after much contemplation, I felt it was wrong to sign the paper stating I agreed with the beliefs of her church. I felt it would be a conflict and a betrayal of my spiritual beliefs, which were complex and defied neat categorization. It seemed to deny my professional code of ethics, which embraced diversity (American Art Therapy Association, 2013; American Counseling Association, 2014). I felt it was my education and expertise that made me a fit clinician and not my religious or secular beliefs. If I signed this paper so I could continue to work with Rachel, how would this impact my integrity? And what message would be communicated to Rachel about caving to another's orientation or will? This discomfort I experienced felt like a parallel process to Rachel's previous trauma: being asked to submit to an act or belief system that was not congruent with my own, which supported diversity. In the end, I did not sign this statement because I did not feel that it was authentic or relevant to the treatment. I felt that, by signing this statement, I would be held accountable to the mission of the church. I did not believe that what was said or not said in treatment should be held to a religious doctrine, because, at times, it is the very things that seem incompatible with religious teachings that are the concerns or struggles that need to be expressed in treatment.

For four months, Rachel's feelings of powerlessness increased as she became resolved to the fact that she would be unable to make any decision other than to terminate treatment. We worked with her anger, issues, and concerns of separation, and the details of termination. As we prepared for our last session, Rachel created Figure B.1 as a response to my invitation that she draw herself "picking an apple from a tree."

The first picture Rachel drew of herself "picking an apple from a tree" (Figure 25.1) is illustrated in my chapter. We compared the first and second drawings, done four

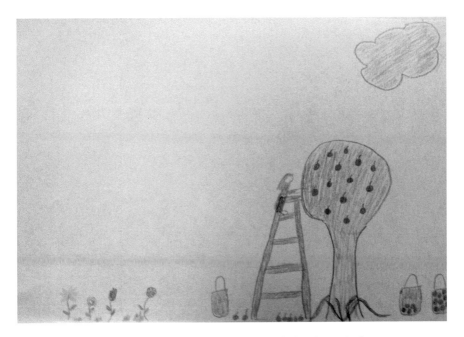

FIGURE B.1 *Picking an Apple from a Tree*, drawn by Rachel at the end of treatment.

years apart. In the most recent picture, she clearly has more support, as demonstrated by the strong and visually substantial ladder. She is within reach of the apple and has a surplus of apples on the ground and in bags to take with her. Her figure, though small, is not distorted or exaggerated as it had been four years earlier, which I believe spoke to a decrease in the distortions and reactivity which were a part of her trauma response. The image of herself appears transparent, reflective of her ongoing development of Self, which had been so significantly disrupted by her previous trauma, or perhaps she felt transparent because her wishes were not being heard and thus she felt partially invisible. Included in her surroundings are flowers and a partially covered sun, which she said reflected both her sadness in leaving and her gratefulness for having worked together, a brighter disposition than when she first entered treatment.

"You will be pleased to see my tree has roots," she exclaimed.

"They look a bit like legs, perhaps insect legs getting ready to pull up and walk away," I said.

Rachel looked at me and smiled.

I wished Rachel the best and reminded her that my door would always be open should she decide that she would like to return.

References

American Art Therapy Association (2013). *Ethical principles for art therapists.* Alexandria, VA: Author.

American Counseling Association (2014). 2014 ACA code of ethics: As approved by the ACA Governing Council. Retrieved from www.counseling.org/resources/aca-code-of-ethics.pdf

---

Cheryl Doby-Copeland

When fidelity and client choice conflict, how do I proceed?

Although my commitment to fidelity advocates telling the child the truth (that the parent is incarcerated), ethical practice dictates honoring the guardian's request, while determining how and when to tell the truth as a treatment goal. In these cases, we decided to use age-appropriate shared language which allowed me not to state that the parent was away in college; I provided reading material on talking to young children about parents who are incarcerated; and we gradually discussed telling the child the truth, particularly when a visit to the prison was planned.

How should I respond when subpoenaed to testify on the termination of parental rights?

To determine how I would testify, I took the following steps, based upon my ethics training (Jobes, 2011):

- Identify the ethical issue.
- Consult the *Ethical Principles for Art Therapists* (AATA, 2013).
- Contemplate potential ethical issues and consequences.
- Review and commit to memory all relevant information.
- Consult with supervisors, colleagues, and the agency's legal counsel on the rights, responsibilities, and vulnerabilities of the parents, children, foster parent.
- Identify and assess all possible courses of action.
- Identify potential consequences of my actions.
- Make a decision based upon the best course of action.
- Implement and fully document the decision.

After meeting with my clinical supervisor, I contacted the agency's general counsel to discuss my concerns about testifying in a hearing that could result in the termination of parental rights for parents with whom I worked for over two years. Despite her relapse, the mother had been one of the most consistent participants in my family art/play therapy sessions. My concerns clustered around the ability of the parents to provide adequate care for their two young children, given their substance use, recent incarceration, and lack of consistent employment. My observations during therapy supported my belief that the children were very comfortable in their parents' presence and the parents were attuned to the children. I reviewed the standardized assessments that I had administered throughout the course of therapy (which supported Monae's progress, growth, and development) and all of my clinical documentation, in order to recall key dates and indicators of Monae's progress in therapy, as I could not bring my clinical process notes into the court room during my testimony. Having clinical case notes or process notes present while testifying could result in *discovery in litigation*, which is the attorneys' right to ask for and receive your notes (Remley & Herlihy, 2007).

On the day of my testimony, I was questioned by the mother's attorney, the father's attorney, each child's guardian *ad litem,* the foster (pre-adoptive) mother's attorney, and the Assistant Attorney General of the Child Protection Division of the court. When asked my opinion of the parents' ability to provide for their children, I did not answer in a negative manner, which would have placed me in the position of endorsing the termination of parental rights. Instead, I said that I was concerned that, without gainful employment, adequate housing, and sobriety, it would be very challenging for either parent to care adequately for the children. Because the foster (pre-adoptive) mother had not participated in the therapy sessions, I simply stated, when asked, that the children appeared to be well fed and very well cared for. In the end, the parents' rights were terminated and both children were adopted.

References

American Art Therapy Association (2013). *Ethical principles for art therapists.* Alexandria, VA: Author.

Jobes, D.A. (2011, February). Contemporary ethics and risk management. Ethics training conducted at St. Elizabeths Hospital, Washington, DC.

Remley, T.P., & Herlihy, B. (2007). *Ethical, legal, and professional issues in counseling.* Upper Saddle River, NJ: Pearson Merrill Prentice Hall.

Karina Donald

Should I re-draw the boundaries of confidentiality?

First, I inquired if there were an alternative mode of transportation that would exclude me. There was none. I asked if there were a social worker to address the situation. No one was available at such short notice. I contacted my online art therapy supervisor about confidentiality, competence, and dual relationships before I made the decision. In this situation, clients' safety was paramount. They had no alternative place to live. I told my clients that their confidentiality might be breached because many persons knew my profession and would connect unrelated young people who were with me to my work. I gave them the option to sit with me or not during the journey. They chose to sit in another part of the ferry, but agreed not to talk about their emergency or about therapy during the journey. When we arrived, they were met by a social worker.

Should I alter my usual approach to self-disclosure?

If the client had continued to ask if I were related to the person she mentioned, I might have asked if the absence of self-disclosure on my part caused her any discomfort and then suggested that she process, through art or verbally, the addressing of personal boundaries (mine, her own) in a meaningful way. It is hoped that this would clarify why the question and the answer were so important to her. If the issue continued to be raised and I sensed that there was a degree of mutual discomfort that made continued work untenable, my last resort would have been to open up a discussion of whether she would prefer being referred to a therapist outside my workplace.

Patricia Fenner and Libby Byrne

What function did the art making fulfil for Tanya?

How might her supervisor address Tanya's insistence that her drawing "tells the whole story" and that "words are not important in art therapy"?

Tanya's supervisor supported her in expressing her experience in words, which revealed layers of shame and despair. Tanya's art functioned not only as a container for her feelings of distress, but also as a site of resistance to articulating her needs. Tanya experienced shame at not having better met the needs of the young people in the hospital's care, which, by implication, she felt was her responsibility. Unrealistic and inappropriate expectations such as these are often encountered in novice therapists and trainees. Feeling empowered to express herself visually provided a kind of surrogate expression of personal potency. Tanya had insisted upon the communicative power of the image as a form of overriding authority; yet, without articulation in this case, Tanya would have been left blinded by the image and with a misguided sense of learning.

Michael A. Franklin

How should I respond to visual free speech in the studio?

My simple response to the teen's attempt to shock me was, "Is this the best you can do? What do you really mean? Show it ... Tell it ... What is behind this 'FUCKYOU' that you insist on displaying? Dig deeper and find out what you really mean and, if you need help, I am here." He took the bait and proceeded to become a self-reflective artist investigating this autobiographical material.

It could be argued that I applied the simple counseling skills of paraphrasing behavioral and visual communication and reflecting it back, before extending him an invitation to artistically sublimate significant yet superficially displaced aggression. Although I was not interested in thinking diagnostically, this language is certainly derived from my clinical, *art as therapy* instincts. Importantly, I did not try to unfold family history or skillfully probe for deeper affect in order to develop psychological insight. Instead, my goal was to understand what was happening in the moment and then, by speaking as one artist to another, move art into more art. Assuming an *art as therapy* perspective, which skates between psychotherapy and studio work, I hoped to question his chaotically discharged impulses and invite aesthetic ego resources to rally towards formed expression (Gerity, 2001). In the studio I do think from an *art as therapy* perspective, yet my interventions are not meant to engage in traditional therapeutic processes.

Reference

Gerity, L.A. (2001). *Art as therapy: Collected papers of Edith Kramer.* London: Jessica Kingsley.

Lisa Raye Garlock

Shirley Mason's artwork: To exhibit or not to exhibit?

We exhibited the work. Considerable time, expense, and commitment had gone into procuring it. Although the context of the exhibit was trauma, there was no way of telling whether Shirley Mason had experienced the significant and sadistic traumas that Schreiber had "documented" in her book. Although we weren't able to do so because of timing, the exhibit would have provided a great opportunity for an ethics seminar and discussion of the case and the artwork.

Community-based artists' studios and art therapy: Is it a good fit?

The learning that takes place when using art materials is broad and the process stimulates and develops both body and mind. Developing skills, individual style, and vision, maintaining a daily practice of creating, and expressing oneself through art materials is high-level work—in contrast to stuffing envelopes all day, an occupation in which people with cognitive disabilities are often placed, without regard to their unique interests and abilities. Facilitated well, the making of this art has therapeutic benefits, despite its commercial purpose.

The question here is really, "Is it ethical for *students* to be at this type of site?" A student does not have the understanding or experience to see that the work is therapeutic, even if the art is ultimately for sale. They need to learn how to do art therapy, rather than art teaching, and making art for commercial purposes is not their goal. An art therapist supervisor can make all the difference, as he or she can train the student to work with the clients therapeutically. While we stopped sending students to one of these settings, other art studios with art therapy supervisors have been excellent training sites for students; they're able to integrate art therapy and artist studio work successfully and put things into perspective.

Exhibiting art created in supervision: A good idea?

The project for interns and supervisors to make art for a show was optional. The continuum between showing and never showing artwork leaves space for each person to decide where on that spectrum he or she would fit comfortably, taking into consideration the context and the purpose of the activity. Personally, my belief is that, as art therapists, it is our professional responsibility to continue to develop and nurture our artist selves; doing so may include exhibiting our artwork. At the very least, we need to be creating our own artwork on a regular basis—learning new skills, making response art related to our clients, and staying fresh artistically and psychologically—in order to best serve our patients.

Elaine S. Goldberg

What should I do when the interpreter is bypassed?

Knowing that my first language is English, father and daughter tested boundaries by switching from Spanish to English, excluding mother, bypassing the interpreter, and ignoring my statement that we would be speaking Spanish throughout the session. I stopped the conversation and asked everyone to speak in Spanish and to allow the interpreter to interpret everything that was said. While this dilemma illustrates how complex family dynamics can be, part of my role is to ensure that every individual's voice can be heard, including that of the interpreter.

Deborah A. Good

How should I respond to my client saying goodbye first?

Caryn's reaction to my medical procedure reflected her sense of insecurity regarding the termination of our relationship due to my impending retirement. After having yelled at me, her shame and her fear of rejection must have been unbearable; to block it out, she imagined that I had yelled at *her*, which allowed her to feel rejected by *my* behavior (i.e., as she would have felt had I become very ill, died, or retired). By choosing to end our relationship, rather than wait for me to announce when our last day would be, Caryn felt more in control. This dynamic concurred with her lifelong history of being hurt, abandoned, and rejected; a pattern she found difficult to relinquish, due to her abuse.

I wrote a letter to Caryn stating that I had hoped that we could have worked out the differences that came between us, but I would respect her desire to end therapy. I told her what an honor it had been to work with her and then gave her three referrals, with contact and website information. I said that I wanted to return her artwork and asked her to let me know the most convenient way to do so. I wished her well and placed a copy of the letter in her client file.

Caryn called the office and arranged to pick up her work on a day when I was out of town.

Six months later, I saw her and her husband at a wedding reception and greeted them when they approached me. Caryn began gushing over me, hugging me, and touching my arms as if she were checking to see if I were OK; it reminded me of the way my dermatologist scans for abnormal skin lesions. Obviously nervous, she spoke incessantly. I did not let her know that I was uncomfortable with her physical touch, but treated her with respect and participated in small talk with her and her husband. Eventually, they left the reception. I thought that having a polite, face-to-face interaction would help Caryn to feel that things were fine between us.

How should I respond to my client having experienced too many changes?

Ralph's case laid heavy on my mind and his comment about me "dumping him" concerned me. I waited four weeks and then called to see if he felt that his new therapist was a good fit. Ralph was very appreciative of the call and said that he had been to one appointment with his new therapist but that he had some concerns. The therapist's voice quivers when he speaks and Ralph said that it reminded him of his facial tic. Because of this, he was not sure that he could continue to work with this therapist, but said that he would try a few more sessions to see if he could use the situation to work through personal issues that were triggered by the therapist's voice. I have not heard back from Ralph, so I assume that he was able to settle into a successful therapeutic relationship.

How should I respond to my client's refusal to terminate?

Betsy retired from her job two weeks before I did. I did speak to her about the discomfort I felt about her disclosing our therapeutic relationship to our pastor. She became emotional and said that she needed someone to know. I acknowledged that this has been very difficult for her and said that I thought that we could respect each other's privacy. Although I referred Betsy to another art therapist, I don't know if she was able to make the transition.

I did not return any of Betsy's phone calls or comment on the card she sent me, but when she cornered me in the hallway of the church, I empathized with her frustrations about job-hunting and congratulated her when she told me that she had found a job. I realize that Betsy joined the choir at my church to remain in contact with me. Should this situation become uncomfortable for me, I will weigh the discomfort against my desire to continue my involvement with the church.

How should I respond when no one saw it coming?

I did visit Carina in the hospital. She was devastated and afraid, and it was evident that she would never to be able to walk or use her hands again. I spoke with her briefly and she was grateful that I came. Most of the time, she cried and told me that she missed me. There was nothing I could do to console her, except to acknowledge her grave situation and her pain.

It was clear to me that visiting Carina brought up a lot of emotional pain for her. It was as though seeing me reminded her of the creativity that she could no longer express. I spoke with my clinical supervisor about how to proceed and after discussing the pros and cons of continuing to visit her, I decided to stop. I didn't think that it was in Carina's best interest for me to continue to see her. Our relationship would never be anything other than that of therapist and client, and I needed to honor the termination that took place before her stroke. Carina's sisters moved her into a nursing home where members of her church frequently visit her. One sister is trying to find a nursing home close to where she lives, so that Carina will be near family. I often think about her and hope that she finds some happiness in what is left of her life.

How should I respond to an impossible termination?

It was impossible to have closure with Noreen before I ended by clinical practice. I spoke with her on the phone when she was on her way to take care of her daughter's remains. When I asked Noreen what she needed, she was adamant that she did not want to go back to the therapist who had referred her to me. At the same time, it did not seem appropriate for Noreen to be left without a therapist during this time of immediate grief. I offered to see her for six sessions, to help her work through the grief of losing her daughter. She insisted on compensating me for my time and we agreed upon an amount. I was acutely aware that our relationship needed to remain professional, without any intimation that a personal relationship between us was possible. Noreen and I agreed upon the professional parameters necessary to complete her therapeutic termination; we decided upon a place to meet, a financial arrangement, the number of sessions, and set a time limit on when the sessions would end.

Noreen completed a photo album of her daughter on her own and reviewed each picture during one of our sessions. Due to unforeseeable circumstances, Noreen had to make several trips out of state to be with her family, canceling several of our appointments. To date, we have completed three of the six sessions we agreed upon. My plan is to meet with Noreen one more time to review our agreement. It would be easy to extend the time allotted for our sessions beyond the end date we had originally agreed upon. To ensure that our relationship boundaries are understood, however, a new end date will be selected at our next appointment. I will inform Noreen that I am unable to extend our time together past that date, clarifying when the termination of our relationship will take place.

David E. Gussak

What happens to confidentiality in a courtroom?

Although the authorization granted by the court gave me the legal right to present my conclusions about the defendant's work during and after the trial—without a signed release form from the defendant—ethically, I felt that I needed to let the defendant know that I respected his work and his right to confidentiality. I demonstrated this by asking the defendant if he would sign an additional form that would grant me permission to present his work in an open forum, in presentations, and in publications. My professional integrity committed me to this action.

Ellen G. Horovitz

How should I deal with counter-transference in telehealth?

I sought the supervision of a trusted colleague. We talked about the case at length, including how my client's comment had made me feel and the ways in which I could broach this subject with her. Despite my colleague's lack of understanding of the parameters of video therapy counseling, his sage advice was useful in aiding me with my counter-transferential issue of feeling like *arm candy*.

Thinking about therapy as an elite offering did not sit well with me. I knew I had to create my own artwork to put this "class notion" to bed. I created the "Interspecies

Proposal," a quilt that incorporates traditional and modern quilting techniques, kiln-fired glass, and hand beading. It shows a kneeling *Ankylosaurus* male offering an *Allosaurus* female a citrine engagement ring while a shocked Stegosaurus witnesses the event. Both the *Allosaurus* and the *Ankylosaurus* are adorned with fancy wardrobes and costume jewelry, while the *Stegosaurus*, an obvious stand-in for me, is plainly garbed and stares shocked at the soon-to-be-engaged couple. Even the art was impacted by the vehicle of video therapy: the quilt incorporates the actions of the *Allosaurus* and the *Ankylosaurus*, while the glass piece behind the couple reflects their issues. The *Stegosaurus* is not reflected in their dialogue but, like the therapist (me), witnesses the event. This quilt allowed me to look at my patient's needs within the context of her cultural and social world, rather than my own. Sharing the finished piece with my colleague enabled me to see my patient's issues in a broader perspective, that is, that her acquisition of me as her therapist was intricately tied to what she thought she wanted (e.g., the engagement and a happily-ever-after life filled with material goods that would make her feel fulfilled and happy). The quilt also seemed to foreshadow future events, as, about a year later, the couple broke their engagement.

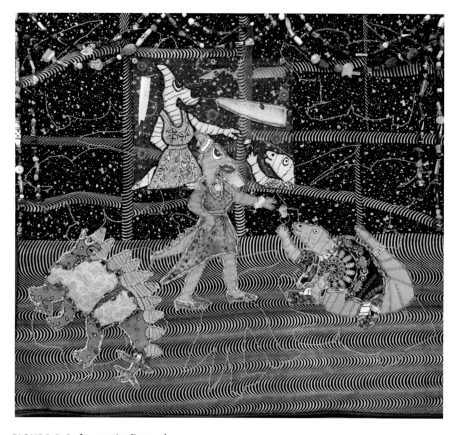

FIGURE B.2 *Interspecies Proposal.*

While I might have brought my reaction up with my patient, I knew that it had to do with my counter-transference and that sharing it would not have aided her. Oftentimes, creating artwork is the only resolution that really works for me, but this isn't surprising, since, in fact, isn't this what we preach and what we do?

Paula Howie

Should I break confidentiality?

My client had made a thinly veiled threat, her mood in group had changed, and she had not been willing to go to the hospital by herself. Though she had engaged in provocative behavior in the past, this seemed to constitute a genuine cry for help. I could not talk her into coming to the emergency room and had no other way to assure her safety. I believed that she was in real danger of harming herself if she stayed home. I decided to break confidentiality.

First, I called her psychiatrist, who encouraged me to contact the sheriff's department and ask someone to go by her home to check on her. I asked the sheriff's department also to take away any guns with which she could harm herself or pills that she could use to overdose. They were familiar with her and knew where she lived, as they had made several calls to her home to check on her in the past. They assured me that they would make sure that she was safe; if they could not guarantee her safety, they would bring her to the hospital. I found out later that they had taken her weapons and she had seen her doctor the next afternoon.

I knew that my client would be angry about my breaking confidentiality not once but twice—by calling her psychiatrist and then calling the sheriff's department. When she came back to group two weeks later, she was angry at first, but this gave way to gratitude that I would be willing to find help for her. I felt as though I were always walking a tightrope with her—allowing her to tell me what was on her mind when she did have suicidal thoughts and making sure that she was safe.

Yuriko Ichiki and Mercedes Ballbé ter Maat

Is it ethical to train teachers or other non-art therapists to use art in psycho-education?

What would be the most ethical way in which to incorporate the MATSP into Japanese schools?

Upon consulting with my co-author, I am now training the teachers in accordance with guidelines for training non-art therapists, produced by the American Art Therapy Association (2013, 2016) and by other art therapists working around the world (Kalmanowitz & Potash, 2010). During training, teachers learn psycho-education applications of art by understanding the use of different art materials, the value and types of directives that can be given to students, considerations related to making art (e.g., space, time, ownership, storage), and how best to understand what is drawn. Teachers are trained to listen and to elicit stories told by students without adding their personal comments or interpretations.

Unlike what I had initially recommended, teachers are now advised to talk with students in private when a concerning image arises. Thus, instead of allowing the student who had drawn "Help" to go home without having addressed the situation, the teacher would now be encouraged to speak privately with the student to find out more about what was meant by "Help." If "Help" had not been about a fight with a friend but had referred to a dangerous situation outside of school that needed immediate intervention, the teacher could have taken appropriate action, such as communicating with the parent. Opportunities to role play enable teachers to practice how to talk with parents and students in a sensitive way. We have concluded that there are ways to train non-art therapists to use the MATSP ethically as psycho-education in Japanese school settings.

To whom does the artwork belong—the student artist or the educational system in which it was created?

As art therapists, we have been taught that the artwork belongs to the person who created it, unless the institution or setting makes it explicit that the artwork is part of the client's medical or clinical record (or, as in our case, the educational record). Although schools are not therapeutic settings and students are not in therapy when they are participating in the MATSP, we believe that the artwork created by students in schools belongs to the students. Even though tests, completed homework, school projects, and "one-line journals" are returned to students at the teacher's discretion, since, typically, they *are* returned, so should art that is created as part of a classroom activity. We suggest that, as part of educating and informing parents about the purpose and value of the MATSP, a statement be added to clarify that the students' artwork belongs to the students and will be returned to them.

Should parents have the right to decide if their children should participate in the MATSP through an informed consent process or is the MATSP part of the required educational school curriculum and, thus, not subject to parental consent?

What are the rights of minors, with regard to confidentiality, in deliberations between parents and school personnel?

With regard to the first question, we believe that the MATSP is part of the school curriculum and, as such, parental consent is not necessary. Just as the "one-line journal" is commonly used by teachers as part of the basic curriculum to engage students in the exploration of their feelings through words, so is the mini art therapeutic drawing.

The second question is more complex. In Japan, parents have legal rights over any school deliberations involving their children. Morally and ethically, however, we contend that student deliberations should be treated as private and confidential unless the student's well-being is threatened. But what about information that does not reach the level of "harmful"? The question of "to tell or not to tell" might more aptly be broken into two questions: "whom to tell" and "what to tell." When we believe that parents should be informed of certain information revealed by their children (information that is not considered "harmful"), we train the teachers to involve the students in deciding how and what information will be shared with their parents.

Teachers must participate in bi-weekly consultation sessions with me, an art therapist, or a school counselor. (In Japan, many school counselors are registered clinical psychologists, trained in administering and interpreting projective drawing tests.) Consultation provides continuous support and training to teachers participating in the MATSP. We encourage teachers to use the MATSP, to explore the meaning of the drawings with the students, to establish conversations with parents as necessary, and to refer students in need to the school counselor for more in-depth, professional support.

References

American Art Therapy Association (2013). *Ethical principles for art therapists.* Alexandria, VA: Author.

American Art Therapy Association (2016). Art therapists training non-art therapists. Retrieved from: www.arttherapy.org/upload/ECTrainingNonATs.pdf

Kalmanowitz, D., & Potash, J. D. (2010). Ethical considerations in the global teaching and promotion of art therapy to non-art therapists. *Arts in Psychotherapy,* 37(1), 20–26.

Catherine Rogers Jonsson

How should I respond to projection and displaced aggression?

I was aware of myself starting to tense up when the man asked if I knew that Hillary Clinton had started ISIS in Afghanistan, a physiological response to a fear of violence. I began to breathe more deeply and focus my attention upon him more acutely. As he became more distraught, I automatically turned my body sideways to him, a non-threatening stance I learned while working in a psychiatric hospital. This also had the advantage of allowing me to see the other clients at the tables, in order to observe their reactions and ensure that they were safe. When he realized that I was not going to argue with him or challenge him in any way, his behavior stopped escalating. He did not become violent. He yelled something at his wife in Dari, the official language of Afghanistan (a derivation of Farsi), and abruptly left the room. His family quickly stood up and followed him out of the room, leaving their artwork behind.

I went to the other clients and asked if everyone was all right. They all seemed to take the incident in stride, but, due to the lack of a common language, I couldn't be sure. To clear the air and help my remaining clients refocus upon their tasks, I initiated some breathing exercises and arm stretches. Everyone returned to art making and attended to the process.

I realized that the man was experiencing displaced aggression, often a symptom of trauma.

Although I am not Hillary Clinton, like her I am a white, privileged American woman who (as group leader) is in a position of power. After this session, the man and his family never returned to the art therapy group. I wish that I could have worked with him and his family again. Perhaps art therapy might have helped them to express the anger, sadness, homesickness, and frustration of living as refugees, cut off from the lives they had led and the homeland they loved.

P. Gussie Klorer

Couldn't I just give her the little fox?

Because I was in private practice and did not have a treatment team with whom to confer, I contracted for supervision with a psychiatrist/psychoanalyst. My counter-transferential feelings were strong and I spent every one of our consultations talking only about Julie, so when I brought up the issue of the toy fox, my supervisor was already familiar with the case. I presented my reasons for wanting to give Julie the fox, then admitted that what I really wanted to give her was the princess figurine that she had played with during every session. Through this consultation I realized what I already knew: that neither the fox nor the princess could possibly meet Julie's needs and would end up being a disappointment. A toy could not fix the sadness that either one of us felt in terminating. My supervisor was also concerned that giving Julie any sand-tray figure of mine would be too symbolically loaded, carrying too much responsibility for a four-year-old. I finally got my supervisor to agree that buying a figurine that was not on my toy shelf would be acceptable, though she wisely noted that this gesture was for my benefit, not the child's. I found a neutral "pretty girl" figurine (a theme that came up often in Julie's play) and wrapped it up to give Julie during her last session. It was somewhat disappointing that she did not get excited about the present. She made no comment and then started playing with something else. I was confronted once again with the reality that a gift can never make up for the feelings of loss that are triggered at termination.

What happens when a therapist disagrees with a decision made on behalf of a client?

Lila came to her next therapy session very angry, as her foster mother had already told her that the judge had said that Lila had to start visits with her mom again and had to get a new therapist. Lila, who knew I wrote reports for, and talked with, the judge, came in, sat down, and shouted, "That is a stupid judge! Why did she say I can't come see you anymore? And why does that stupid judge think I have to see my mom? I'm not going!" I had to maintain professional neutrality, so I could not vent my own feelings about the decision. Over the next two weeks, as I helped her to articulate her feelings, I explained to Lila that judges have to listen to a lot of different people in the courtroom and sometimes they make decisions we don't like. As Lila was adamant that she did not want to go to another therapist, I assured her that, although it might take a while to get to know the person, I was sure that Lila would like her new therapist. At our last session, Lila brought me a painting that she made as a goodbye gift. I told her what a beautiful painting it was and that I would think of her every time I looked at it. Lila said she really liked coming to therapy and though she liked making things, she knew the main point was to talk about how she felt so that I could tell the judge. As we were talking, I made Lila a goodbye picture and a card. Since her foster family took her on hikes, I drew a picture of her hiking to the top of a mountain. I told her how special she is and to keep using words to tell people how she feels, even when it feels like they don't listen. For her last project, Lila decided to decorate a box in which to keep the card I was making for her. She would not read the card in front of me, but took it in the waiting room to read with her foster mother.

May a client and a therapist ever become friends?

In weighing whether to set up a visit with Lila, I pondered the pros and cons. I could not be her therapist and I did not want to intrude into the boundaries of her current therapy. How would she perceive a visit? What was the purpose of the visit? Though I really wanted to see her, I could not set up a visit to meet my needs. The foster mother told me that Lila missed me and talked about me often. Would it be good for her to know that I remembered her, too, and still cared about her? The foster mother and I discussed it and determined that a visit would be good for Lila. We set up an after-school visit in my office and her foster mother explained that it was just a friendly visit, not a therapy appointment. I framed and hung in the waiting room the picture Lila had made me so that she would know that I still thought about her. She excitedly pointed it out to her foster mother when they came in.

"I missed you!" Lila said as she hugged me. "I missed you, too," I said, hugging her back. Because I was no longer her therapist, I did not delve into her feelings or ask questions other than those that one would typically ask a 10-year-old (regarding school, sports, vacation). We were meeting as if we were old friends. I told her, "Lila, you know I can't be your therapist anymore, so we are just going to have a visit, okay?" Her foster mother chimed in, "Gussie is your friend now." Lila told me all about her summer vacation, checked out my new office to be sure that all the expected items were still on my shelves, had a snack, and then gravitated to the sand tray and started playing while the foster mother and I talked. We hugged again at the end. The visit seemed to satisfy her need to know that I was still there and still cared about her. We did not set up any more visits. I still get updates on Lila periodically from her social worker and her foster mother. It is possible that I will see her again in a few years. I encouraged her to move on so she is no longer dependent upon me, but the relationship that we had was genuine and did not go away because a judge made a ruling.

Barbara Mandel

What factors should be taken into consideration when providing art materials for clients' use? What happens when those factors conflict with each other?

Given the secure setting, the small number of group members, and the large amount of information we had about the boys, I decided that it was possible to provide opportunities to support the important developmental tasks of the boys' age group (e.g., industry, choice, autonomy) by taking precautions that would limit potential risk. My co-therapist and I provided them with clear safety instructions and then demonstrated appropriate tool use and safe ways in which to handle objects that might be rough or pointed. Safety goggles and gloves were provided. As the four boys took apart the old appliances, each of us carefully monitored their activities, while providing enough space to foster a sense of mastery and encourage creativity. The boys' enthusiasm was palpable! Deconstructing and reconstructing the appliances as artwork expanded their notion of art and seemed to build confidence and competence. Suddenly, they had become artists, engineers, and inventors!

Are uneven cultural exchanges ethical?

We felt humbled by the Guatemalan children's efforts, by their generosity, and by the opportunity to be exposed to a traditional sewing method that has been passed on for generations. While equal exchanges are ideal, to decline the *bolistas* would have risked offending the children. We gratefully accepted them.

Martina E. Martin

How do I hold the therapeutic frame while experiencing strong counter-transference?

Shortly after the altercation with my client, I noticed that the client's attendance at the program began to suffer. He started coming less and less often and, when he did attend, he was in so much physical pain that he barely said a word. As I was leaving work a month later, I ran into him in the lobby and noticed that something about him seemed different. He had a glow about him that I had never seen before and he did not appear to be in pain. Even though I was in a rush to leave, I took a few minutes to sit with him and, as soon as I sat down, he burst into tears. He thanked me for my patience and willingness to tolerate his hard questions and, more importantly, he thanked me for not giving up on him. He acknowledged those times when his actions pushed others away, but he remained astounded by the fact that, in spite of his anger, I never stopped trying to connect with him. He was happy to report that he became a Christian during the previous week's Spirituality group and that, for the first time in his life, he truly felt at peace. I thanked him for his kind words and offered a few more words of encouragement. Less than a week later, we were informed that he had passed away.

Emery Hurst Mikel

How do I maintain confidentiality on a home visit?

I was only two years out of school and this was my first experience making home visits. I had seen Mrs. Goodrich for a few months and had a good relationship with her. I had met Sara once before, briefly. Something felt odd about answering Sara, but I wasn't sure what. I knew I couldn't divulge information about my client, but wondered if I could mention her decline. I stammered that Sara would have to check with the family, smiled, and moved down the hallway. I was tempted to tell Sara about her friend's deterioration, so she could see Mrs. Goodrich once more before she died; I was worried that the family might be too distracted to do so.

I raised the issue in supervision, where I was able to admit that one reason I felt conflicted was that I knew it wasn't my place to make that decision; I couldn't possibly know what the family would want to share with others. Also, although Sara knew me, anyone could have been within earshot of our conversation—something especially important to be aware of in public spaces such as apartment buildings and assisted living facilities. Even if I had met a colleague in an empty hallway, it would not have been right to speak about my client. Apartment doors are not soundproof. If it were necessary to share information, we would need to move to a more secure location.

If someone had asked me that day if Mrs. Goodrich were my client, the best response I have heard, and now use, is "I can neither confirm nor deny that." If I always said "no" when someone was not my client but gave a different answer when someone was my client, it would be just as identifying as saying "yes." I should also wait for the person to leave before approaching my client's door. It wouldn't be very ethical to say the line above and then walk right to Mrs. Goodrich's door with someone watching me!

So, looking back, I wish I'd said nothing to Sara, something similar to the line above, or "I'm sorry, I have to go"—all of which can be said pleasantly and with a smile, but also with conviction.

Abbe Miller

How should I proceed when the boundary between supervision and therapy starts to slip?

Aware of the powerful impact of her disclosure, I made a mental note of Principle 8.5 of the American Art Therapy Association's *Ethical Principles for Art Therapists* (2013), assuring Ciara that she could continue this journey, while emphasizing that extra support (personal therapy) was indicated. A heartfelt verbal conversation ensued, led by my supervisor/program director self; widened and held by my clinical skills of compassion and attunement. It was up to her to continue the conversation non-verbally in the painting process. I suggested that Ciara choose a soothing color to re-engage with

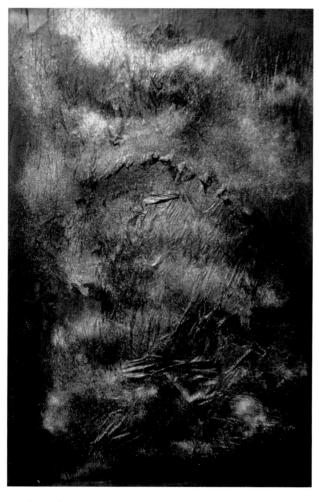

FIGURE B.3 *Soothing Blue.*

the painting in a way that would help her settle rather than re-trigger her. She layered blue with silver glitter over the entire surface, appearing to center.

Reference

American Art Therapy Association (2013). *Ethical principles for art therapists.* Alexandria, VA: Author.

Anne Mills

Should I terminate with this client?

I felt that terminating with an ill and depressed client would be abandonment, which is unethical. Since it seemed apparent that the client did not have long to live and was unable to travel, I offered to provide in-home sessions, an offer that was appreciated but not accepted.

Should I clarify or renegotiate the status of the therapeutic relationship?

A risk management expert recommended saying to the client, "I need brief updates if you are not attending. If you can't provide them, and can't attend, let's get you to a provider who *can* provide services under those circumstances. I care too much to do otherwise."

Should I seek the patient's written permission to participate in the email collaboration of my client's other providers?

HIPAA allows treatment professionals on a team to communicate about their work with the client using "reasonable means" without a written consent form. Since the client was identified by only his initials, the psychiatrist felt that normal, unencrypted email constituted "reasonable means" by which to communicate. I was aware that I felt honored to be included in the "conversation" and wanted to participate. Although the email seemed, to me, to be against the client's wishes, I knew that good collaboration among medical professionals was valuable and rare. My offer to help the doctors utilize an encrypted email, such as Hushmail, was not accepted. I felt uncomfortable reading the emails, but wondered if doing so was justified, given my concern for my client's safety

How should I respond to colleagues' questions about my fee?

Talking with colleagues about fees could be a risky practice for art therapists who are contractors or in private practice because, in the US, the discussion of fees by competitors might be considered price fixing and, therefore, be subject to antitrust laws and criminal and civil suits at the federal and state level. Although laws such as the Sherman Anti-trust Act of 1890 were intended to prevent monopolies from controlling business practices and colluding in fixing prices, and to ensure competition in the marketplace to benefit consumers, it is generally agreed that these laws apply to psychotherapists just as they do to multinational corporations. Businesses that agree to charge a certain price for a service are price-fixing, which is generally illegal. If businesses are found to be exchanging information with each other about their fees, they could be violating antitrust laws, because it could appear as if they have fixed prices or want to influence the prices a competitor will set. If a private practitioner advertises his or her prices, but did not discuss them with competitors or encourage competitors to match the price, it would not seem to be price fixing, as other therapists would be free to disregard those prices when setting their own. However, this is the kind of thorny issue that an attorney could help clarify. Because of these issues, I have omitted my fee from this version of my contract, but I do so with regret, since financial issues have ethical import and, therefore, should be discussed.

When situations such as those in the dilemma present themselves, it is easy to forget the risk involved or to feel that a private discussion is acceptable. Since my former supervisee was paying for my time, part of me felt as if I should simply share my budget, as a resource. Since he lived far away and, thus, would not be my competitor, I wondered whether we could discuss fees without even the appearance of violating any anti-trust laws. I also considered talking about the different processes by which we arrived at our fees—it not being uncommon for male psychotherapists to set fees equal to their therapists' or supervisors' fees when starting out. I must admit to feeling a bit intimidated and angered by the psychologist who seemed to be a self-appointed art therapist. If we lived in a state with title protection, I would have had a firm foundation upon which to inquire about his educational background, since, in the US, a Master's degree in Art Therapy is considered to be entry level to the profession. I chose to explain the potential risks of competitors engaging in discussions about setting fees.

It's my money—isn't it?

When the need for a late payment fee became apparent, I didn't know how other therapists handled it. I've since learned that the most common approach is a $20 fee on any unpaid balance after 30 days, and that there is value in doing that which is most commonly done. Instead, I instituted a policy of charging compound interest at 1% above prime rate. I stated in the contract that "Interest will be charged on any overdue balances," but did not specify details. The policy and the failure to state it in writing made it confusing and time-intensive to administer, and caused client dissatisfaction, particularly when large balances had been allowed to accrue. I have since instituted a policy of not allowing balances to accrue beyond the value of three sessions. Initially, I informed clients of the amount owed by email, reminding them that, after 30 days, the interest charge would be instituted. I have since learned that presenting clients with statements or invoices in session is a clearer, more effective way to get payment.

Challenges such as these have led me to make my payment policy increasingly explicit, as shown in lines 102, 103, and 142 of the contract, as well as in conversations with my clients.

What constitutes an emergency?

Have you, an art therapist who is also a client in psychotherapy, ever had an emergency that prevented you from attending your psychotherapy session? Would you late-cancel if you had the symptoms of a contagious illness such as the flu or if your children were ill and no one was available to watch them? What if you needed to go to the hospital because a family member was dying? What if a natural disaster had affected transportation systems? I asked myself whether I would have late-cancelled if I were in a situation similar to that of my client.

Asking myself, "What's best for this person's progress in therapy?" my rational mind said, "Be firm, charge for the late cancellation," but my emotional mind fretted, "No, don't charge! Don't encourage her to attend if she's sick; you might catch something! Besides, she has money issues! Remember when you charged that other client? He got offended and terminated prematurely!" Too quickly, I told the client over the phone that she was excused from our session at no charge. I did not truly examine her story or the symptom in the next meeting. A wiser, more balanced option might have been to address all the elements of the situation, including my skepticism about this emergency, the possibility of her nausea being psychologically based, and the deeper meaning of the interaction. The topic could have been re-opened in subsequent meetings, but it was not, and a therapeutic opportunity was lost.

Laurie Mowry-Hesler

What difference would a few decades make?

What would a current, more ethical, case conceptualization and treatment plan for Reggie entail?

Based upon codes in effect as I write this, social services would be engaged to evaluate the safety of the home, the mother's willingness to receive treatment for herself, and the family's eligibility to receive in-home services to improve the living conditions and care of the children, whether at home or in a family shelter. If the conditions were not met, the children would be placed, together, with a family member or in a specialized foster home within their community. Home-based services would be offered either to the placement home or to the mother, either at home or in a shelter.

An art therapist/licensed professional counselor (LPC) on a home-based service team would be assigned to work with the entire family in the home and to engage other community services to support the treatment of each family member. The goal would be to maintain attachments among siblings, mother, and grandmother through therapy, education, and/or visitation. Reggie, as well as his two-year-old brother, would be assessed for attachment and/or trauma issues. Art therapy would be recommended for treatment and self-expression. In addition to substance abuse intervention, family and/or family art therapy would be indicated for the mother and possibly the grandmother, whether the children were in their care or in foster care. The goal would be to maintain attachment, improve parenting skills, family dynamics, and communication, to promote the well-being and autonomy of the entire family and to preserve the family unit. In the event that the mother was unable to care for her children, continued contact with the children would be supported through collaborative efforts with social services and home-based services unless or until parental rights were terminated.

Iryna Natalushko

If I anticipate that I will have only one session with a client who has complex needs, including a trauma history, what, ethically, should I try to accomplish?

In this situation, I have learned to treat any session as a final one and to make it as efficient, effective, and safe for closure as possible. At the same time, my intention is to help a client learn to regulate emotion at a time of ongoing stress; provide brief psycho-educational information; support the unfolding of as tangible a therapeutic outcome as possible given the time; as well as to help screen for contributing earlier trauma and encourage those with complex trauma histories to see a professional at a later time when resources become available.

Penelope Orr

Can one, ethically, teach art-making interactions online?

There wasn't any research for me to reference, other than looking at how art is taught online. Watching a video and then creating a piece of art and sending it to the teacher, however, does not meet the requirements of an art therapy curriculum. I studied online counseling guidelines and watched examples of online video meetings in order to assess what was—and was not—therapeutic and how that might apply to art therapy.

I decided to require students in the Materials class to create art individually and also within a group that is formed where they live; this allows them to reflect upon the differences between making art in isolation and within a group. In other classes, I provide experientials which enable students to try out different levels of interaction, such as creating mail art and sending it to other class members; creating online art/collaging together; and creating art individually, eliciting feedback about it from other class members, then working on it again. I also ask students to conduct art therapy assessments and, respecting confidentiality, to share the images and their ideas with the class so that they can practice giving appropriate feedback and analysis.

The Group class meets in online video chat, creating art together and trying to discover how best to position the art making so that others can see what you are doing and you can see what they are doing. We discuss how creating art in person in a group differs from creating art online in a group, and the benefits and drawbacks of each. Students have to keep a visual journal throughout the program, which they share individually with their professors. Students are required to complete traditional in-person internships and practica under supervision. The combination of these activities, along with the students' reflections upon the nature of each, helps us to gain an understanding of the interactions surrounding the art-making process in art therapy.

Mavis Osei

If, in a country with no full-fledged academic art therapy training program, an art educator has taken the art therapy courses available, would it be more—or less—ethical for that teacher to ignore opportunities to use art "therapeutically"?

It may be important to remember that, at present, there are not only no art therapy training programs in Ghana, but also no national or regional art therapy associations, no art therapy standards of practice or codes of ethics, and no formally recognized occupation called "art therapist." Therefore, the ethical position of a Ghanaian art teacher in the situation described above is not comparable to that of an art teacher who works in a country in which formal art therapy training programs are plentiful, or at least accessible, and, despite that, decides—having taken only a couple of art therapy courses—to use art therapeutically in the classroom. Being astride the fields of art education and art therapy, Ghanaian teachers will draw upon their knowledge of both, as appropriate, to enhance their teaching and their students' learning. If, some day, a formal training program in art therapy—and a certification program for those it has trained—is developed, I believe that it is likely that they would be among the first to apply.

Unnur Ottarsdottir

How can I prepare professionals to be able to provide strong enough emotional containment for clients and students who make memory drawings?

Tasks completed:

• I submitted grant applications to the Icelandic Centre for Research for a three-year project that included putting memory drawing research into a firm theoretical context, writing and publishing about it, developing an educational training program and curriculum for professionals interested in applying the method, introducing the research findings to professionals, and conducting further research on the subject. However, the applications were unsupported.

• Eighteen years passed before I decided that there were sufficient resources available to safely begin to introduce the findings of my memory research. With Wammes, Meade, and Fernandes's (2016) introduction of their memory drawing research findings, it was apparent that other researchers were now working in this area and that they, too, carried the responsibility of introducing their findings and putting them into context, which meant that they could be contacted for further information. However, I claim that an important art therapeutic context is missing in their research, which I have included.

• I wrote a paper about memory drawing, which has been published in the open access journal *ATOL: Art Therapy OnLine* (Ottarsdottir, 2018). The publication includes the quantitative memory drawing research in connection with an art educational therapeutic case study and detailed, contextualized reviews of literature regarding memory of pictures and drawings; art therapy in schools; and art therapy in relation to memories of trauma.

• I gave a keynote lecture on memory drawing research at the 20th Nordic Art Therapies Conference, held in Iceland in 2018.

Tasks being conducted:

• Writing this chapter and, thereby, introducing the memory drawing research within the context of art therapy theories and methods, as well as addressing associated ethical concerns.

Tasks that lay ahead:

• To further introduce memory drawing research in lectures, publications, and workshops.
• To provide supervision for educators or other non-therapists who may apply memory drawing in a school setting.
• To create a memory drawing curriculum for students in teaching, psychotherapy, and art therapy departments at universities.
• To seek cooperation with such educational institutions, with the aim of educating students about memory drawing.
• To apply, once again, to the Icelandic Centre for Research for a grant; this time, updating progress made in the area of memory drawing research.

References

Ottarsdottir, U. (2018). Processing emotions and memorising coursework through memory drawing. *ATOL: Art Therapy OnLine*, 9(1). Retrieved from http://journals.gold.ac.uk/index.php/atol/article/view/486/pdf

Wammes, J.D., Meade, M.E., & Fernandes, M.A. (2016). The drawing effect: Evidence for reliable and robust memory benefits in free recall. *The Quarterly Journal of Experimental Psychology*, 69(9), 1752–1776.

Sojung Park

Does a gift policy also need translation according to culture?

In Korea, it is not uncommon for a client to bring their therapist homemade food or a cup of coffee, bought, along with their own, on the way to a session. How would I handle this situation? The first thing I would do is to ban myself from reading about, or interpreting, this specific behavior from a Western perspective. Instead, I might recognize that I have become a person to whom the client wishes to extend her *jeong* (with the possibility of entering her psychological *jip-an*). I would probably still draw a line, explaining that I'd accept the gift only that one time, but I would use my judgment regarding the appropriateness of the "gift," based upon the cultural norm.

From a Korean perspective, the therapy, itself, is inseparable from *jeong*. Just as Korean students can be confused between *jeong* and the therapeutic boundary, so can clients. Knowing that the therapist's act of drawing a therapeutic line can be perceived as a refusal of *jeong*, as well as a rejection of the client, I find myself extremely careful and sensitive whenever I believe that the therapeutic boundary needs to be addressed.

Jordan S. Potash

How can I best support a client's community arts initiative?

In resolving this dilemma, my first step was to identify potential role conflicts. As my client was the organizer of the event, but not the direct supervisor of the facilitators, we would have limited interaction. Thus, it seemed unlikely that he would be at risk for exploitation (ATCB Principle 2.3.4) or that my participation would impede the therapeutic relationship (AATA Principle 1.4). Would my presence show him that I supported his endeavors or would it remind him of the challenging times that had led to the initiation of our work together? To answer this question, a crucial component of the decision-making process was to have a conversation with him, thereby promoting client autonomy. One aspect of the discussion was to acknowledge our clinical relationship, while affirming that any interaction we might have at the event would be within a non-clinical context.

We also discussed our expectations of working together at that event, including the extent to which we might interact and whether either of us would be letting others know that we had a therapeutic relationship. (I would not be.) As we identified our respective roles and acknowledged any role differentiation—for example, the fact that, as the person responsible for giving volunteers guidance, my client would be in a superior position to me—we arrived at shared expectations of each other, thereby maintaining fidelity in our relationship.

I also sought supervision and professional consultation in an effort to determine if my participation could support my client's artistic achievements while maintaining my objectivity and therapeutic stance. I wanted to make sure that my participation was rooted in the value of beneficence; that is, that my presence could promote the welfare of both my client and the community. As an art therapist who was well known in the community, my presence could lend the event credibility, which in turn could support its standing within that community, thereby furthering my client's goals. In the end, I agreed to participate in the event, along with other colleagues from my agency. Together, our presence demonstrated an agency initiative to support a community arts and well-being project.

Sangeeta Prasad

Is it necessary to institute, in a more informal cultural environment, the strict boundaries regarding confidentiality and informed consent that are such an important feature of therapeutic work in the US?

When I was asked, in the late 1980s, to write an article on art therapy for a leading newspaper in India, I felt honored and submitted an article that included a case study. I then received a phone call from the editor, asking to photograph the children creating artwork. When I asked the parents and the school administration if a reporter could come to photograph the children, everyone agreed; in fact, they seemed proud and delighted. As a young art therapist, I felt as if asking them to sign a formal release form would give them the impression that—within an environment where transactions always took place verbally—I could not trust their (spoken) word. When the article was published, many of the teachers and parents reported that they liked it; none of the parents voiced any objections to the photograph or what I had written.

If this were to happen today, I would do things very differently. Over the years I have come to realize how important it is to gain consent whenever we use images created in art therapy. One incident, in particular, taught me this. Someone I knew in hospital management told me that a reporter once wrote an article about volunteers providing art, music, and other activities to children undergoing cancer treatment. The published article was accompanied by a photograph of a child who was undergoing treatment. The child's family was very upset, since they had not told other members of their family or their community about their son's cancer treatment. This is a good example of why—even in a country in which there are no formal policies, regulations, or laws governing informed consent—the individual's right to give permission for the use of his or her art, or a photo of him- or herself creating art, must be respected. We cannot even fathom how far-reaching the effects of a breach of privacy might be.

In this day and age, when an image on social media can be reused by others without permission, it can be damaging not only to the person who created it, but also to the person who shared it. Recently, artwork that had been created in India was reused, for the purpose of advertising an expressive arts therapy program completely unrelated to the work in India! This underlines, yet again, the importance of requesting permission and, if it is granted, acknowledging the source.

> 2.2.2 Art therapists shall not make or permit any public use or reproduction of a client's art therapy sessions, including verbalization and art expression, without express written consent of the client or the client's parent or legal guardian.
>
> 2.2.3 Art therapists shall obtain written informed consent from a client, or when applicable, a parent or legal guardian, before photographing the client's art expressions, making video or audio recordings, otherwise duplicating, or permitting third-party observation of art therapy sessions.
>
> *Art Therapy Credentials Board, 2018*

Reference

Art Therapy Credentials Board (2018). *Code of ethics, conduct, and disciplinary procedures.* Greensboro, NC: Author.

Michael Pretzer

As a male art therapist, how should I respond to the apparent boundary crossing of a female client?

Having a 16-year-old female client use part of my body as her canvas threw me into what I will call controlled panic. Part of my mind shouted "Breach of ethics," while another part yelled back, "Think about your client!" I weighed my objections against the client's history of male emotional and sexual abuse and parental rejection. I decided to let her paint on my hand. Afterward, the image seemed to seep into my skin like a stain. I scrubbed the painting off in the men's room.

I had concluded that allowing her to paint on me was not an ethical violation. Later, however, I realized the implication of washing the image down the drain. I had destroyed a client's artwork without her knowledge or consent. Standard 2.1.9 of the Art Therapy Credentials Board's *Code* (2018) states: "Whenever possible, a photographic representation should be maintained … for all work created by the client that is relevant to document the therapy if maintaining the original artwork would be difficult." Assuming that I had obtained written consent from the client's legal guardian, the proper action would have been to explain to the client that I planned to photograph her painting and then to wipe it off my hand. I also should have told her that I would store the photograph with her confidential clinical record. These actions would conform not only to the ATCB *Code*, but also to the AATA *Code* (2013): "The client is notified in instances when the art therapist and/or the clinical agency retain copies, photographic reproductions or digital images of the artwork in the client file as part of the clinical record" (Principle 4.1.a).

References

American Art Therapy Association (2013). *Ethical principles for art therapists*. Alexandria, VA: Author.

Art Therapy Credentials Board (2018). *Code of ethics, conduct, and disciplinary procedures*. Greensboro, NC: Author.

Pamela Reyes H.

How do I weigh the patients' right to privacy against the institution's desire to exhibit their art?

The way in which I confronted this dilemma was not by flatly refusing to organize expositions of the works of my patients. These requests often came from team members interested in what we were doing in the art therapy workshops; the patients' art generated a sense of fascination in them, due to the strangeness, intensity, or subtlety of some of the images. What I did to resolve this dilemma was to share with my patients the requests of the health team, to present the potential problems and benefits of exhibiting their work, and to respect their right to choose whether they wanted to participate. Sometimes we were able to perceive a therapeutic objective to the organization of expositions, in that it led us to analyze, in the art therapy workshop, what the patients did or did not want to show of themselves to others (family, health team, or community). Only in this way could I balance the requirements of the institutions with the care of the privacy of my patients. Slowly, the health teams with which I worked started to understand the different levels of art in health and of therapy through art.

Mary Roberts

How should I respond when I hear: "He seems to be doing well, considering his emotional state"?

No student should receive accommodations beyond the scope of the policies outlined in the Student Handbook, unless the student has pursued an official accommodation through the Disabilities Office or all students receive the accommodation. For instance, the deadline for an assignment may be extended for all students, but not just for one student. Ethical concerns arise when faculty make accommodations for students individually and not in accordance with ethical practices and with the program's policies and procedures as described in the Student Handbook. A faculty member who makes exceptions in individual circumstances opens herself to ethical violations related to questions of integrity and the equitable application of justice.

When tempted to treat a student differently from the others, it would be important for faculty to clarify issues that might be related to their multiple roles (i.e., being a faculty member who is also an art therapist), as well as to explore any counter-transference related to the student in question.

How should I proceed when a student failed her initial courses and no action plan had been initiated?

Meet with the student to address learning difficulties and perhaps suggest testing for the presence of learning disabilities, which would make additional resources available to her. Recommend an academic action plan that addresses learning difficulties and documents a time frame within which the student agrees to meet technical standards and minimum academic competencies before moving on to the internship semester. Consider a leave of absence.

Meet with faculty to devise a systemic way in which to report student progress in an on-going, timely, clear, detailed manner.

What should be done when a student who is in good academic standing exhibits a lack of investment in her internship?

Although doing well academically, the poor judgment and lack of integrity exhibited by the student in abandoning her responsibilities to her internship without communicating with her site supervisor or faculty placed the welfare of her clients at risk. Since supervisors are legally responsible for the actions of their supervisees, she also placed her site supervisor and the art therapy program at risk. The disclosure of mental illness did not occur until well after the missed days at her internship and her site supervisor was never notified of the student's struggles with mental illness. AATA's ethical principle 1.5, Responsibility to Clients, is relevant in this regard: "Art therapists refrain from engaging in an activity when they know or should know that there is a substantial likelihood that their personal problems will prevent them from performing their work-related activities in a competent manner" (American Art Therapy Association, 2013).

Due to the poor judgment and lack of integrity she exhibited in the way she interacted with her internship placement, as well as her noncompliance with program policies, procedures, and ethical principles, the student was invited to withdraw from the art therapy program. She readily accepted the invitation. Site supervisors were immediately encouraged to report student absences and insufficient student progress to the art therapy program faculty supervisor and administrator.

How do we allow an individual with a mental illness to become an art therapist? How do we disallow an individual with a mental illness to become an art therapist?

The student's decision to openly disclose to faculty her struggles with mental illness enabled them to discuss concerns during a faculty meeting early in the semester and to track her progress in weekly faculty meeting reports. Through continued monitoring, it was determined that the student would be placed on academic probation and provided with an action plan, which meant that the program could require the student to demonstrate proof of consistent attendance in therapy, assist and support the student in identifying appropriate self-care measures, and monitor the completion of unfinished work. The student did increase investment in coursework and internship, resulting in her meeting GPA requirements.

Reference

American Art Therapy Association (2013). *Ethical principles for art therapists.* Alexandria, VA: Author.

Mary Ellen Ruff

How should I respond to an ethical dilemma that occurred while working with a group?

Scott's stepmother's behavior in the family group became so disruptive that, in order to protect that group, I asked that she discontinue her participation altogether. This was the right thing for the group, the right thing for Scott, and probably the right thing for his stepmother as well. Her erratic presentation led me to recommend that she seek her own treatment. Although I was concerned that she might be unprepared to hear that, she was receptive to the recommendation.

How should I respond to an ethical dilemma that occurred while working with a family?

This situation created a tremendous amount of stress for me, personally and professionally. I chose to testify on my client's behalf, in opposition to my agency. Although I was able to feel good about the decision I made to follow my personal and professional ethics, it created an untenable dynamic at work and, eventually, I decided to resign from my position. Throughout the legal proceedings, I was portrayed by my agency's attorney as inexperienced, unprofessional, and lacking in boundaries. I was able to weather that storm only by virtue of good supervision, confidence in my own ethics, and the belief that I had done the right, albeit difficult, thing.

How should I respond to an ethical dilemma while working with a couple?

I found working with Ellen and Keith to be particularly difficult. I felt allegiance to both of them individually and as a couple. I tried to focus upon what had brought them to therapy in the first place (their grief), but, as it so often does, therapy evolved into the exploration of deeper, underlying relationship issues. It wasn't my place to divulge Ellen's secret—I felt clear about that; however, I felt pulled by my positive regard for Keith. I decided that I needed to continue to hold Ellen's information—thereby creating a space in which Ellen and Keith could explore their relationship—and to wait. Ellen never told Keith about her infidelity within the context of our work together and, as far as I know, they are still together. I feel as though I made the right decision at the time, and I would probably still make the same decision today, but I have often thought of Keith and his living in the dark about Ellen's infidelity. I had to suspend my personal feelings about the situation and to keep the focus upon their evolution as a couple. I could empathize with each of them, but my work with them was as a couple, and I needed to see the whole as greater than the sum of its parts.

Jane Scott

What should I do when I discover that information about a crime has been disclosed on a sheet of drawing paper?

I decided to bring John's letter to my administrator, to honor the chain of command and ask for help with this ethical situation. To be honest, as a brand new art therapist, I was hoping that I would not have to deal with the repercussions of reading the note. Couldn't I just throw it away and pretend never to have seen it? This was serious stuff! Ultimately, the note was given to the police and sealed in a file as evidence. I had to speak with a gang intervention agency representative as well. It was a difficult experience but I learned the true meaning of ethics: to do what is right even when no one is watching and even when it isn't comfortable. It is normal to feel nervous, upset, or conflicted over reporting situations; what matters is making the final decision, to protect our clients.

The ethical issue in this scenario happens often in detention. Adolescents have little insight into the legality of their disclosures—evidenced by the number of incriminating posts, photos, and videos on social networks such as Facebook and YouTube. Whether or not the disclosure is intentional, as an art therapist working in a court system, we are bound to report certain information and/or artwork. Other times, it can be up to our clinical judgment. As the seasoned psychologist at my Center said while supervising me, "It's tough when the client has to face the reality of the boundaries of confidentiality. The most important thing is to have informed consent." Clients need to know clearly what will be reported and what will not.

The lesson of this ethical dilemma is that, as much as we sometimes do not want to get involved in legal cases or are afraid to turn in evidence or to make a report, it is our ethical obligation in these situations to step up. When in doubt, ask for help. Turn to another professional at your job whom you trust and who shows sound ethical judgment and consult with that individual in confidence. In detention settings, part of the job is being willing to stand strong when feeling intimidated.

Gwendolyn M. Short

How should I respond when staff members limit freedom of expression in art therapy?

I took a three-pronged approach. First, I engaged the staff by inviting them to participate in the group, rather than hovering over the boys as they worked. This seemed to increase their understanding of art therapy—and they became so involved in the process that they did not focus as much upon the boys. Second, I carved out a portion of the final hour to meet individually with each boy, which gave them some privacy in which to express themselves and explore their artwork without fear of reprimand by staff. Third, I decided to talk both individually and in small groups with staff about what the opportunity to draw whatever one wanted to draw in art therapy (including drug paraphernalia) might actually accomplish.

Elizabeth Stone

When a religious patient creates transgressive imagery in art therapy, how should I respond?

Evoking the multicultural dimension of this experience might have helped raise the question of Nadima's own level of comfort about having breached her religious tenets, which would have introduced an ethical component into a clinical situation. The student could have observed aloud that Nadima seemed to have adapted very quickly to a Western approach to art expression and asked whether that posed any conflicts for her due to her own religious beliefs. Optimally, empathic attunement toward discovering whether Nadima felt coerced into "adapting" so seamlessly to her new surrounding culture could have helped her sort out her feelings. She might have then felt reassured, knowing that the intern understood her cultural taboos and dilemmas, whether she chose to create unbridled or more circumspect pictorial expressions in the future.

In addressing this dilemma, I found Standards 7.2 and 7.5 of AATA's ethics code (2013) to be particularly useful, as well as Standard 1.2.4 of the ATCB's ethics code (2018).

When the presence of a painting on the art therapist's wall poses an ethical dilemma. how should I proceed?

I decided to replace the piece, because a painting of a nude figure might have been offensive to some, even if most of my Muslim patients were rather liberal-minded. I felt it better to err on the conservative side and not risk replaying the kind of situation described in the previous vignette, where a patient might have felt compelled to fit into her surrounding culture.

Addendum

Months after writing the previous paragraph, I happened to mention to Maggie Mortifée, the artist, the ethical dilemma that I had had and the way in which I had resolved it. Clearly disappointed that her painting had been removed and replaced by a large but inoffensive mountainous landscape by Edith Kramer, I told her that I, too, missed her lovely nude. Suddenly, I had reopened my dilemma. In taking the painting down, I had removed it not only from *my* sight, but also from that of the cancer patients (and other patients) who had come to know it over the months. The creation of the piece had had a therapeutic component for the artist; might it not have one for those who view it? I found the painting abstract enough to be less than explicit. What did I do? I decided to look for a new home for it on a less prominent wall. It now resides in an alcove of my waiting room, out of direct view of anyone sitting in one of the chairs, but possible to see by walking toward the area where I keep my printer.

Editor's note: Given the cultural considerations described so well by the writer, the question of whether to include in this book a photograph of Mlle. Mortifée's lovely painting raised yet another ethical dilemma. Given this cautionary note, the author and I thought that the following page might serve as another kind of "alcove" for the painting. What are your thoughts?

References

American Art Therapy Association (2013). *Ethical principles for art therapists*. Alexandria, VA: Author.
Art Therapy Credentials Board (2018). *Code of ethics, conduct, and disciplinary procedures*. Greensboro, NC: Author.

Todd C. Stonnell

Disclosing burnout to patients: To tell or not to tell?

Depending, of course, upon the needs of the patient and the strength of the therapeutic relationship, I have found that it has been helpful, during times such as this, to err on the side of transparency. For individuals who are prone to impulsive and

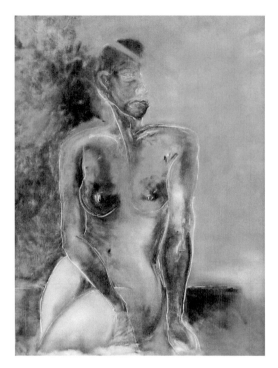

FIGURE B.4 *Femme Sans Titre* by Maggie Mortifée. We regret that the brilliant turquoise and gold tones of the original painting could not be reproduced here.

compulsive behaviors, seeing us in a state of burnout could convey the message that it is "okay" for someone to work him- or herself to the bone and then show up the next day and do the same thing. I have to wonder if our untreated burnout reinforces their belief that they should never slow down and rest or simply be still.

I aim to be more open about my current space with patients, especially if I am feeling distracted during the session; this can be approached in a manner which encourages the patient to explore what it feels like to be *knocked out of balance* or *stressed-out*. This, in turn, might lead to a conversation about how we can affect the recalibration needed. Another important component to consider is the prospect of patients perceiving changes in our behavior as a direct consequence of their interactions with us; in other words, they may think that they caused our current mindset. Having a clear conversation that clarifies misunderstandings can maintain the health of the therapeutic alliance. It can also offer the patient a chance to say (to him- or herself, if not directly to us): *"Phew. It's not me, it's you."* (And don't we all just love to hear that?)

I created "Flowerbomb" (see Figure B.5) as I reflected upon how hard I tend to be on myself in response not only to burnout, but also to other significant areas of my life. I realized that compassion for myself is not something that comes easily and

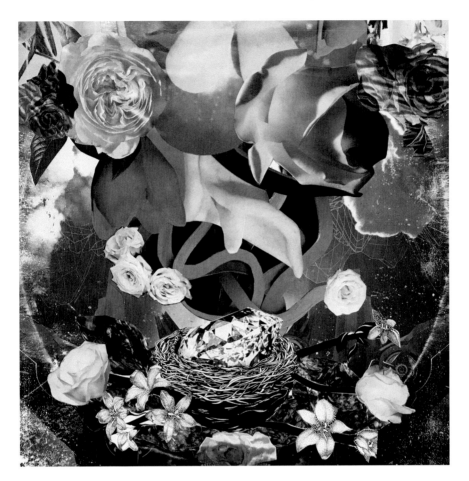

FIGURE B.5 *Flowerbomb.*

I must really work hard to allow it to stick. Compassion is a vital part of dealing with burnout, as it softens the edges of the judgment that accompanies this decline in energy and motivation. It is during this time that I seek the internal strengths and resources that can protect me, while also remembering that they deserve to be nurtured as well.

Sharon Strouse

To attend or not to attend?

I was caught off guard when April showed me her ticket to the Kristin Rita Strouse Foundation Yellow Dress Speaker Event. I had not advertised our event to the private clients who came to my studio; I felt that it would be inappropriate to promote our foundation and sell tickets. April came across our information at a suicide survivors support group. I thanked her for her support and told her that the speaker's story of loss and healing would be intense. I encouraged her to be conscious of good self-care that evening.

On the heels of that conversation, April reminded me that Justin's first year anniversary was coming up and that she was having a special memorial service. Justin's headstone would be placed, followed by a reception at home with family and friends. She asked me to come. I immediately noticed the juxtaposition of the invitation to attend her son's memorial service with the mention of her up-coming attendance at a public event honoring our daughter and the work of our foundation. I paused, sensing a professional boundary. April's anniversary event was personal. I would have entered her home and socialized with her family and friends. Would it be in April's best interest for me to come or for me to keep a clear boundary between us? The Preamble to the American Art Therapy Association's *Ethical Principles for Art Therapists* (2013) highlights the importance of fidelity: "Art therapists accept their role and responsibility to act with integrity towards clients, colleagues and members of their community. Art therapists maintain honesty in their dealings, accuracy in their relationships, faithfulness to their promises and truthfulness in their work." This value is further clarified in principle 1.3: "It is the professional responsibility of art therapists to avoid ambiguity in the therapeutic relationship and to maintain clarity about the different therapeutic roles that exist between client and therapist." I thanked April profusely for wanting to include me in this special event, and I graciously declined her invitation.

Reference

American Art Therapy Association (2013). *Ethical principles for art therapists.* Alexandria, VA: Author.

Tally Tripp

What can I take away from hearing: "I asked you to help me remodel the kitchen, not renovate the entire house!"?

Therapists can "only be where the client is." That is, the client must determine when he or she is ready to dig deep and when to stay on the surface. In the case of Ellen, I knew that the attachment wounds and severe lack of attunement throughout her childhood were at the root of her current problems maintaining intimate relationships. It was equally clear that dealing with this interpersonal trauma story would be a painful and difficult journey.

For a few sessions, I recommended that we slow down the pace to modulate the overwhelming feelings and reduce the likelihood of her being flooded with emotion. I suggested that, once stable, we could work with the underlying issues of trauma and neglect that were negatively impacting her life. I warned her that this would be a challenge, but I believed we could do the work required for healing. But neither slowing down nor healing trauma were concepts on Ellen's agenda. She became extremely angry that I could not just move forward and magically "fix" the problem in her current relationships. She was angry that I was controlling the pace of our work. We were stuck. I wanted to slow down the pace and work with the early trauma. She wanted to rush forward and heal the current symptoms. Unable to resolve this deadlock, Ellen began missing sessions and talking about termination.

Ultimately, we terminated treatment because it became clear that we were working at cross-purposes. In my view, I could not help Ellen and attend to the "reason" she was referred to me because there was so much more to the picture. In our final session, she was able to share her disappointment, tearfully telling me, "I asked you to come in and just remodel the kitchen, but you felt you had to renovate the entire house!"

I learn every day from my clients. Ellen taught me that, despite all the knowledge a therapist may have, we must "stay in the kitchen" and be true to the contract. Art therapy can add so much to an on-going treatment, but we must honor our clients' needs and expectations for a successful result.

Jennifer Vivian

Teachable moments: How and when should I speak up?

When the nurse bypassed the parent to address me, I replied that the practitioner should be speaking with the family; that sharing the family's private medical information with me—and in a public hallway, where anyone could hear—was inappropriate. At the time, I wished that I had spoken to the family beforehand about what they would want me to do if this—or other similarly disquieting—situations arose. Since then, I have raised the subject with the other Indigenous people with whom I have worked. There have been times when clients have asked me to act as a liaison between themselves and other practitioners and, in those cases, I have to be particularly clear about my boundaries. I am sorry that the possibility of a practitioner not speaking directly to an Indigenous person even exists.

The many meanings of love: Is our response to the term "love" culturally considerate?

In contrast to the Eurocentric idea of love as something exclusionary and intimate, the local Indigenous perspective is that love is something that brings one joy; a positive experience. Therefore, I did not address this situation in the way that I might have if I were working from a psychodynamic perspective; regarding it as a possible concern. As my time with this child progressed, the identification as an artist was strengthened, and our therapeutic relationship grew, the word "love" was dropped. If I had challenged this word when it had first appeared and not been open to what it meant to the child, I believe that the outcome might have been different.

The role of honesty in building the therapeutic alliance: How much would you share with your client?

In honoring the sacred teachings of honesty and wisdom, I shared with this client my own personal experience of how art making had helped me in my life. I tried to keep things as general as possible, but to honor the sacred teaching of love, to lead with the heart. I knew that I would have to be genuine with, and to trust, this person, in order for the therapeutic alliance to develop. I chose to make art alongside this person, but did not focus my attention on my own artwork during the session. The opportunity to look at my work afterwards allowed me to gain insight into counter-transferential issues. In sharing myself in this way, I honored the concept of healing as a community endeavor, rather than as one that involved only an individual. It also underlined my position as one who sought not to be an authority figure, but to offer help, through building a therapeutic art-making practice.

In deciding how to respond to these three ethical dilemmas, I reached out to my relationships within the community—while maintaining confidentiality—asking if they would tell me, in general terms, about their concepts of love and of healing. Their responses were invaluable.

Diane Waller

Is it ethical to maintain in a group someone who seems to need the group but has violated its boundaries and behaved aggressively, albeit symbolically?

I decided to deal with the matter by doing some teaching about group dynamics, focusing upon the reasons for having the rules that had been so clearly stated and reinforced throughout the group. I used the incident as a teaching tool for emphasizing how essential boundaries and containment were within a powerful intervention such as an art psychotherapy group; that, if rules were ignored, the group became unsafe for everyone. This calmed down the situation and took the pressure off individuals, but did not deal with the incident itself, so I asked the group for advice on how we should manage it—but said that excluding Marta was not an option. Indeed, I tried to involve Marta in the decision making, without much success. She seemed puzzled about being able to remain in the group. Though her anger had subsided, she could not own up to the impact of her actions in getting the key to the room late at night and interfering with her small group's work. She denied its importance. She dismissed the import of crushing the doll, saying, "It is only a plastic thing…" I decided not to persist in questioning her. I realized that the group was not the place for Marta to try to relive the original trauma and that she would have to stay in the group at a level that was safe for her—and for other people. Although she remained in a quiet and somewhat sulky mood for the remainder of the week, she did not leave the group.

Unfortunately, Marta's defenses were so great that, at our very first contact, she had not been able to share with me the anxiety that had led her to ask me to look at and comment upon her artwork. Had I done as she'd wished, I might have understood that she was not in a fit psychological state to undertake a workshop that demands considerable emotional and psychological insight from its participants. I could have calmly and kindly advised her to seek help and given her some further information. *Was I wrong not to follow my gut feeling, not to look at her artwork, not to try to dissuade her from joining the group? Was I wrong to assume that Marta had experienced a severe trauma and that her desperate action in violating the group's boundaries was a move towards being able to start the painful process of reliving the trauma of abuse?* I don't think I was wrong and I believe that, by returning to theoretical aspects of group psychotherapy to help process this incident, I limited the harm that was done. Had I removed Marta from the group, I feel that this would have harmed her and that the group would have been left feeling guilty and unaware of the importance of maintaining a safe, contained space. I believe that I was correct in not persisting in trying to persuade Marta to explore her actions and her feelings, thus enabling her to remain in her own safe, psychological space. This was one of my most stressful experiences in conducting art therapy groups and one from which I have learned a very great deal about the need for careful vetting of participants and for reinforcing "group rules" throughout.

Shirin Yaish

What do we do when the experiences shared by others feel so overwhelming that we question whether our supports are sufficient to the task?

I felt that I needed to reach for what felt right in the depth of my soul, in that central point within me. I turned to my art materials. In fact, I chose to make a *mandala*, a Sanskrit word for "circle." Carl Jung, who painted mandalas (1972) and asked his patients to create them, regarded the form as, among other things, a representation of wholeness. So, that evening I created my own *mandala* and the next day I went back to the group and introduced its members to the concept of the *mandala*.

Reference

Jung, C.G. (1972). *Mandala symbolism*. Princeton, NJ: Princeton University Press.

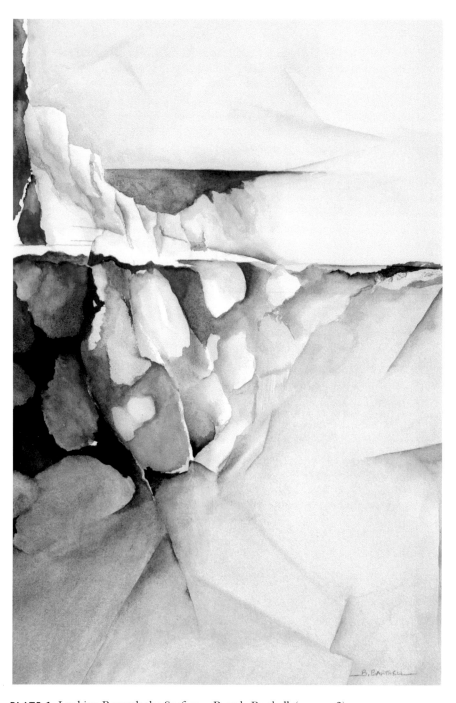

PLATE 1 Looking Beneath the Surface – Brenda Barthell *(see page 2).*

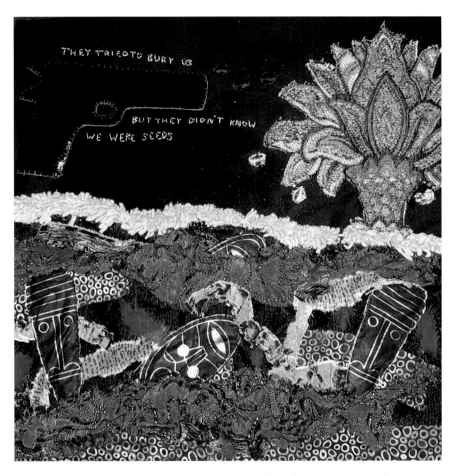

PLATE 2 Uprising: They tried to bury us but they didn't know we were seeds – Martina E. Martin *(see page 39)*.

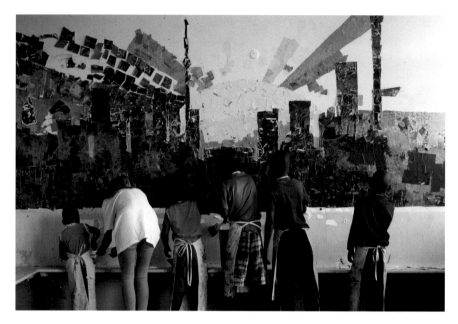

PLATE 3 Children creating a mural of the Hillbrow skyline *(see page 69)*.

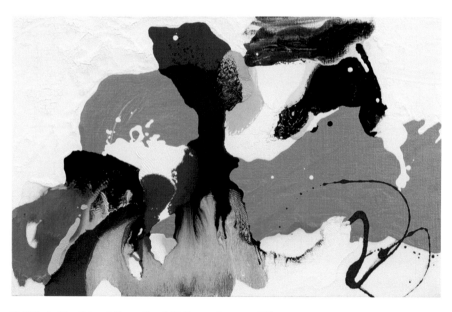

PLATE 4 Confidentiality – Sarah Vollman *(see page 89)*.

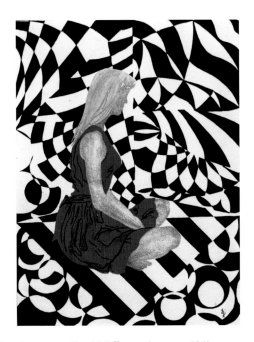

PLATE 5 Conflicting Interests – Bani Malhotra *(see page 131)*.

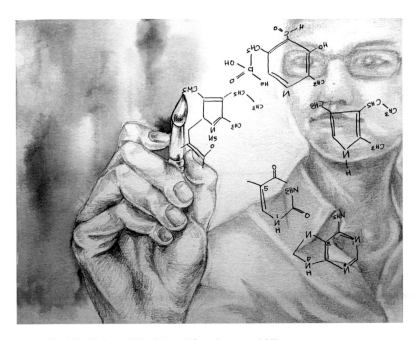

PLATE 6 Multiple Roles – Min Kyung Shin *(see page 189)*.

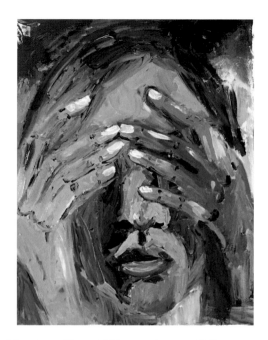

PLATE 7 Scope of Practice – Hannah Wittman *(see page 233).*

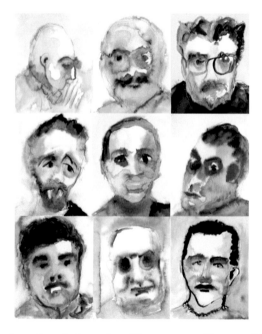

PLATE 8 Male art therapists ask themselves: "Are we agreeable enough? Are we open enough? Are we nurturing enough?" – Michael Pretzer *(see page 312).*

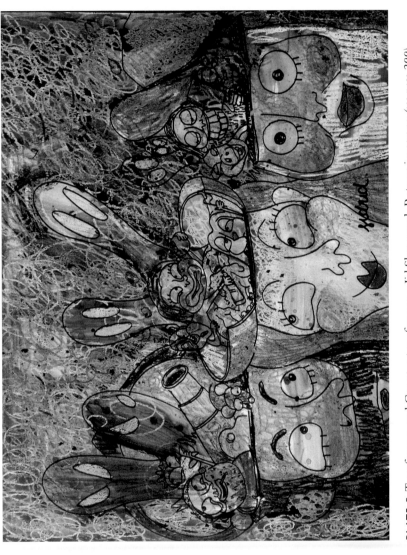

PLATE 9 Transference and Counter-transference – Jid Shwanpach Ratanapinyopong (*see page 299*).

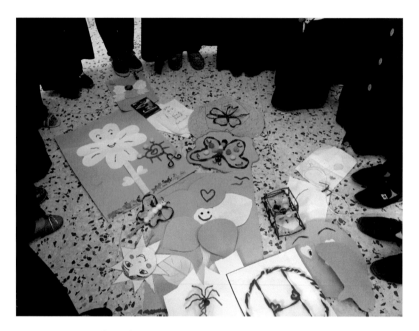

PLATE 10 Experiential art therapy training (initial session) *(see page 323).*

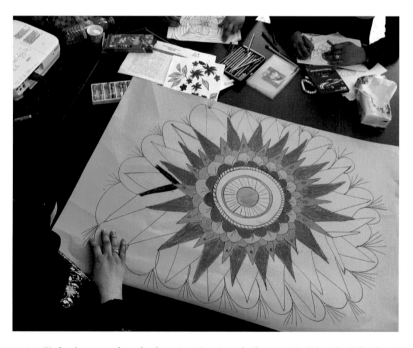

PLATE 11 "I don't remember the last time I enjoyed silence as I did today"(final session) *(see page 330).*

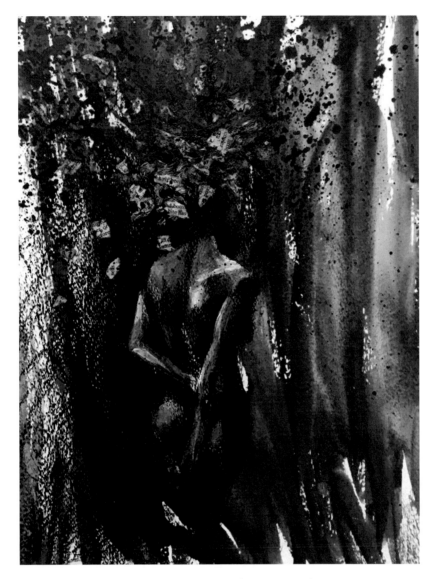

PLATE 12 The Abuse of Power – Kristina Nowak *(see page 359).*

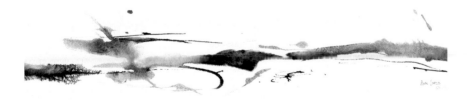

PLATE 13 Drawing to a Close – Anne Corson *(see page 371).*

INDEX

Aba-Afari, S. 205
abuse 183–5, 382
abuse of power 359–60
accreditation 72–3
Acquaye, R. 205
addiction 316–21
adolescents 124–9, 230, 296
adults 37–41, 45, 55–61, 91–103, 111–17,
        140–53, 161–87, 235–52, 259–65,
        292–307, 316–31, 352–7, 379–88
age groups *see* client age groups
ageism 62, 65
Alfonso, M.R.A. xiii, 27–34, 396–8
Alter-Muri, S. 144
Ambrogi, R. 108
American Art Therapy Association 6, 134,
        191–2, 210–11, 276, 292–3, 308–9
American Psychological Association
        (APA) 91–2
Andrews, C. 168
anorexia nervosa 149
anxiety 342
apps 242–52
Argentina 50–4
Arhin, E.L. 205
armour 326–7
art educational therapy (AET) 266–72
art envy 262
art making by art therapists 2, 39, 64, 89, 113,
        131, 145, 189, 233, 299, 303–4, 309,
        312, 359, 371, 412, 437, 441

art making by art therapy students 77, 136,
        332–51
art making by clients 64, 97, 127–8, 140–6,
        184–6, 249–50, 263, 266–72, 293–6,
        382–7, 402, 407
art objectivity 194
Art Therapy Credentials Board (ATCB) 6,
        106–7, 134, 274–5, 285–6, 374
Art Therapy International Work Assessment
        (ATIWA) 43–4
artist/scientist role relation 198–200
Asociación Chilena de Arteterapia 148
aspirational values 6, 56–60, 192, 220, 297, 404
assisted living facilities and hospices 63–7
assumptions 36–7
asylum seekers 351–7
attention deficit disorder (ADD/ADHD) 274
Australia 332–8
Australian and New Zealand Arts Therapy
        Association xxi
autism spectrum disorder 274
autonomy 57–9, 65–6, 125, 156, 220–1,
        227, 418

Ballbé ter Maat, M. xiv, 50–4, 279–84,
        398–9, 413–15
Bardot, H. xiv, 43–8, 399–400
Bares, K. 168
Barthell, B. 2
bartering 115
baseball group 228–9

beginning treatment 4, 12–21
beneficence 57–9
bereavement 301–7
Berman, H. xiv, 68–75, 400
bias and discrimination 9–10, 43–8, 65,
    177, 366
Bitter, J.B. 78, 81
Blandy, D. 296
board game group 228
Bolin, P. 296
Bollas, C. 74
borderline personality disorder 382
Boston, C.B. xiv, 173–80, 400–1
boundaries
    peers 317
    staff 173–4, 254–8
    students 340–1
    studio 294–7
    therapeutic 44–5, 56–7, 78–80, 112–16,
        178, 254–8, 301–7, 310–11, 340, 346,
        373–7, 383–4, 420, 429–30
boundary violation see multiple roles
Bragge, A. 333
Breakthrough app 243–7
British Association of Art Therapists xxi, 71
Brownlee, K. 195
Bryan, B. 168
Burgard, E.L. 194
burnout 318–20, 435
Byrne, L. xiv, 332–8, 406–7

Cain, S. 77
Canada 83–8
cancellation see late cancellation
Carolan, R. xiv, 198–203, 401
Cartwheel Foundation 27–8
Case, C. 333
case management 161–6, 172, 219–24
Casement, P. 323
certification bodies xxi
chae-myun (face-saving) 79–80
children 69–70, 153–60, 164–5, 219–24,
    226–31, 266–72, 274, 279–84,
    373–7, 414
Chile 147–52
choice see autonomy

client age groups:
    adolescents 124–9, 230, 296
    adults 37–41, 45, 55–61, 91–103,
        111–17, 140–53, 161–87,
        235–52, 259–65, 292–307, 316–31,
        352–7, 379–88

children 69–70, 153–60, 164–5, 219–24,
    226–31, 266–72, 274, 373–7
    older adults 62–6
client choice see autonomy
closing a clinical practice 379–88
co-leading 174
co-therapy 97, 101
Cogan, D.M. xv, 55–61, 401–2
Cohen-Liebman, M.S. 104–5
collaboration 14–16, 149–50, 215, 259–65
collectivism 76–8
combat service members and their
    families 91–6
Community Art Counsellors (CAC) 70–2
community-based art studios 70–4, 142–3,
    195, 293–7, 408
community-based treatment 27–34, 55–6,
    60–1, 71–4, 151–2, 157–8

conditions addressed by the chapter
    writers:
    abuse 66, 183–5, 382
    addiction 316–21
    anxiety 342
    autism spectrum disorder 274
    dementia 65
    depression 149, 248–9, 384–6
    developmental delays 157
    dissociation 184–5, 236, 260, 380, 387
    eating disorders 149, 181–7
    grief and loss/bereavement 301–7, 381
    homelessness 161–6
    job-related injuries 167–72
    learning difficulties 153–60
    post-traumatic stress disorder (PTSD) 91,
        98, 124, 235–6, 380, 382, 387
    schizophrenia and psychosis 148–9, 219,
        226, 254, 363
    self-injury 125–6, 182–4, 363–4, 367
    severe and persistent mental illness
        (SPMI) 55–61
    suicidality 94–5, 137, 262, 296, 367
    trauma 59–60, 182–7, 235, 241, 257,
        259–65, 322–31, 353–7, 438
confidentiality xxiii–xxiv, 64–5, 95, 107,
    113–14, 118–23, 126–7, 136, 157–8,
    211–12, 276–7, 283, 287–8
conflicting values 58–60, 76–80
Confucianism and collectivism 76–7
consent see informed consent
containment 267–72, 340–1
contract see private practice contract
corrections personnel 169–70

Corson, A. 371
counter-transference 3–4, 40–1, 171, 250,
    329, 374–5, 441–2
  see also transference
couples art therapy 122–3
courage 360–9
courts 104–10
courts *see* forensic facilities
creativity 165, 231, 275–6, 293, 296, 316–17,
    407, 434
credentials xxi, 14, 133–4
Crenshaw, D. 376
Csapo, K. 271
cultural awareness/considerations 4–5, 44–7,
    50–4, 76–81, 83–8, 112–16, 133–6,
    138–9, 177, 253–8, 275–8, 323
curator of public art therapy gallery 140–6
curiosity 342–3
Cutcher, D.J. xv, 167–72, 402

Dalley, T. 333
dance 31, 34
DASS (Depression Anxiety Scale) 248–9
Dean, M.L. xv, 181–7, 402–4
decision-making process *see* ethical decision-
    making process
demeaning comments 177–8
dementia 65–6
Department of Defense (DoD) 91–2
depression 149, 248–9, 384–6
depth-oriented art-based
    learning 340–3
detention facilities *see* juvenile detention
    centers
development 274
Di Maria, A. xiii, xxiii, 3–11
diagnosis 108–9
dilemma resolutions *see* resolutions
displaced aggression 356
disruptive behavior 101, 255–7, 294–5
dissociation 184–5, 236, 260, 380, 387
diversity 186
diversity training 177
Doby-Copeland, C. xv, 207, 219–24,
    404–6
document retention 16
Donald, K. xv, 111–17, 406
Dowd, E.T. 319
drawing xxii, 267–72, 384
dual relationships *see* multiple roles
duties 175
duty to report 6, 95, 126–8, 137, 362–6,
    413, 433

eating disorders 149, 181–7
educational settings:
  training programs 46–7, 68, 70–4,
    78–80, 133–9, 210–18, 254–8,
    285–91, 339–50
  university 71–3, 133, 205–6, 210–12, 254,
    294–5, 333–4
educator (multiple role) 125, 204–8,
    212–14, 229–31
Edwards, D. 342
el duende one-canvas process painting
    (EDPP) 339–50
elder abuse 66
electrical injuries 167–9
Eliot, T.S. 91
Elman, B.D. 319
employment injuries *see* job-related injuries
ending treatment *see* terminating treatment
Engelstatter, G. 168
ethical decision-making process 3–11, 221–3
  beliefs, biases and blind spots 9–10
  clientele/setting/mode of treatment 6–7
  films 10–11
  graphic 4–5
  laws/ethics codes/informed consent 5–6
  type of setting 5
  theoretical orientation/training/
    experience 7
  values/traits/tendencies 7–9
  work place norms 5
ethical dilemma resolutions *see* resolutions

ethical issues associated with:
  abuse of power 360–9
  access to training 68–75, 147, 204–8,
    273–8, 285–91, 425
  art making by art therapists 2, 39, 64, 89,
    113, 131, 145, 189, 233, 299, 303–4,
    309, 312, 359, 371, 412, 437, 441
  art making by art therapy students 77, 136,
    332–51
  art making by clients 64, 97, 127–8, 140–6,
    184–6, 249–50, 263, 266–72, 293–6,
    382–7, 402, 407
  autonomy 57–9, 65–6, 125, 156, 220–1,
    227, 418
  bartering 115
  beginning treatment 4, 12–21
  beneficence 57–9
  bias and discrimination 9–10, 44–8, 65,
    177, 366
  boundaries (therapeutic) 44–5, 56–7,
    78–80, 112–16, 178, 254–8, 301–7,

310–11, 340, 346, 373–7, 383–4, 411, 417, 420, 429–30, 440
burnout 171, 318–20, 402, 435
closing a clinical practice 379–87, 409–10
collaboration 14–16, 149–50, 215, 259–65
confidentiality xxiii–xxiv, 20, 64–5, 95, 107, 113–14, 118–23, 126–7, 136, 157–8, 211–12, 276–7, 283, 287–8, 406, 413–14, 428
conflicting values 58–60, 78–80, 91–6
counter-transference 40–1, 171, 250, 329, 374–5, 441
cultural awareness/considerations 43–9, 50–4, 76–81, 83–8, 112–16, 133–6, 138–9, 177, 253–8, 275–8, 323
disclosure of crimes 126–8, 433
duty to report 6, 66, 95, 126–8, 137, 362–6, 413, 433
exhibiting client art work 140–6, 148–9, 158, 194, 368
fidelity 58, 156, 220–1
financial issues 17–19, 135, 181–2, 365–6, 421
furor curandis 149
gift-giving and receiving 64, 80, 115, 178, 221, 304, 373–4, 376, 416
grading artwork created by art therapy students 213–14
informed consent xxiii–xxviii, 6, 13, 65–6, 70, 144, 220, 276–7, 283, 294, 414, 434
isolation 125
justice 58–60
language interpreters (use of) 97, 103, 135–6
laws and legal issues 5–6, 12–13, 59, 104–10, 222–3, 243, 374–5
multiple roles 37–42, 80, 114–5, 125, 159, 172, 191–6
    artist 194–5
    case manager 161–6, 172, 219–24
    curator of public art therapy gallery 140–6
    educator 125, 204–8, 210–18, 225–31, 425
    expert witness/testifying in court 104–10, 222–3, 404, 433
    Hospital Review Board member 60, 401
    Institutional Review Board (IRB) member 201, 401
    mandated reporter 6, 66, 95, 126–8, 137, 362–6, 413, 433
    minister 36–42
    non-clinical engagement 194–5
    relationship with self 198–200
    researcher 84, 198–203, 266–72, 425
    role differentiation 193–4
    shared expectations 193
    supervision 332–8, 339–50
natural disaster aid 27–35, 151–3
nonmaleficence 59–60
ownership of the art 282, 414
power dynamics 32, 341–2, 361, 396–7
private practice 12–21
religion/spirituality 37–42, 116, 182–7, 402–3
response art 332–8, 406
safe space/place 72, 93–4, 113–14, 136, 157, 177, 253–8, 355, 364
scope of practice 201, 274, 401
self-disclosure 37–8, 56–7, 63, 87, 115–16, 302–6, 318–20, 406
solitary confinement 125
supervision 74, 137, 177, 223, 274, 287, 289, 334, 339–50, 360–9
technology 14, 16, 17, 173, 242–52, 285–91, 411, 421
terminating treatment 19, 373–7, 379–88
time limits 53–4, 305, 398
third-party payers 168, 170–1, 181–7, 402
touch xxii, 63, 116, 135, 221, 305, 310–11, 317–18, 429
training art therapy students 46–7, 68, 70–4, 78–80, 133–9, 210–18, 254–8, 285–91, 339–50
training non-art therapists 45–6, 253–8, 280–2, 322–31, 413
transference 3–4, 51–2, 60, 99–100, 260, 382
visual free speech 165, 227, 231, 292–8, 407, 418, 434
work place norms 4, 5, 360–9
Ethical Self-Exam 7
ethics codes 5–6
Ethics Formula Evaluation Test (EFET) 178–9
Europe 133 9
evaluation 13, 108, 213–14, 355
exhibiting client art work 140–6, 148–9, 158, 194, 368
exhibitions 58–9, 143, 408
expert witness 104–6, 108, 222–3

factors that can influence ethical
decision-making 3–11
fairness *see* justice
family/couples art therapy 27–34,
51–4, 120–3
fees and payment 17–19, 135, 421
Fenner, P. xv, 332–8, 406–7
Fernandes, M.A. 271
fidelity 58, 156, 220–1
films 10–11
financial issues 17–19, 135, 181–2, 365–6,
421–23
Fish, B. 341
Fonagy, P. 70
forensic art therapy 104–10
forensic facilities:
courts 104–10
juvenile detention centers 124–9
prisons 44–5, 150–1
France 133–9
Franklin, M.A. xv, 292–7, 313, 407
fraud 365–6
furor curandis 149–50

Gadamer, H. 334
galleries *see* exhibiting client art
gambling addiction *see* addiction
games 228
Gantt, L. 236, 241
Garlock, L.R. xvi, 140–6, 407–8
Gaza 322–31
gender 99–100, 308–14
Genogram Analytics App 249
Gerhardt, P. 362
Ghana 204–8
gift-giving and receiving 64, 80, 115, 178,
221, 305, 373–4, 376, 416, 427
Gil, E. 376
Glime, O. 205
Goldberg, E.S. xvi, 97–103, 408–9
Goldstein, H. 192
Gombilla, E. 205
Good, D.A. xvi, 379–88, 409–11
Goren, E. 340–1
grading art by art therapy students 213–14
grief and loss/bereavement 301–7, 381
group art therapy 45–8, 53–4, 56–60, 70–1,
76–81, 118–20, 150–2, 157, 164–5,
173–5, 225–31, 253–8, 322–31,
365–6, 440
Gussak, D. xvi, 104–10, 219, 411

Halverson, G. 195
harm reduction *see* nonmaleficence
Havsteen-Franklin, D. 333

Health and Care Professions Council xxx, 253
Health Professions Council of South Africa
72–3
Hendriksen, J.O. 334
Herman, J. 59
hidden trauma 169–70
Higgitt, A. 70
HIPAA 17, 19–20, 243, 289, 394
Hoggett, P. 74
home-based services 158–9
homelessness 161–6
honesty xxvi–xxvii
Hong Kong 191–6
hope 343–9
Horovitz, E.G. xvi, 242–52, 411–13
hospices *see* assisted living facilities and
hospices
Hospital Review Board 60, 401
hospitals 55–61, 94–5, 97–101, 137, 167–8,
173–85, 254–5, 259–62, 267–70,
335–6, 366–8
Howie, P. xvi, 91–6, 413
human rights 292–3
humility xxvi–xxvii
Hurley, R. 168

Iacuzzi, C.M. 7
Iceland 266–72
Icelandic Art Therapy Association 266
Ichiki, Y. xvii, 279–84, 413–15
iCouch 248
identity 176
image 201–2
imaginative problem-solving *see* creativity
immigrant families 51–4
immigrant populations 6, 97–103, 398
India 273–7
indigenous people 27–35, 83–8
individual therapy 36–42, 55–67, 91–110,
167–72, 181–7, 235–41, 266–72,
301–7, 373–88
information release 20, 126–8
informed consent xxiii–xxviii, 5, 6, 12, 13,
65–6, 70, 144, 220, 276–7, 283, 294,
414, 434
see also private practice contract
injuries *see* job-related injuries
Instinctual Trauma Response (ITR)
model 236–40
institutionalization 55–6
integrity *see* fidelity
intent 43–4
international work 43–8
internet addiction *see* addiction
internship placements 136

interpreters *see* language interpreters
isolation 125–6
Italy 254–7
Iyer, J. 207

Japan 279–84
jeong (a heart to care for others) 78–9
jip-an (within the house) 79–80
job-related injuries 167–72
Jobes, D.A. 223
Jonsson, C.R. xvii, 351–7, 415–16
Jordan 322
Jordan, J.R. 307
Jung, C.G. 141, 309
justice 58–60
juvenile detention centers 124–9

Kapitan, L. 221
Karamanol, A. xxii
Kaynouna Arab Art Therapy Center xxi, 322
Kawai, H. 279
Kim, B.C. 79
Klorer, P. Gussie xvii, 373–7, 416–18
knowledge 199–202
Koney, J.N.A. 205
Koomson, E. 205
Korea 76–81
Kosminsky, P.S. 307
Kramer, E. 3–4, 225, 231, 296

labeling *see* diagnosis
Langer, S.K. 199
language interpreters 97–103, 135–6
late cancellation 18–19
law enforcement personnel 169–70
laws and legal issues 5–6, 12–13, 59, 104–10,
    222–3, 243, 374–5
    see also private practice contract
learning difficulties 153–60
Lefika La Phodiso 69–74
Lett, W. 342
Levinas, E. 152
LGBTQ+ 37, 176, 400–1
location tracking 19
loss 301–7

McNiff, S. 340
Malchiodi, C. 170
maleness 309–14
Malhotra, B. 131
mandala making 330
Mandel, B. xvii, 225–31, 418
Marshall-Tierney, A. 332
Martin, M.E. xvii, 36–42, 418–19
masculinity 309–14

Mason, S. 142
material culture 296
materials 9, 10, 227, 255, 262, 276, 355,
    368, 418
Meade, M.E. 271
memory drawing 267–72, 425–7
men 308–14
Mikel, E.H. xvii, 62–6, 419
military setting 91–6
military specific ethical issues 92
Miller, A. xvii, 339–50, 420–1
Mills, A. xviii, 12–21, 389–95, 421–3
Milofsky, L. xviii, 360–9
Mini Art Therapeutic Session Project
    (MATSP) 280–4, 413–15
minister 38–41

modes of treatment:
    co-therapy 97, 101
    collaboration 14–16, 149–50, 215, 259–65
    community-based 27–34, 55–6, 60–1, 71–
        4, 151–2, 157–8
    family/couples art therapy 27–34, 51–4,
        120–3, 432–3
    forensic art therapy 104–10
    group art therapy 45–8, 53–4, 56–60,
        70–1, 76–81, 118–20, 150–2, 157,
        164–5, 173–5, 225–31, 254–8,
        322–31, 365–6, 355, 432
    individual art therapy 36–42, 55–67,
        91–110, 167–72, 181–7, 235–41,
        266–72, 301–7, 373–88
    rehabilitation 61, 101, 124–5, 148, 151,
        220, 277, 335, 366
    telehealth/telemedicine 242–52
    trauma therapy 235–41, 259–65
McInally, F., cover artist
Moon, B. 277, 340
Moon, C.H. 334
moral courage 360–9
Mowry-Hesler, L. xviii, 153–60, 423–4
multiple roles 37–42, 80, 114–15, 125, 159,
    172, 191–6
    case manager 161–6, 172, 219–24
    curator of public art therapy gallery
        140–6
    educator 125, 204–8, 212–14, 229–31
    mandated reporter 66, 126–7
    minister 36–42
    non-clinical engagement 194–5
    relationship with self 198–200
    researcher 198–203
    role differentiation 193–4
    shared expectations 193
    supervision 332–8, 339–50

Naropa Community Art Studio
    (NCAS) 292–7
Natalushko, I. xviii, 235–41, 424
National Research Council 66
natural disasters *see* sites of natural disasters
Neff, K. 369
non-academic issues 210–18
non-clinical engagement 194–5
nonmaleficence 59–60
nonverbal communication 99–100
notes *see* record keeping
Nowak, K. 359

objectivity *see* art objectivity
objectivity myth 200–1
Obu, P. 205
older adults 62–6
online training 285–91
online working *see* telehealth/telemedicine
open studio format 175
Orr, P. xviii, 219, 285–91, 424–5
Osei, M. xviii, 204–8, 425
Ottarsdottir, U. xix, 266–72, 425–7
ownership of artwork 282

Paivio, A. 271
Palawan 27–34
Palestine 322–31
Paper 53 App 249–50
parental rights 222–3
Park, S. xix, 76–81, 427
Patrick, A. 6
Peligah, Y.S. 205–6
permissions xxiii–xxviii
Philippines 27–8
physical closeness *see* touch
post-traumatic stress disorder (PTSD) 91, 98,
    124, 235–6, 380, 382, 387
Potash, J.S. xxx, 191–6, 427–8
power dynamics 32, 341–2, 360–70, 396–7
Prasad, S. xxx, 273–8, 428–9
pre-session summary 243–7
prejudices *see* bias and discrimination
Pretzer, M. xix, 308–14, 429–30
Primeau, M. 168
prisons 45, 150–1
privacy *see* confidentiality; safe space
private practice 12–21, 113–14, 135, 147–53,
    160, 167–72, 181–7, 242–52, 266–72,
    301–7, 379–88
private practice contract 12–21, 389–95,
    421–3
  collaboration 14–16
  credentials 14

document retention 16
fees and payment 17–19
HIPAA 19–20
information release 20
late cancellation 18–19
location tracking 19
presenting 13–14
referrals 19
release forms for collaborators 15–16
telehealth 14
termination 19
unsecured email 17
professional identity 81
projection 356
promotional use of art *see* exhibiting client
    art work
protective clothing *see* smock
psychiatric facilities 55–61, 97–103, 173–80
puppetry 226
Purswell, K. 342

racism 32, 38–9, 68, 177, 366
Ratanapinyopong, J. Shwanpach 299
record keeping 274–5
referrals 19, 260–1, 263, 379, 381, 386–7,
    409–10
Reflective Art Experiences and Discussion
    Questions 21, 23, 34, 42, 48, 54, 61,
    67, 75, 81, 87, 96, 103, 109, 117, 123,
    128, 139, 146, 152, 160, 166, 172, 180,
    187, 196, 203, 208, 217–18, 223–4,
    231, 240, 252, 258, 265, 272, 278, 284,
    291, 297, 307, 314, 320–1, 331, 337,
    350, 357, 377, 387–8
refugee camps 322–31
refugees 351–7
rehabilitation 61, 101, 124–5, 148, 151, 220,
    277, 335, 366
reliability 202
religion/spirituality 37–42, 116, 138, 182–7,
    365, 434
religious discrimination 185–6, 366, 402
reporting 362–5
researcher 198–203
residential treatment settings 57, 155–6,
    226–9, 316–21, 376
resolutions to ethical dilemmas:
  Alfonso, M.R.A. 396–8
  Ballbé ter Maat, M. 398–9, 413–15
  Bardot, H. 399–400
  Berman, H. 400
  Boston, C.B. 400–1
  Byrne, L. 406–7
  Carolan, R. 401

Cogan, D.M. 401–2
Cutcher, D.J. 402
Dean, M.L. 402–4
Doby-Copeland, C. 404–6
Donald, K. 406
Fenner, P. 406–7
Franklin, M.A. 407
Garlock, L.R. 407–8
Goldberg, E.S. 408–9
Good, D.A. 409–11
Gussak, D. 411
Horovitz, E.G. 411–13
Howie, P. 413
Ichiki, Y. 413–15
Jonsson, C.R. 415–16
Klorer, P. Gussie 416–18
Mandel, B. 418
Martin, M.E. 418–19
Mikel, E.H. 419
Miller, A. 420–1
Mills, A. 421–3
Mowry-Hesler, L. 423–4
Natalushko, I. 424
Orr, P. 424–5
Osei, M. 425
Ottarsdottir, U. 425–7
Park, S. 427
Potash, J.S. 427–8
Prasad, S. 428–9
Pretzer, M. 429–30
Reyes H., P. 430
Roberts, M. 430–2
Ruff, M.E. 432–3
Scott, J. 433–5
Short, G.M. 434
Stone, E. 434–6
Stonnell, T.C. 435–7
Strouse, S. 437–8
Tripp, T. 438–9
Vivian, J. 439–40
Waller, D. 440–1
Yaish, S. 441
respect 65
response art 332–8
retirement 379–88
Reyes H., P. xix, 147–53, 430
Rhyne, J. 384
Ridley, C. 9
Robbins, A. 340
Roberts, M. xix, 210–18, 430–2
Robinson, L. 66
Rubin, J.A. xiii, xxii–xxix, 174
Ruff, M.E. xx, 118–23, 432–3
Ryu, E. 79

Saah, G.E. 205
safe space/place 72, 93–4, 113–14, 136, 177, 253–8, 271, 355, 425
safety 125, 157, 364
schizophrenia and psychosis 148–9, 219, 226, 254, 363
schools 157–8, 229–31, 266–77, 279–84
scientific method 198–202
scope of practice 112, 201, 401
Scott, J. xx, 124–9, 433–4
self-assessment 43–4
self-compassion 10, 369
self-disclosure 37–8, 56–7, 63, 115–16, 318, 302–5, 320
self-injury 125–6, 182–4, 363–4, 367
selfies 327–9

settings:
  assisted living facilities and hospices 63–7
  community-based art studios 70–4, 142–3, 195, 293–7
  educational settings
    training programs 46–7, 68, 70–4, 78–80, 133–9, 210–18, 254–8, 285–91, 339–50
    university 71–3, 133, 205–6, 210–12, 254, 294–5, 333–4
  forensic facilities
    courts 104–10
    juvenile detention centers 124–9
    prisons 44–5, 150–1
  group homes 164–5
  home-based services 158–9, 302
  hospitals 55–61, 94–5, 97–101, 137, 167–8, 173–85, 254–5, 259–62, 267–70, 335–6, 366–8
  military settings 91–6
  psychiatric facilities 55–61, 97–103, 173–80
  refugee camps 322–31
  residential treatment 57, 155–6, 226–9, 316–21, 376
  schools 157–8, 229–31, 266–77, 279–84
  shelters 163
  sites of natural disasters 27–34, 151–2
severe and persistent mental illness (SPMI) 55–61
sexual harassment 366–7
Shin, M. Kyung 189
Short, G.M. xx, 161–6, 434
Siegel, D. 236
sites of natural disasters 27–34, 151–2
smock 136–7
social injustice 38–9, 68–70, 74

solitary confinement 125–6, 128
soup kitchens 163
South Africa 68–74
South African National Arts Therapists Organisation 71
South Korea 76–82
space journey group 227–8
special education schools 157–8
special needs children 153–60, 274
spirituality *see* religion/spirituality
Spring, D. 384
standards *see* boundaries
stereotypes *see* stigma
stigma 145
Stone, E. xx, 133–9, 434–5
Stonnell, T.C. xx, 316–21, 435–7
stress 318–20
Strouse, S. xx, 301–7, 437–8
studio environment *see* community-based art studios
Stulmaker, H. 342
subpoenae 222–3
substance addiction *see* addiction
substance use 210–11
suicidality 94–5, 137, 262, 296, 367
Sun, S. 78, 81
supervision 74, 133–9, 177, 223, 274, 287, 289, 334, 339–50, 360–9
sustainability 33, 46, 73, 397
Swedish National Association for Art Therapists 357
Sweden 351–7
systemic failures 170

Taber, K. 168
Tagbanua 27–34, 396–8
Taleff, M. 7
Talwar, S. 207
Tanay, E. 108
technology *see* online training; telehealth/ telemedicine
telehealth/telemedicine 242–52
terminating treatment 19, 373–7, 379–88
testimony 104–10
thematic groups 226–9
theoretical orientations 7
therapeutic boundaries 44–5, 56–7, 78–80, 112–16, 178, 301–7, 373–7, 383–4
therapeutic language 81
therapist art making *see* art making by art therapists
third-party payers 167–72, 181–7, 402–3
time limits 53–4, 305, 398
Tinnin, L. 236, 241
torture 91–2

touch xxii, 63, 116, 135, 221, 305, 317–18
training 7
training art therapy students 46–7, 68, 70–4, 78–80, 133–9, 210–18, 254–8, 285–91, 339–50
training non-art therapists 45–6, 253, 280–2, 322–31, 413
transference 3–4, 51–2, 60, 99–100, 260, 382
see also counter-transference
translators *see* language interpreters
trauma 59–60, 182–7, 235, 257, 322–31, 353–7
trauma history 237–40
trauma therapy 235–41, 259–65
treatment *see* modes of treatment
treatment integrity 157
triangles 384
Tripp, T. xx, 259–65, 438–9
Typhoon Yolanda 27–34

UK 253–4
Ukraine 235–41
Ulman, E. 10
university 71–3, 133, 205–6, 210–12, 254, 294–5, 333–4
unsecured email 17

validity 202
values 4–7, 56; *see also* aspirational values
van der Kolk, B. 31, 260, 388
Vedantam, S. 9
violations 91–2
visual free speech 165, 231, 275–6, 293–7, 316–17
Vivian, J. xxi, 83–8, 439–40
Vollman, S. 89
Von Franz, M.L. 327

Waller, D. xxi, 253–8, 440–1
Wammes, J.D. 271
Welfel, R.R. 10
well-being *see* beneficence
West Indies 111–17
white privilege 68, 308, 313–14
whiteness 50–1
Winnicott, D. 71
Wittman, H. 233
work place norms 361–9
work place injuries *see* job-related injuries

Yaish, S. xxi, 322–31, 441
Yalom, I.D. 174

Zakour, A. 25

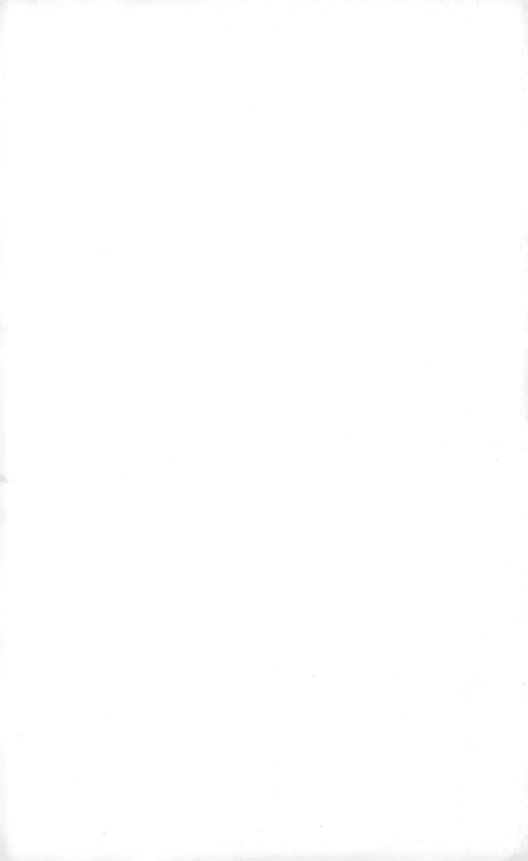